Neuroanatomy

NEUROANATOMY

A Review with Questions and Explanations

Richard S. Snell, M.D., Ph.D.

Emeritus Professor of Anatomy, George Washington University
School of Medicine and Health Sciences, Washington, D.C.

Little, Brown and Company   Boston / Toronto / London

Library of Congress Cataloging-in-Publication Data

Snell, Richard S.
   Neuroanatomy : a review with questions and explanations / Richard
S. Snell.
      p.   cm.
   Includes index.
   ISBN 0-316-80246-8
   1. Neuroanatomy.   2. Neuroanatomy—Examinations, questions, etc.
I. Title.
   [DNLM: 1. Nervous System—anatomy & histology—examination
questions.   WL 18 S671n]
QM451.S65   1992
611′.8′076—dc20
DNLM/DLC
for Library of Congress   91-44528
                                                                          CIP

Printed in the United States of America

MV-NY

To those students who have difficulty retaining factual information for neuroanatomy examinations

Contents

Preface

Neuroanatomy: A Review with Questions and Explanations is for medical, dental, and allied health students who are preparing for examinations. The neuroanatomy is presented in a condensed form with simple diagrams. This book is specifically designed for those students who are overwhelmed by factual detail and who are trying to learn sufficient information to pass examinations. At the end of each chapter are numerous National Board type questions, which are followed by answers, and, where appropriate, brief explanations. (The K type questions have been retained.)

The book begins with an introductory chapter dealing with the organization of the nervous system and the basic structure of neurons, nerve processes, synapses, and nerve fibers. This is followed by chapters dealing with the neuroglia, degeneration and regeneration of nervous tissue, peripheral nerves, and peripheral nerve endings. The text then considers the different parts of the central nervous system and their connections. Special chapters deal with simplifying and describing the connections of the cranial nerves and the structure and function of the autonomic system. The numerous tables assist in the memorization of the distribution of the cranial nerves and the sympathetic and parasympathetic parts of the autonomic system.

The purpose of the questions is threefold: (1) to focus the student's attention on areas of importance, (2) to enable the student to find out his areas of weakness, and (3) when answered under examination conditions, with the factual material not in view, to provide the student with a form of self-evaluation.

I wish to express my sincere thanks to Ira Alan Grunther, AMI, for his excellent artwork. Finally, to the staff of Little, Brown and Company I express my gratitude and appreciation for their assistance throughout the preparation of this book.

R.S.S.

Neuroanatomy

1 Nervous System and Neurons

SUGGESTED PLAN FOR REVIEW OF CHAPTER 1

1. Understand the organization of the nervous system and realize that nerve fibers can run from one part to another without interruption. Throughout this text emphasis is placed on getting the reader to understand the spatial relationships of different parts of the nervous system. Once you have mastered this, it is easier to appreciate how nerve fibers travel from one part to another. If you also learn the functions of the parts, then it is much easier to learn the nervous connections between them. In other words, you begin to be able to visualize the connections in your mind's eye rather than having to learn facts like a parrot.

2. Learn the types of neurons and know examples of each type.

3. Review the cell biology of a neuron so that you may more easily understand the function of a nerve cell and its processes. Pay particular attention to the structure of the plasma membrane as it is related to its physiology.

4. Understand axon transport.

5. Synapses are very important, so learn the detail. Include in your review the different types of neurotransmitters and their actions (see pp. 9 and 257).

6. Learn the structure of myelinated and nonmyelinated nerves. Understand how the physiology of conduction is related to the structure of nerve fibers.

NERVOUS SYSTEM

The nervous system and the endocrine system control the functions of the body. The nervous system exerts its control by means of specialized cells that rapidly pass signals to different parts of the individual. The nervous system receives input signals from the external and internal environments by means of sensory receptors. Once inside the nervous system, the signals are integrated with one another and either are transmitted to bring about muscle contraction or glandular activity or are stored in the memory for future use. Learning occurs as the result of the continual adaptation of the connections of the nervous system as the body is exposed to new sensations.

Organization. The nervous system is divided into two main parts, the **central nervous system,** consisting of the brain and spinal cord, and the **peripheral nervous system,** consisting of the cranial and spinal nerves and their ganglia. The **autonomic nervous system** is an important subdivision of the nervous system, which innervates involuntary structures, such as the heart, smooth muscle, and glands.

The basic units of the nervous system are the nerve cells, which are specialized to conduct nerve impulses over long distances at great speeds. The **neuron** is the name given to the nerve cell and all its processes (Fig. 1-1). Neurons possess a **cell body** or **perikaryon** and processes called **neurites.** The long processes of a nerve cell are called **axons,** or **nerve fibers;** the short processes are **dendrites.**

The central nervous system is composed of large numbers of neurons supported by specialized tissue called **neuroglia.** In the peripheral nervous system, the nerve fibers and the nerve cells in ganglia are supported by delicate areolar tissue.

The interior of the central nervous system is organized into **gray** and **white matter.** Gray matter consists of nerve cells embedded in neuroglia. White matter consists of nerve fibers embedded in neuroglia.

NEURONS

Types of Neurons. Neurons may be classified according to the number and mode of branching of the neurites (Fig. 1-1):

Unipolar neurons are those that have a single neurite that divides a short distance from the cell body into two branches, one proceeding to a peripheral structure and the other entering the central nervous system. Examples of this form of neuron are found in the posterior root ganglion.

Bipolar neurons possess an elongated cell body, which gives rise to a single neurite at each end. Examples of this form of neuron are found in the retina and the sensory ganglia of the cochlear and vestibular nerves.

Multipolar neurons are those in which a number of neurites arise from the cell body. With the exception of the long process, the axon, the neurites are dendrites. Almost all the neurons of the central nervous system are of this type.

Neurons may also be classified by their size:

Golgi type I neurons have long axons that may be 1 meter long in extreme cases. The axons of these neurons form the long fiber tracts of the brain and spinal cord and the nerve fibers of peripheral nerves. The pyramidal cells of the cerebral cortex, the Purkinje cells of the cerebellar cortex, and the motor anterior gray column cells of the spinal cord are Golgi type I neurons.

Golgi type II neurons have a short axon that terminates near the cell body or is absent. The short dendrites give these cells a star-shaped appearance. This type of neuron greatly outnumbers the Golgi type I neurons, and they are found in large numbers in the cerebral and cerebellar cortex and in the retina.

Fig. 1-1

(A) A neuron. (B) Different types of neurons classified according to the number, length, and mode of branching of the neurites.

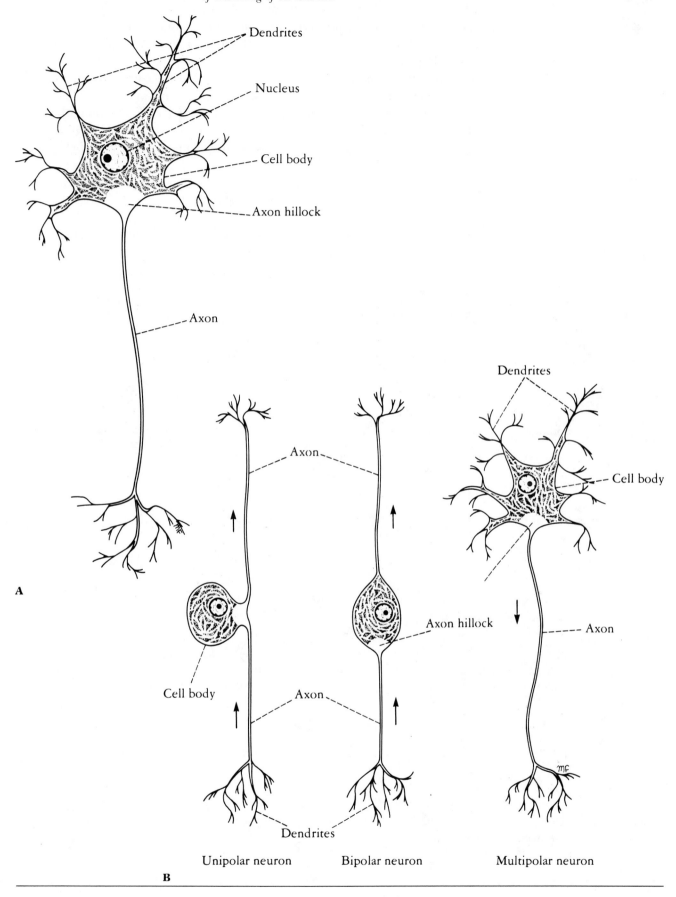

Dendrites

Nucleus

Cell body

Axon hillock

Axon

A

Axon

Dendrites

Cell body

Cell body

Axon

Axon hillock

Axon

Axon

Cell body

Dendrites

Unipolar neuron

Bipolar neuron

Multipolar neuron

B

Structure of a Neuron. The nerve cell body consists of a mass of cytoplasm in which a nucleus is embedded and is surrounded by a plasma membrane (Fig. 1-2.) The cell body produces the organelles that are passed out into the axon and dendrites; it also synthesizes the transmitter substances that are transported in the axoplasm down the axon. The plasma membranes of the dendrites and cell body possess receptors that are stimulated by transmitter substances from other neurons. When the receptors are stimulated electrical currents begin to flow through the membrane so that the resting potential of the dendrites or cell body is raised or lowered. The altered potential, which spreads along the nerve fiber as the nerve impulse, if greater enough will induce similar changes in rapid succession along the plasma membrane of the axon.

NUCLEUS. The nucleus is large and pale with widely dispersed fine chromatin granules. There is usually a prominent nucleolus.

CYTOPLASM. The cytoplasm possesses granular and agranular endoplasmic reticulum and the following organelles and inclusions.

Fig. 1-2   *Fine structure of a neuron cell body.*

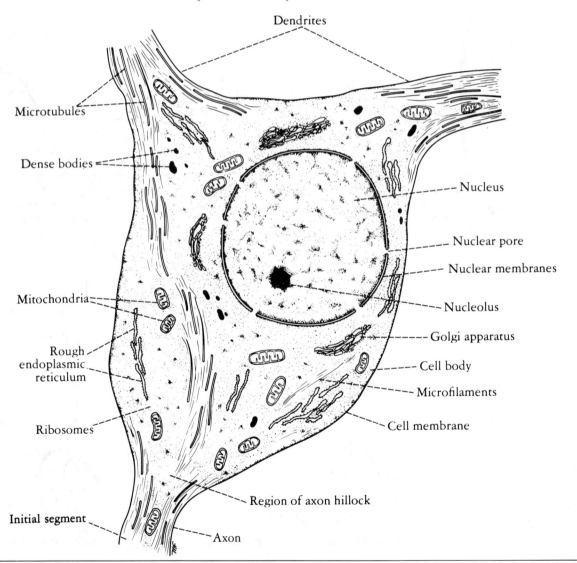

Nissl Substance. This is granular material and is composed of rough-surfaced endoplasmic reticulum. It is found throughout the cytoplasm of the cell body except the region where the axon emerges; this area is known as the **axon hillock.** It also extends into the proximal parts of the dendrites. The Nissl substance synthesizes protein.

Golgi Apparatus. This is composed of clusters of flattened cisternae and small vesicles made up of smooth-surfaced endoplasmic reticulum. It is found close to the nucleus. The Golgi apparatus adds carbohydrate to the protein molecules brought to it, packages products for export from the cell, and forms cell membranes.

Mitochondria. These are found scattered throughout the cytoplasm of the cell body and the dendrites and axons. They are vesicular structures having an outer membrane that surrounds the mitochondrion and an inner membrane that is folded to form cristae. Mitochondria are responsible for cellular respiration and are the chief sites for the formation of chemical energy.

Neurofibrils. These are found running parallel to one another through the cell body and into the neurites. Each consists of a bundle of microfilaments measuring about 7 nm in diameter. The function of the filaments is not known, although the presence of actin and myosin within them would suggest that they may give contractile assistance to transport mechanisms.

Microtubules. These are found scattered in among the microfilaments and are found in the cell body and the neurites. Each tubule measures about 20 to 30 nm in diameter. Microtubules are thought to transport substances from one part of the neuron to another with the assistance of the microfilaments. A ratchet mechanism, consisting of proteins projecting out from the tubules, assisted by the contracting microfilaments, is thought to transport substances to and from the cell body.

Lysosomes. These are membrane-bound vesicles measuring about 8 nm in diameter. They are formed from the Golgi apparatus. They contain hydrolytic enzymes. Lysosomes exist in three forms: (1) **primary lysosomes,** which have just been formed, (2) **secondary lysosomes,** which contain partially digested material **(myelin figures),** and (3) **residual bodies,** in which the enzymes are inactive and which have evolved from secondary lysosomes.

Centrosome. This is found in immature nerve cells that are undergoing cell division. Occasionally they are found in mature nerve cells where their function may be associated with the formation of microtubules.

Lipofuscin. This is a yellowish-brown pigment found in the cytoplasm. It is a metabolic by-product that accumulates with age.

Melanin Granules. These are found in the cytoplasm of nerve cells in the substantia nigra of the midbrain. They may be associated with the catecholamine-synthesizing function of these cells.

Glycogen. This carbohydrate is seen as electron-dense rosettes in the cytoplasm and serves as a source of energy.

Lipid. This occurs as droplets in the cytoplasm and is a source of energy.

PLASMA MEMBRANE. The plasma membrane is about 8 nm thick and separates the cytoplasm from the exterior. It is composed of an inner and outer layer of protein molecules, separated by a middle layer of lipid. Certain protein molecules lie within the lipid layer spanning its entire width. The molecules provide the membrane with hydrophilic channels through which inorganic ions may enter and leave the cell. Carbohydrate molecules are attached to the outside of the plasma membrane forming the cell coat, or **glycocalyx.**

The plasma membrane forms a semipermeable membrane that allows diffusion of certain ions through it, but restricts others. In the resting state (unstimulated state) the K⁺ ions diffuse through the plasma membrane from the cell cytoplasm to the tissue fluid (Fig. 1-3). The permeability of the membrane to K⁺ ions is much greater than to Na⁺ ions, so that the passive efflux of K⁺ is much greater than the influx of Na⁺. This results in a steady potential difference of about 80 mV, which can be measured across the plasma membrane since the inside of the membrane is negative with respect to the outside. This potential is known as the **resting potential.**

Excitation of the Plasma Membrane of the Nerve Cell Body. Stimulation of a nerve cell by electrical, mechanical, or chemical means produces a rapid change in membrane permeability to Na⁺ ions, which diffuse through the plasma mem-

---

Fig. 1-3   *The creation of the action potential by the arrival of a stimulus from a single presynaptic terminal. Note that the action potential generated at the initial segment will only occur if the threshold for excitation is reached at the initial segment.*

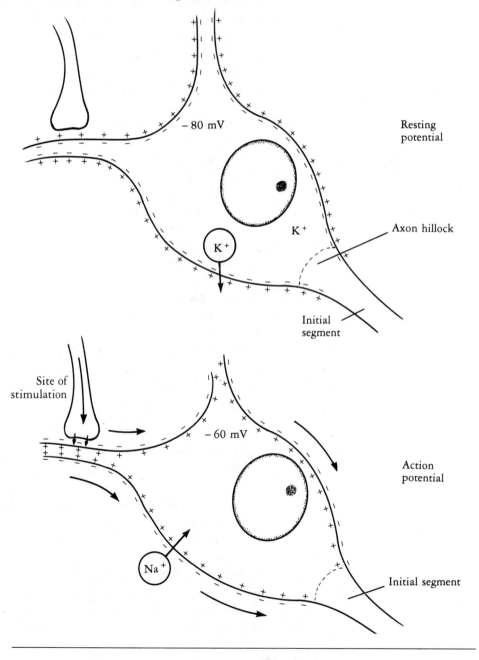

---

brane into the cell cytoplasm from the tissue fluid (Fig. 1-3). This results in the membrane becoming progressively depolarized. The sudden influx of Na$^+$ ions followed by the altered polarity produces the so-called **action potential.** This potential is, however, very brief, lasting about 5 msec, for very quickly the increased membrane permeability for Na$^+$ ions ceases and that for K$^+$ ions increases, so that the K$^+$ ions start to flow from the cell cytoplasm and so return the localized area of the cell to the resting state.

Once generated, the action potential spreads over the plasma membrane, away from the site of initiation, and is conducted along the axon as the **nerve impulse.** This impulse is self-propagated, and its size and frequency do not alter (Fig. 1-6). Once the nerve impulse has spread over a given region of plasma membrane, another action potential cannot be elicited immediately. The duration of this nonexcitable state is referred to as the **refractory period.**

It should be noted that the greater the strength of the initial stimulus, the larger will be the initial depolarization and the greater the spread into the surrounding areas of the plasma membrane. If multiple excitatory stimuli are applied to the surface of a neuron, then the effect can be **summated.** For example, subthreshold stimuli may pass over the surface of the cell body and be summated at the root of the axon and so initiate an action potential.

Inhibitory stimuli are believed to produce their effect by causing an influx of Cl$^-$ ions through the plasma membrane into the neuron, thus producing hyperpolarization and reducing the excitatory state of the cell.

Nerve Cell Processes. Nerve cell processes or neurites may be divided into dendrites and an axon (Fig. 1-2).

DENDRITES. These are the short processes of the cell body and are extensions of the cell body to increase the surface area for the reception of axons from other neurons. They conduct the nerve impulse toward the cell body. Dendrites often branch extensively, and in some neurons the smaller branches bear projections called **dendritic spines.**

AXON. This is the name of the longest process of the cell body. It arises from the axon hillock. It has a smooth surface and is uniform in diameter. Axons may be very short, as in many neurons of the central nervous system, or very long, as in peripheral nerves. The diameter of axons varies with different neurons. The plasmalemma bounding the axon is called the **axolemma.** The cytoplasm of the axon is called the **axoplasm.** The axoplasm possesses no Nissl substance or Golgi apparatus. Just before their termination, axons often branch extensively. The distal ends of the branches are commonly enlarged and are called **terminals or boutons terminaux.**

The **initial segment** of the axon is the first 50 to 100 μm after it leaves the axon hillock of the nerve cell body (Fig. 1-2). This is the most excitable part of the axon and is the site at which an action potential originates. It is important to remember that under normal conditions an action potential does not originate on the plasma membrane of the cell body, but always at the initial segment.

It is usual to state that an axon always conducts impulses away from the cell body. The axons of sensory posterior root ganglion cells are an exception; here the long neurite, which is indistinguishable from an axon, carries the impulse toward the cell body (see unipolar neurons, p. 2).

Axon Transport. Materials are transported from the cell body to the axon terminals by a process called **orthograde transport,** and to a lesser extent in the opposite direction, a process called **retrograde transport.**

Fast orthograde transport of 100 mm per day refers to the transport of proteins and neurotransmitter substances or their precursors. **Slow orthograde transport** of 1 to 3 mm per day refers to the transport of axoplasm and includes microfilaments and microtubules.

Retrograde transport explains how the cell bodies of nerve cells respond to changes in the distal end of the axons. Pinocytotic vesicles arising at the axon terminals can be returned quickly to the cell body. Worn out mitochondria are returned to the cell body for breakdown by the lysosomes.

The microtubules and the microfilaments of the axoplasm are involved in the transport mechanism (see p. 5).

SYNAPSES

The nervous system consists of a large number of neurons that are linked together to form functional conducting pathways. Where two neurons come into close proximity and functional interneuronal communication occurs, the site of such communication is called a **synapse.** The definition has also come to include the site where a neuron comes into close proximity with a skeletal muscle cell and where communication occurs.

Synapses are of two types: chemical and electrical. Most synapses are chemical, in which a chemical substance, the **neurotransmitter,** passes across the narrow space between the cells and becomes attached to a protein molecule in the postsynaptic membrane called the **receptor. Chemical synapses** are either excitatory or inhibitory. Once stimulation or inhibition has taken place, the neurotransmitter is broken down by an enzyme or it is taken up by the presynaptic axon terminal.

Electrical synapses are ordinary gap junctions between two neurons. They permit the spread of activity from one neuron to another and thus ensure that a group of neurons performing an identical function act together. Since there is no chemical transmitter, there is a minimal delay in getting the information across between the cells.

Ultrastructure of Chemical Synapses. The apposed surfaces of the terminal axonal expansion and the neuron are termed the **presynaptic** and **postsynaptic membranes,** respectively, and are separated by a **synaptic cleft** 20 nm wide. The presynaptic and postsynaptic membranes are thickened, and the underlying cytoplasm shows increased density. On the presynaptic side, the dense cytoplasm is broken up into groups, and on the postsynaptic side, the density often extends into a **subsynaptic web.** Close to the presynaptic membrane are presynaptic vesicles, mitochondria, and lysosomes in the cytoplasm. On the postsynaptic side of the synapse, the cytoplasm often contains parallel cisternae.

The presynaptic terminal contains many small presynaptic vesicles that contain the neurotransmitter. The vesicles fuse with the presynaptic membrane and discharge the neurotransmitter into the synaptic cleft by a process of exocytosis.

Types of Synapses. The most common type of synapse is that which occurs between an axon of one neuron and the dendrite or cell body of the second neuron. The axon may have a terminal expansion (bouton terminaux) or a series of expansions (bouton de passage) so that the axon makes several contacts as it passes through the dendritic tree. In other types, the axon synapses on the proximal segment (initial segment) of another axon, or there may be synapses between terminal expansions from different neurons. Depending on the site of the synapse they are called **axodendritic, axosomatic,** or **axoaxonic.**

Neurotransmitters at Synapses. The presynaptic vesicles and the mitochondria play a key role in the release of neurotransmitter substances. The vesicles contain the neurotransmitter substance that is released into the synaptic cleft, and the mitochondria provides adenosine triphosphate (ATP) for the synthesis of new transmitter substance.

The majority of neurons produce and release only one type of transmitter at all their nerve endings. However, a few neurons release an excitor transmitter, such as glutamate, at one synapse and a neuropeptide at another synapse. Different neurons may produce and release different transmitter substances. For example, acetylcholine is widely used by different neurons in the central and peripheral parts of the nervous system, whereas dopamine is released by neurons in the substantia nigra. Glycine, another transmitter, is found principally in synapses in the spinal cord.

The following are chemical substances known to act as neurotransmitters and there are probably many more yet to be discovered: acetylcholine, norepinephrine, epinephrine, dopamine, glycine, serotonin, gamma-aminobutyric acid (GABA), enkephalins, substance P, and glutamic acid.

Action of Neurotransmitters. All neurotransmitters are released from their nerve endings by the arrival of the nerve impulse. Once in the synaptic cleft they achieve their objective by raising or lowering the resting potential of the postsynaptic membrane for a brief period of time.

The receptor proteins on the postsynaptic membrane bind the transmitter substance, thereby increasing the membrane permeability. In the case of excitatory synapses the permeability to most ions is increased, but with inhibitory synapses there is an increase in permeability to chloride ions. At an excitatory synapse the postsynaptic membrane is depolarized, whereas at an inhibitory synapse the postsynaptic membrane is hyperpolarized.

The excitatory and the inhibitory effects on the postsynaptic membrane of the neuron will depend on the summation of the postsynaptic responses at the different synapses. If the overall effect is one of depolarization, the neuron will be excited and an action potential will be initiated at the initial segment of the axon and a nerve impulse will travel along the axon. If, on the other hand, the overall effect is one of hyperpolarization, the neuron will be inhibited and no nerve impulse will arise.

NERVE FIBERS

A nerve fiber is an axon (or a dendrite) of a nerve cell. Two types of nerve fibers exist in the central and peripheral parts of the nervous system: myelinated and nonmyelinated fibers.

Myelinated Nerve Fibers. A myelinated nerve fiber is one that is surrounded by a myelin sheath (Fig. 1-4). The myelin sheath is not part of the neuron but is formed by a supporting cell. The supporting cell in the central nervous system is the oligodendrocyte and in the peripheral nervous system is the Schwann cell.

The myelin sheath is segmented, the segments being separated at regular intervals by the nodes of Ranvier. In the central nervous system, each oligodendrocyte can form and maintain myelin sheaths for as many as 60 nerve fibers (axons). In the peripheral nervous system, there is only one Schwann cell for each segment of a single nerve fiber.

Myelination of Peripheral Nerve Fibers. This process begins during late fetal development and during the first postnatal year. The nerve fiber first grooves

Fig. 1-4

(A–D) Cross sections of a myelinated nerve fiber showing the different stages in the formation of myelin. (E) Longitudinal section of a mature myelinated nerve fiber showing a node of Ranvier.

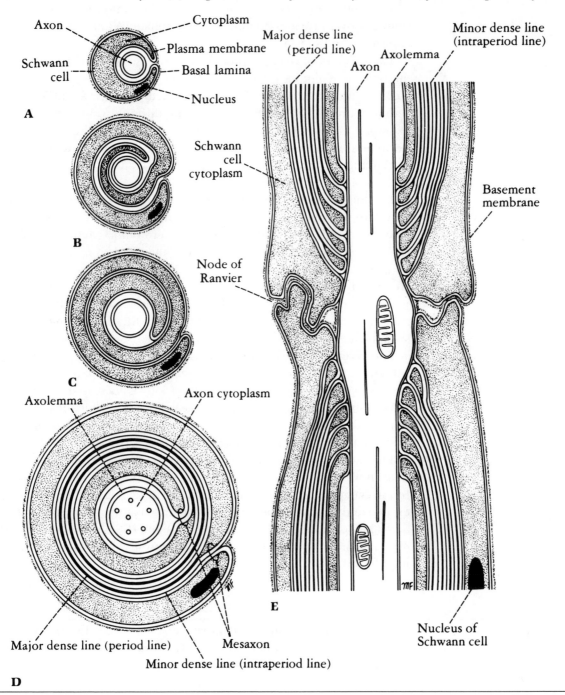

the side of a Schwann cell and then sinks further into the cell. In this manner the plasma membrane of the Schwann cell forms a **mesaxon,** which suspends the axon within the cell. The Schwann cell now rotates on the axon so that the plasma membrane becomes wrapped repeatedly around the axon in a spiral. The cytoplasm recedes from the spirals into the Schwann cell body, and the cytoplasmic surfaces of the plasma membrane in the elongating mesaxon come into apposition to form the **major dense lines** seen on electron micrographs of transverse sections. The external surfaces of the plasma membrane of the mesaxon also come together to form the **minor dense lines.** The fused outer protein layers of the outer plasma membranes form a thin **intraperiod line.** At the node of Ranvier, two adjacent Schwann cells terminate and the plasma membrane of the axon is exposed.

The **incisures of Schmidt-Lanterman** are seen in longitudinal sections of myelinated nerve fibers. These are localized areas of Schwann cell cytoplasm that have persisted between the plasma membrane of the mesaxon. These small areas in fact form a continuous spiral of cytoplasm from the outermost region of the Schwann cell to the region of the axon. This spiral pathway provides a route for the passage of metabolites from the surface region of the Schwann cell to the axon.

Myelination of Central Nerve Fibers. Myelination begins in the vestibular and spinocerebellar tracts during late fetal development and the process continues in the central nervous system after birth. The pyramidal tracts and the fasciculus gracilis and cuneatus, for example, are not completely myelinated at birth.

The plasma membrane of the oligodendrocyte becomes wrapped around the axon to form the myelin (Fig. 1-5). The nodes of Ranvier are situated in the intervals between adjacent oligodendrocytes. A single oligodendrocyte may be connected to the myelin sheaths of as many as 60 nerve fibers. It is believed that myelination in the central nervous system takes place by the growth in length of the mesaxon of the oligodendrocyte, the mesaxon wrapping itself around the axon. The incisures of Schmidt-Lanterman are formed in the same manner as in the peripheral nervous system.

Nonmyelinated Peripheral Nerve Fibers. These are usually small-diameter nerve fibers (less than 1 μm in diameter). Each axon indents the plasma membrane of the Schwann cell so that it lies within a trough. Fifteen or more axons may lie within their own troughs on a single Schwann cell; sometimes an axon will share a trough. In some Schwann cells the troughs may be deep so that a mesaxon is formed from the Schwann cell plasma membrane. The Schwann cells lie close to one another along the length of the axons and there are no nodes of Ranvier. In regions where there are synapses or where transmission occurs, the axon emerges from the trough of the Schwann cell, thus exposing the axon.

Nonmyelinated Central Nerve Fibers. These fibers run in small groups and are not particularly related to the oligodendrocytes.

Conduction in Nerve Fibers. In the resting unstimulated state, a nerve fiber is polarized so that the interior is negative to the exterior. The potential difference across the axolemma is about 80 mV and is called the **resting membrane potential.** As has been explained previously, this so-called resting potential is produced by the diffusion of sodium and potassium ions through the plasma membrane and is maintained by the sodium-potassium pump. The pump involves active transport across the membrane and requires ATP to provide the energy.

A nerve impulse (action potential) is initiated at the initial segment of the axon. A nerve impulse is a self-propagating wave of electrical negativity that passes along the surface of the plasma membrane (axolemma). The wave of electrical negativity is initiated by an adequate stimulus being applied to the surface of the neuron. Under normal circumstances this occurs at the initial segment of the axon, which is the most sensitive part of the neuron. The stimulus alters the permeability of the membrane to Na^+ ions at the point of stimulation. Now Na^+ ions rapidly enter the axon (Fig. 1-6). The positive ions outside the axolemma quickly decrease to zero. The membrane potential therefore is reduced to zero and is said to be **depolarized.** A typical resting potential is 80 mV, with the out-

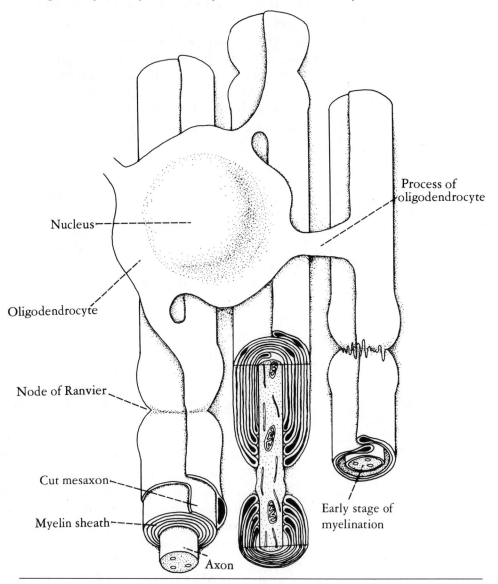

Nucleus

Process of oligodendrocyte

Oligodendrocyte

Node of Ranvier

Cut mesaxon

Early stage of myelination

Myelin sheath

Axon

side of the membrane positive to the inside; the action potential is about 40 mV, with the outside of the membrane negative to the inside.

The negatively charged point on the outside of the axolemma now acts as a stimulus to the adjacent positively charged axolemma, and in less than 1 msec the polarity of the adjacent resting potential is reversed (Fig. 1-6). The action potential now has moved along the axolemma from the point originally stimulated to the adjacent point on the membrane. It is in this manner that the action potential travels along the full length of a nerve fiber.

As the action potential moves along the nerve fiber, the entry of the Na^+ ions into the axon ceases and the permeability of the axolemma to K^+ ions increases. Now K^+ ions rapidly diffuse outside the axon (since the concentration is much higher within the axon than outside) so that the original resting membrane potential is restored. The permeability of the axolemma now decreases and the status quo is restored by the active transport of the Na^+ ions out of the axon and the K^+ ions into the axon. The outer surface of the axolemma is again electrically positive compared to the inner surface.

Fig. 1-6

The ionic and electrical changes that occur in a nerve fiber when it is stimulated.

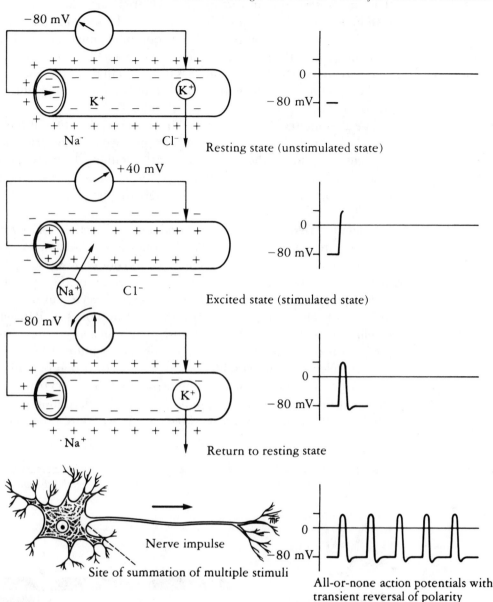

Resting state (unstimulated state)

Excited state (stimulated state)

Return to resting state

Nerve impulse

Site of summation of multiple stimuli

All-or-none action potentials with transient reversal of polarity

For a short time after the passage of a nerve impulse along a nerve fiber, while the axolemma is still depolarized, a second stimulus, however strong, is unable to excite the nerve. This period of time is known as the **absolute refractory period.** This period is followed by a further short interval during which the excitability of the nerve gradually returns to normal. This latter period is called the **relative refractory period.** It is clear from this that the refractory period makes a continuous excitatory state of the nerve impossible and it limits the frequency of the impulses.

Sodium and Potassium Channels. The so-called sodium channels and potassium channels through which physiologists believe the sodium and potassium ions diffuse through the plasma membrane have not been identified. It is possible that some of the protein molecules that extend through the full thickness of the plasma membrane may serve as channels. Each channel is thought to be controlled by an electrically charged gate that can open or close the channel.

In the nonstimulated state, the gates of the potassium channels are wider open than those of the sodium channels, which are nearly closed. This allows the potassium ions to diffuse out more readily than the sodium ions can diffuse in. In the stimulated state, the gates of the sodium channels are at first wide open; then the gates of the potassium channels are opened and the gates of the sodium channels are nearly closed again. It is thus seen that it is the opening and closing of the sodium and potassium channels that is thought to produce the depolarization and repolarization of the plasma membrane.

The absolute refractory period, which occurs at the onset of the action potential when a second stimulus is unable to produce a further electrical change, is thought to be due to the inability to get the sodium channels open. During the relative refractory period, when a very strong stimulus can produce an action potential, presumably the sodium channels are opened.

Conduction Velocity in Nerve Fibers. The conduction velocity of an axon is much greater in large-diameter axons than in small-diameter axons. In nonmyelinated axons, the action potential passes continuously along the axolemma, progressively exciting neighboring areas of membrane (Fig. 1-7). In myelinated axons, the presence of a myelin sheath serves as as perfect insulator and prevents the flow of ions to any extent. However, at the nodes of Ranvier there is no myelin, and ionic flow is possible. Consequently, in a myelinated axon, the action potential is conducted from node to node, i.e., it jumps from node to node, a process called **saltatory conduction** (Fig. 1-7). The action potential at one node sets up a current in the surrounding tissue fluid that quickly produces depolarization at the next node. This jumping of the depolarization process along the length of the axon in myelinated fibers is a much more rapid mechanism than

Fig. 1-7   (A) A stimulated myelinated axon (saltatory conduction). (B) A stimulated nonmyelinated axon.

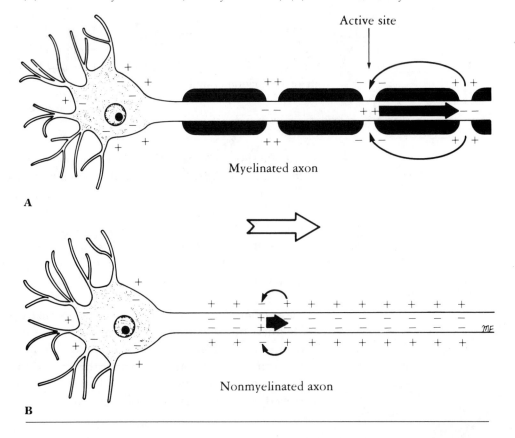

Active site

Myelinated axon

A

Nonmyelinated axon

B

is found in nonmyelinated fibers. Furthermore, since the ionic exchange across the axolemma is practically restricted to the nodes, less energy is required to conduct the nerve impulse.

The conduction velocity in large myelinated fibers may be as high as 120 meters per second and as small as 0.5 meters per second in small unmyelinated fibers.

NATIONAL BOARD TYPE QUESTIONS

Select the **best** response.

1. The interruption of the individual myelin sheath segments along a peripheral axon is called a:
   A. Incisure of Schmidt-Lanterman.
   B. Paranode region.
   C. Major dense line.
   D. Node of Ranvier.
2. The larger the diameter of a myelinated axon:
   A. The thinner is its axolemma.
   B. The greater is its conduction velocity.
   C. The greater is its sensitivity to local anesthetic blockade.
   D. The greater is its sensitivity to painful stimulation of the skin.
3. Which of the following types of synapses make up the majority within the central nervous system?
   A. Axoaxonic.
   B. Axodendritic.
   C. Dendrodendritic.
   D. Electrical synapses.
4. Which of the following is **not** true regarding axons?
   A. They may be extremely long compared to dendrites.
   B. When of large diameter they are myelinated.
   C. Recurrent collaterals do not function in feedback inhibition.
   D. The ending may be either a synapse or a motor end-plate.
5. Which of the following nervous system structures myelinates earliest?
   A. Pyramidal tracts.
   B. Posterior sensory roots of the spinal cord.
   C. Anterior motor roots of the spinal cord.
   D. Superior cerebellar peduncle.
   E. Medial longitudinal bundle.
6. In the most typical synapses, small vesicles containing neurotransmitter substance are found in the:
   A. Dendrite.
   B. Soma of neuron.
   C. Bouton.
   D. Axon.
   E. Synaptic cleft.
7. In a typical multipolar motor neuron, the part of the neuron providing the greatest surface area for synaptic reception is the:
   A. Axon.
   B. Cell body.
   C. Dendritic processes.
   D. All of the above.
   E. None of the above.

8. Which one of the following is associated with the major dense line in the myelin sheath?
   A. Inner mesaxon.
   B. Basal lamina.
   C. Apposition of the outer cytoplasmic surface of the plasma membrane in the mesaxon.
   D. Fusion of the inner cytoplasmic surface of the plasma membrane in the mesaxon.
   E. Outer cytoplasmic layer of the plasma membrane.

9. Which of the following is **not** a typical feature of the axon?
   A. Usually one per neuron.
   B. May be myelinated.
   C. Cylindrical in shape.
   D. Usually short with acute angle branching.
   E. Smooth contour without many synapses.

10. Which one of the following terms does **not** properly describe the large anterior horn cell?
    A. Lower motor neuron.
    B. Inhibitory.
    C. Golgi type 1.
    D. Alpha efferent.
    E. Multipolar.

11. Which one of the following statements concerning the axon is **not** true:
    A. The action potential is produced by the sudden influx of Na^+ ions into the axoplasm.
    B. The initial segment of the axon is the first millimeter after it leaves the cell body.
    C. The spread of the action potential along the plasma membrane of the axon is known as the nerve impulse.
    D. The axon hillock is situated at the point where the axon leaves the cell body of the neuron.

In each of the following questions, answer:
A. If only (1), (2), and (3) are correct.
B. If only (1) and (3) are correct
C. If only (2) and (4) are correct
D. If only (4) is correct
E. If all are correct

12. Axons can be traced along their pathways in the central nervous system by using methods that rely on:
    (1) Retrograde transport of proteins.
    (2) Degeneration of an axon cut off from its cell body of origin.
    (3) Anterograde transport of newly synthesized proteins.
    (4) The presence of Nissl substance in the axon.

13. The recycling of membranes of synaptic vesicles (that have released their neurotransmitter into the synaptic cleft) may involve:
    (1) Coated vesicles.
    (2) Rough endoplasmic reticulum.
    (3) Presynaptic membrane.
    (4) Postsynaptic membrane.

14. To qualify as a neurotransmitter a substance must:
    (1) Have a defined method of inactivation or disposal.
    (2) Reproduce the effect of neural presynaptic stimulation.

(3) Be shown to be synthesized within the neuron.

(4) Be an amino acid or a peptide.

15. The release of a neurotransmitter involves:

(1) Fusion of vesicles with the presynaptic membrane.

(2) An increase in the presynaptic permeability to Ca^{++}.

(3) Rupture of the vesicles.

(4) Arrival of an action potential at the axon terminal.

In each of the following questions, answer:

A. If only (1) is correct

B. If only (2) is correct

C. If both (1) and (2) are correct

D. If neither (1) nor (2) is correct

16. (1) The gray matter consists of nerve cells embedded in neuroglia.

(2) The white matter consists of nerve cells and nerve fibers embedded in neuroglia.

17. (1) An example of a unipolar neuron is seen in a posterior root ganglion.

(2) An example of a bipolar neuron is found in the sensory ganglion of the cochlear nerve.

18. (1) Golgi type 2 neurons have long axons.

(2) Golgi type 1 neurons greatly outnumber Golgi type 2 neurons.

19. (1) The Nissl substance is composed of smooth-surfaced endoplasmic reticulum.

(2) The Nissl substance synthesizes protein.

20. (1) Melanin granules are found in the cytoplasm of nerve cells in the substantia nigra of the midbrain.

(2) Microtubules are thought to play a role in the transport of substances from one part of the neuron to another.

21. (1) The resting potential is brought about by the diffusion of sodium and potassium ions through the plasma membrane.

(2) In the resting state, the resting potential is about 80 mV, the inside of the membrane being negative with respect to the outside.

22. (1) Plasma membrane channels are possibly protein molecules that extend through the full thickness of the membrane.

(2) In the stimulated state the gates of the sodium channels are at first closed.

23. (1) Saltatory conduction occurs most often in nonmyelinated axons.

(2) The conduction velocity in large myelinated nerve fibers may be as high as 120 meters per second.

24. (1) Fifteen or more nonmyelinated axons may lie within a single Schwann cell.

(2) In a Schmidt-Lanterman incisure the continuous spiral of cytoplasm from the outermost region of the Schwann cell to the axon provides a passage for metabolites.

25. (1) The subsynaptic web lies beneath the postsynaptic membrane.

(2) The synaptic cleft measures about 20 nm wide.

26. (1) A dendrite conveys a nerve impulse away from the nerve cell body.

(2) The dendritic spines are small projections of the plasma membrane and are artefacts produced by the process of fixation of the neuron.

27. (1) As a general rule neurons produce and release many different kinds of transmitter substances at their nerve endings.

(2) Most dendrites expand in width as they extend out from the nerve cell body.

28. (1) Lipofuscin granules are found in young immature nerve cells.

(2) Microfilaments contain actin and myosin and probably assist in nerve cell transport.

29. (1) The volume of cytoplasm within the nerve cell body is often much less than that in the axon and dendrites.

(2) The axolemma is the name given to the plasma membrane of the axon.

30. (1) The processes of a nerve cell body are called neurites.

(2) Mitochondria present in the axons provide ATP for the synthesis of transmitter substances.

ANSWERS AND EXPLANATIONS

1. D

2. B: The axolemma is of uniform thickness irrespective of the diameter of the axon; the larger the diameter of the axon, the sensitivity to local anesthetic agents becomes less; small-diameter nerve fibers (delta type A fibers) conduct painful impulses from the skin.

3. B: Axodendritic and axosomatic synapses are commonly found in all regions of the central nervous system.

4. C: In certain areas of the central nervous system (e.g., the thalamus and cerebral cortex), recurrent collateral branches of an axon exert inhibitory influences on the neuron that gave rise to the axon.

5. C: Myelination occurs first in the anterior motor roots of the spinal cord at about the fourth month of fetal life and this takes place before the posterior sensory roots. In the central nervous system, myelination begins in the medial longitudinal bundle at about 6 months and in the cerebellar connections at about 7 months. The pyramidal tracts start to myelinate at birth and are not complete until the second or third year.

6. C

7. C: The dendritic processes and their spines provide an enormous surface area for synaptic contact.

8. D: For details concerning the process of myelination, see pages 9 and 11.

9. D: Dendrites are usually short with acute angle branching.

10. B

11. B: The initial segment of the axon is restricted to the first 50 to 100 μm after it leaves the nerve cell body.

12. A: (1) Retrograde transport of proteins. Horseradish peroxidase is injected into the region of the axon under investigation. The enzyme is absorbed into the axon and travels by retrograde transport to the cell body of the axon. (2) An axon or a dendrite when cut off from its cell body undergoes degeneration and this process may be studied microscopically (see Chap. 3). (3) Anterograde transport of newly synthesized proteins. A radioactively labelled amino acid is injected into the region of the nerve cell body. It becomes incorporated into the proteins within the cell body and is transported anterogradely to the axon terminals. (4) Nissl granules are confined to the nerve cell body (except the area of the axon hillock) and the proximal parts of the dendrites.

13. B

14. A: Amines are also neurotransmitters. For example, norepinephrine, epinephrine, dopamine, and serotonin are neurotransmitters.

15. E

16. A: White matter consists of nerve fibers embedded in neuroglia.

17. C

18. D

19. B: Nissl substance is composed of rough-surfaced endoplasmic reticulum.

20. C
21. C
22. A: In the stimulated state of a neuron, the gates of the sodium channels are at first wide open.
23. B: Saltatory conduction occurs in myelinated fibers when the nerve impulse jumps (*saltare*—to jump) from one node of Ranvier to the next.
24. C
25. C
26. D: (1) A dendrite conveys a nerve impulse toward the nerve cell body. (2) Dendritic spines are structural projections of the plasma membrane of the dendrite,
27. D: (1) As a general rule a neuron releases only one type of transmitter at its nerve endings. However, there are a few examples where a neuron releases an excitor transmitter, such as glutamate at one synapse and a neuropeptide at another synapse. (2) A dendrite narrows in width as it extends out from the nerve cell body.
28. B: (1) Lipofuscin granules are found in the cytoplasm of some nerve cells in the elderly.
29. C
30. C

2 Neuroglia

SUGGESTED PLAN FOR REVIEW OF CHAPTER 2

1. Understand that the neuroglial cells far outnumber the nerve cells in the central nervous system and that they provide support for the nerve cells.
2. Learn the structure and function of each of the four types of neuroglial cells and know where each type is located.
3. Understand the difference between active and inactive microglial cells.
4. Be able to define what is meant by ependymocytes, tanycytes, and choroidal epithelial cells.
5. Understand the extracellular space in the central nervous system and learn where it opens into.
6. Be able to define the blood-brain barrier.

INTRODUCTION

The neurons of the central nervous system are supported by nonexcitable cells called neuroglial cells (Fig. 2-1). Neuroglial cells are generally smaller than neurons and outnumber them 5 to 10 times. There are four types: (1) astrocytes, (2) oligodendrocytes, (3) microglia, and (4) ependyma.

ASTROCYTES

Astrocytes have small cell bodies with numerous branching processes. Many of the processes end as expansions on capillary blood vessels (perivascular feet), on ependymal cells, and on the pia mater. Large numbers of astrocytic processes are interwoven at the outer and inner surfaces of the central nervous system, where they form the **outer** and **inner glial limiting membranes.** Thus the outer glial limiting membrane is found beneath the pia mater and the inner glial limiting membrane is situated beneath the ependyma lining the ventricles of the brain and the central canal of the spinal cord.

Large numbers of astrocytes are found around the initial segment of most axons and in the bare segments of axons at the nodes of Ranvier. Axon terminals at many sites are separated from other nerve cells and their processes by an envelope of astrocytic processes.

Two types of astrocytes can be identified, fibrous and protoplasmic.

Fibrous astrocytes are found mainly in the white matter where their long pro-

Fig. 2-1

Different types of neuroglial cells.

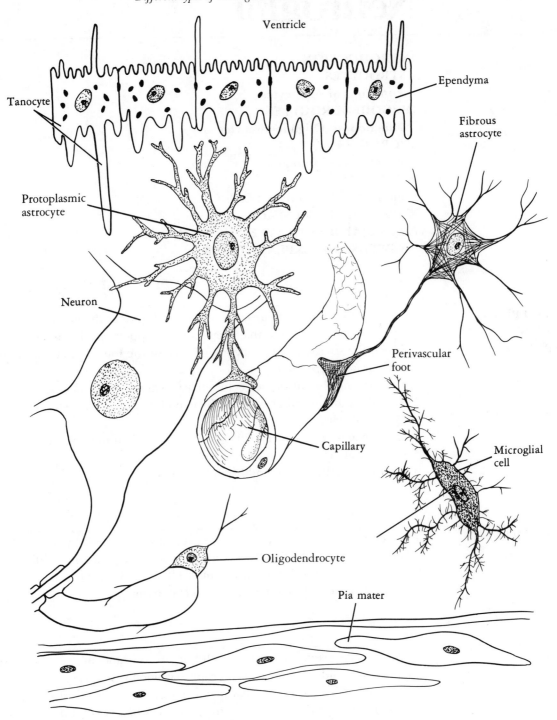

cesses pass between the nerve fibers. The cell bodies and their processes contain many filaments in their cytoplasm.

Protoplasmic astrocytes are found mainly in the gray matter where their short branching processes pass between the nerve cell bodies. The cytoplasm of these cells contains fewer filaments than that of the fibrous astrocytes.

Functions of Astrocytes

1. They form a supporting framework for the neurons, and in the embryo they serve as a scaffolding for the migration of immature neurons.

2. They cover the synaptic contacts between neurons and may serve as insulators preventing axon terminals from influencing neighboring and unrelated neurons.
3. They absorb glutamate and gamma-aminobutyric acid (GABA) secreted by the nerve terminals, thus limiting the influence of these neurotransmitters.
4. They absorb excess K^+ ions in the extracellular fluid.
5. They store glycogen within their cytoplasm. The glycogen can be broken down into glucose and released to surrounding neurons in response to norepinephrine.
6. They serve as phagocytes by taking up degenerating synaptic axon terminals.
7. Following the death of neurons due to disease, they proliferate and fill in the spaces previously occupied by the neurons, a process called **replacement gliosis.**
8. It is possible that metabolites are transported from blood capillaries by the astrocytes to the neurons through their perivascular feet. The fact that astrocytes are linked together by gap junctions would enable ions to pass from one cell to another without entering the extracellular space.
9. They may produce substances that have a trophic influence on neighboring neurons.

OLIGODENDROCYTES

Oligodendrocytes have small cell bodies and a few delicate processes; there are no filaments in their cytoplasm. Oligodendrocytes are found in rows along myelinated nerve fibers and surround nerve cell bodies. The processes of a single oligodendrocyte join the myelin sheaths of several nerve fibers. However, only one process joins the myelin between two adjacent nodes of Ranvier.

Functions of Oligodendrocytes
1. They are responsible for the formation of the myelin sheath of nerve fibers in the central nervous system, much as the myelin of peripheral nerves is formed from Schwann cells. Because oligodendrocytes have several processes, unlike Schwann cells, they can each form several internodal segments of myelin on the same or different axons. A single oligodendrocyte can form as many as 60 internodal segments.
2. Oligodendrocytes that surround nerve cell bodies (satellite oligodendrocytes) probably have a similar function to the satellite or capsular cells of peripheral sensory ganglia. They are thought to influence the biochemical environment of neurons.

MICROGLIA

Microglial cells are the smallest of the neuroglial cells; they are scattered throughout the central nervous system. Their small cell bodies give rise to branching processes with spinelike projections.

Functions of Microglia. In the normal central nervous system, the microglia is inactive and the cells are sometimes called **resting microglial cells.** In inflammatory and degenerative lesions of the nervous system, the microglial cells become active and proliferate and become phagocytic. These active cells are joined by monocytes that migrate into the tissue from the blood capillaries and form new microglial cells.

EPENDYMA

Ependymal cells are cuboidal in shape and possess microvilli and cilia. They form a single layer of cells that line the cavities of the brain and the central canal of the spinal cord.

There are three groups of ependymal cells:

1. **Ependymocytes,** which line the ventricles of the brain and the central canal of the spinal cord and are in contact with the cerebrospinal fluid. Their adjacent surfaces have gap junctions, but the cerebrospinal fluid is in free communication with the intercellular spaces of the central nervous system.
2. **Tanycytes,** which line the floor of the third ventricle overlying the median eminence of the hypothalamus. These cells have processes that have end feet on blood capillaries.
3. **Choroidal epithelial cells,** which cover the surfaces of the choroid plexuses. The sides and bases of these cells are thrown into folds, and near their luminal surfaces the cells are held together by tight junctions that encircle the cells. The tight junctions prevent the leakage of cerebrospinal fluid into the underlying tissues.

Functions of Ependymal Cells

1. The cilia of the ependymal cells assist in the circulation of the cerebrospinal fluid within the cavities of the brain and the central canal of the spinal cord.
2. Tanycytes are believed to transport blood-derived hormones in the cerebrospinal fluid into the capillaries of the median eminence of the hypothalamus and thus may influence the control of the anterior lobe of the pituitary gland.
3. The choroidal epithelial cells have a secretory function and take part in the formation of cerebrospinal fluid.
4. The microvilli on the free surfaces would indicate that they also have an absorptive function.

EXTRACELLULAR SPACE

The extracellular space is the narrow interval that exists between the neurons, the neuroglial cells, and the blood capillaries and is filled with extracellular fluid. The extracellular space is in almost direct continuity with the cerebrospinal fluid in the subarachnoid space externally and the cerebrospinal fluid in the ventricles of the brain and the central canal of the spinal cord internally. The extracellular space thus provides a pathway for the exchange of ions and molecules between the blood and the neurons and glial cells. The plasma membrane of the endothelial cells of most capillaries is impermeable to many chemicals, and this forms the **blood-brain barrier.**

NATIONAL BOARD TYPE QUESTIONS

In each of the following questions, answer:
A. If only (1), (2), and (3) are correct
B. If only (1) and (3) are correct
C. If only (2) and (4) are correct
D. If only (4) is correct
E. If all are correct

1. Which of the following statements concerning fibrous astrocytes is (are) correct?
    (1) They have small cell bodies.

(2) They are found mainly in the white matter.

(3) Their cell bodies and their processes contain many filaments in the cytoplasm.

(4) They do not contribute to the inner glial limiting membrane.

2. Which of the following statements concerning oligodendrocytes is (are) correct?

(1) They are found in rows along nonmyelinated fibers.

(2) They are responsible for the formation of myelin in the central nervous system.

(3) They have large cell bodies.

(4) They surround nerve cell bodies.

3. Which of the following statements concerning microglial cells is (are) correct?

(1) In the normal nervous system they are nonactive.

(2) The resting microglial cells are thought to be derived from mesoderm.

(3) In an inflammatory lesion, monocytes from the blood participate in the formation of new microglial cells.

(4) They have no branching processes.

4. Which of the following statements concerning ependymal cells is (are) correct?

(1) They possess microvilli and cilia.

(2) They are in contact with the cerebrospinal fluid.

(3) They are cuboidal in shape.

(4) Many of them have long basal processes.

In each of the following questions, answer:

A. If only (1) is correct

B. If only (2) is correct

C. If both (1) and (2) are correct

D. If neither (1) nor (2) is correct

5. (1) Astrocytes form perivascular feet.

(2) Astrocytic processes are found in large numbers around the bare axolemma at the nodes of Ranvier.

6. (1) Astrocytes play no part in replacement gliosis.

(2) Astrocytes may function as electrical insulators around neurons.

7. (1) The processes of a single oligodendrocyte join the myelin sheath of a single nerve fiber.

(2) One cytoplasmic process of an oligodendrocyte provides the myelin for one internode.

8. (1) Tanycytes are special ependymal cells that line the third ventricle.

(2) Tanycytes are involved in the control of endocrine glands.

9. (1) Choroidal epithelial cells form a covering for the choroid plexuses and play no part in the formation of the cerebrospinal fluid.

(2) Choroidal epithelial cells are joined together by tight junctions.

10. (1) The extracellular space surrounds the neurons and the glial cells.

(2) The extracellular space communicates with the ventricles of the brain and the central canal of the spinal cord.

11. (1) Neuroglial cells have larger cell bodies than neurons.

(2) The extracellular space in the central nervous system does not communicate with the synaptic cleft between two neurons.

12. (1) Astrocytes take part in the absorption of GABA secreted by nerve terminals.

(2) The extracellular space is filled with fluid that drains into the lymph vessels of the central nervous system.

1. A: (4) Fibrous astrocytes do contribute to the inner glial limiting membrane.
2. C: (1) Oligodendrocytes are found in rows along myelinated nerve fibers. (3) Oligodendrocytes have small cell bodies.
3. A: (4) Microglial cells, especially active cells, have many branching processes.
4. E
5. C
6. B: (1) At sites of degeneration of nervous tissue, astrocytes multiply and fill in the space previously occupied by neurons.
7. B: (1) Oligodendrocytes possess many processes and each can form several internodal segments of myelin on the same or different nerve axons.
8. C
9. B: (1) Choroidal epithelial cells have a secretory function and take part in the formation of cerebrospinal fluid.
10. C
11. D: (1) Neuroglial cells have smaller cell bodies than neurons. (2) The extracellular space does communicate with the synaptic cleft between two neurons.
12. A: (2) The central nervous system does not possess lymph vessels.

3

Degeneration and Regeneration of Nervous Tissue

INTRODUCTION
DEGENERATION OF NERVES IN THE PERIPHERAL NERVOUS SYSTEM
DEGENERATION OF NERVES IN THE CENTRAL NERVOUS SYSTEM
REGENERATION OF NERVES IN THE PERIPHERAL NERVOUS SYSTEM
REGENERATION OF NERVES IN THE CENTRAL NERVOUS SYSTEM
TRANSNEURONAL DEGENERATION
NEURONAL DEGENERATION ASSOCIATED WITH SENESCENCE
PLASTICITY OF THE CENTRAL NERVOUS SYSTEM FOLLOWING
    INJURY
NATIONAL BOARD TYPE QUESTIONS
ANSWERS AND EXPLANATIONS

**SUGGESTED PLAN
FOR REVIEW
OF CHAPTER 3**

1. This material is important for clinical practice so the details outlined must be known.
2. The process of degeneration is rapid whereas regeneration is a slow process. Regeneration is only attempted in the central nervous system but quickly ceases.
3. Degeneration: Learn the changes that take place in the nerve fibers and then the changes that take place in the nerve cell bodies. Note that the process is similar in both the peripheral and central nervous systems. However, note the differences.
4. Regeneration in peripheral nerves: Learn the detailed histology of this process in the nerve fibers and then learn the changes that occur in the nerve cells during recovery.
5. Attempted regeneration of nerve fibers in the central nervous system: Because today so much research is being devoted to investigating why regeneration in the central nervous system ceases within 2 weeks, the attempted histological changes that do occur must be learned.
6. Be able to define the following terms: wallerian degeneration, band fiber, retrograde degeneration, anterograde transneuronal degeneration, chromatolysis, and neuroma.
7. Understand plasticity of the central nervous system.

INTRODUCTION

The survival of the cytoplasm of a neuron depends on its being connected, however indirectly, with the nucleus. The nucleus plays a key role in the synthesis of proteins, which pass into the cell processes and replace proteins that have been metabolized by the cell activity. Thus, the cytoplasm of axons and dendrites will undergo degeneration quickly if these processes are separated from the nerve cell body.

In contrast to the rapid onset of degeneration, the process of regeneration may take several months. Regeneration in the peripheral nervous system may be very successful. However, in the central nervous system, regeneration is attempted but the process ceases after about 2 weeks.

DEGENERATION OF NERVES IN THE PERIPHERAL NERVOUS SYSTEM	When a nerve is cut, the axon is no longer in continuity with the nerve cell body and the distal segment undergoes simultaneous degeneration from the site of the lesion to its termination. Degeneration also extends proximally for a short distance as far as the first node of Ranvier. The process of degeneration is called **wallerian degeneration.**

During the first day the axon becomes swollen and irregular, and by the third or fourth day it becomes broken up into fragments (Fig. 3-1). Meanwhile the myelin sheath slowly breaks down into short segments and then finally degenerates completely. The surrounding Schwann cells proliferate and fill the en-

Fig. 3-1 *The process of degeneration and regeneration in a divided nerve.*

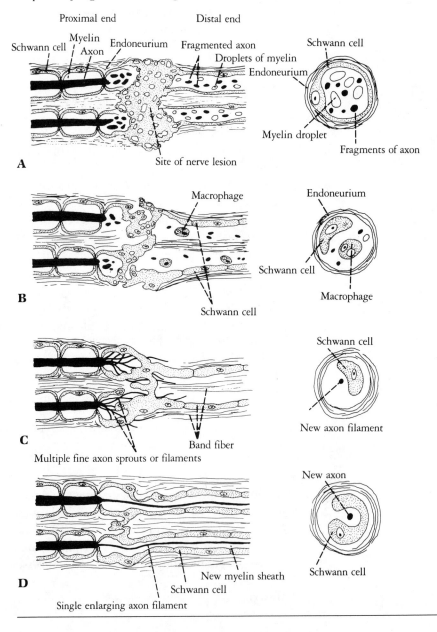

doneurial sheath. The axonal and myelin debris is phagocytosed by the Schwann cells and tissue macrophages. The Schwann cells now become arranged in parallel cords. Each endoneurial sheath and the contained cords of Schwann cells are known as a **band fiber.**

Accompanying injury to the axon, changes may take place in the cell body, and are referred to as **retrograde degeneration.** The first changes that take place occur within the first 2 days following injury and reach their maximum within 2 weeks. The Nissl material breaks up and becomes fine and granular and dispersed throughout the cytoplasm, a process known as **chromatolysis.** The nucleus moves from its central position toward the periphery of the cell, and the cell body swells and becomes rounded due to osmotic changes. The amount of chromatolysis and swelling of the cell is greatest when the injury to the axon is close to the cell body. Synaptic contacts with the plasma membrane on injured motor neurons withdraw and processes of astrocytes enter the synaptic clefts. Sometimes death of the neuron occurs, while on other occasions, when there is only minor injury to the distal end of the axon, very little change may take place in the cell body.

After the macrophages have removed the debris, the neuron is replaced with fibrous tissue produced by local fibroblasts.

| **DEGENERATION OF NERVES IN THE CENTRAL NERVOUS SYSTEM** | In the brain and spinal cord, degeneration of the axons and myelin sheaths follows a similar pattern to that seen in the peripheral nerves. The debris is removed by the phagocytic activity of the microglial cells. Most of the latter cells are monocytes that have emigrated from the blood vessels. The phagocytic process in the central nervous system takes place more slowly than in the peripheral nervous system. The part played by the oligodendrocytes in this process is not known. The changes that take place in the nerve cell bodies in the central nervous system following injury are similar to those seen in the peripheral nervous system. However, chromatolysis is rarely seen and cell death is common. |

After the debris has been removed by the microglial cells, the local astrocytes proliferate and replace the neuron with astrocytic processes and collagen fibers.

| **REGENERATION OF NERVES IN THE PERIPHERAL NERVOUS SYSTEM** | The following regenerative processes take place if the proximal and distal stumps of the severed nerve area are in close apposition. The Schwann cells proliferate and fill in the space within the endoneurial tubes of the proximal stump as far proximally as the next node of Ranvier and in the distal stump as far distally as the end-organs. Any small gap that exists between the proximal and distal stumps is filled in by proliferating Schwann cells. |

Each proximal axon end sends out many fine filaments with bulbous tips. These grow along the clefts between the Schwann cells and cross from the proximal to the distal nerve stump. Many filaments enter the proximal end of each endoneurial tube and grow distally in contact with the Schwann cells. Filaments from many different axons may enter a single endoneurial tube. However, only one filament persists, the remainder degenerating. The remaining filament now grows distally to reinnervate a motor or sensory end-organ and increases in diameter to about 80 percent of its original diameter.

As soon as the axon has reached the end-organ, the adjacent Schwann cells start to lay down a myelin sheath. This process starts at the site of the nerve injury and extends in a distal direction. By this means, the nodes of Ranvier and the Schmidt-Lanterman incisures are formed.

The rate of growth of the regenerating axon in a peripheral nerve is of the order of 2 to 4 mm daily. From a practical standpoint, if we include the delay incurred by the axons as they cross the site of injury, an overall regeneration rate of 1.5 mm daily should be remembered.

In a mixed peripheral nerve containing motor, sensory, and autonomic nerve fibers, the results after regeneration are less satisfactory than following the recovery from a lesion of a pure motor or a pure sensory nerve. The explanation is that regenerating fibers from the proximal stump may be directed to an incorrect destination in the distal stump, i.e., motor fibers entering sensory endings or vice versa, or motor fibers supplying incorrect muscles. Even if by chance the regenerating axon should reach the correct end-organ, the conduction velocity will not be as great as the original axon, since the diameter reaches only about 80 percent of its original diameter.

In crush nerve injuries, where the axon is divided but the endoneurial sheath remains intact, the result of regeneration may be very satisfactory. If a peripheral nerve is divided and the ends are not sutured together, the ends may retract, leaving a gap of several millimeters. Under these circumstances, the gap becomes filled with fibrous tissue, or adjacent structures, such as muscles, may bulge into the gap. The outgrowing axonal filaments grow out into the surrounding connective tissue and form a tangled mass or **neuroma.** None of the filaments may enter the distal stump and no recovery takes place.

Accompanying the regenerative changes in the axon, the nerve cell body shows evidence of returning to normal. The nucleolus moves to the periphery of the nucleus and there is a reconstitution of the original Nissl structure, indicating that RNA and protein synthesis is being accelerated in preparation for the regeneration of the axon. There is a decrease in the swelling of the cell body and a return of the nucleus to its central position.

REGENERATION OF NERVES IN THE CENTRAL NERVOUS SYSTEM

In the central nervous system there is an attempt at regeneration of the axons, as seen by the sprouting of the axons and the formation of filaments. However, the process ceases after about 2 weeks. The reason for this is not understood, although the following suggestions have been made: (1) the absence of endoneurial tubes in the central nervous system, which may be necessary to guide the regenerating axons, (2) the failure of oligodendrocytes to serve in the same manner as Schwann cells, (3) the laying down of connective tissue (scar tissue) by astrocytes, and (4) the absence of nerve growth factors in the central nervous system or the presence of nerve growth inhibiting factors that may be produced by the neuroglial cells.

The failure of axons to regenerate in the brain and spinal cord following injury means that permanent disability will follow.

TRANSNEURONAL DEGENERATION

In the central nervous system if one group of neurons is injured, then a second group farther along the pathway, serving the same function, may also show degenerative changes. This phenomenon is called **anterograde transneuronal degeneration.** For example, if the axons of the ganglion cells of the retina are cut, not only do the distal ends of the axons that pass to the lateral geniculate bodies undergo degeneration, but the neurons in the lateral geniculate bodies with which these axons form synapses also undergo degeneration. In some instances, a third set of neurons may be involved in the degenerative process in the visual cortex.

NEURONAL DEGENERATION ASSOCIATED WITH SENESCENCE

It has been estimated that in old age a person may have lost up to 20 percent of the original number of neurons. This may account to some extent for the loss of efficiency of the nervous system that is associated with old age.

PLASTICITY OF THE CENTRAL NERVOUS SYSTEM FOLLOWING INJURY

Axon regeneration in the brain and spinal cord is minimal following a lesion and yet considerable functional recovery often occurs. This is especially the case if the lesions are small. Several explanations exist for the functional improvement, and more than one mechanism may be involved.

1. Following a lesion, the function of adjacent nerve fibers may be interrupted as the result of compression by edema fluid. Once the edema subsides a substantial recovery may take place.
2. Nonfunctioning neurons may take over the function of damaged neurons.
3. Following a lesion to branches of a nerve, all the neurotransmitter may pass down the remaining branches, producing a greater effect.
4. Following a lesion of an afferent neuron, an increased number of receptor sites may develop on a postsynaptic membrane. This may result in the second neuron responding to neurotransmitter substances from neighboring neurons.
5. The damaged nerve fiber proximal to the lesion may form new synapses with neighboring normal neurons.
6. The normal neighboring nerve fibers may give off branches distal to the lesion, which then follow the pathway previously occupied by the damaged fibers.
7. If a particular function, as for example, the contraction of voluntary muscle, is served by two nervous pathways in the central nervous system and one pathway is damaged, the remaining undamaged pathway may take over the entire function. Thus it is conceivable that if the corticospinal tract is injured, the corticoreticulospinal tract may take over the major role of controlling the muscle movement.
8. It is possible with intense physiotherapy for patients to be trained to use other muscles to compensate for the loss of paralyzed muscles.

NATIONAL BOARD TYPE QUESTIONS

Select the **best** response.

1. Following transection of the ulnar nerve:
   A. The nerve fibers in the distal stump degenerate.
   B. Myelin is phagocytosed.
   C. Schwann cells form longitudinal bands.
   D. All the above.
   E. None of the above.
2. The rate of regeneration in a peripheral nerve is:
   A. 5–10 mm/day.
   B. 1–4 mm/day.
   C. 20 mm/day.
   D. 11–15 mm/day.
   E. 16–19 mm/day.
3. Regeneration in a peripheral nerve can be limited by:
   A. The length of segment of peripheral nerve lost (gap).
   B. Neuroma formation.
   C. Infection of the wound.

D. The presence of muscle between the cut ends.

E. All of the above.

4. Which one of the following best describes chromatolysis in the cell body in response to axon damage?

A. The nucleolus disappears.

B. There is a peripheral shift of the nucleus.

C. Deafferentation of the neuron surface may occur.

D. The cell undergoes marked swelling.

E. The rough endoplasmic reticulum becomes dispersed.

5. From a practical standpoint, peripheral nerve regeneration can be enhanced by reuniting:

A. The axolemma.

B. The endoneurium.

C. The perineurium.

D. The Schwann cell layer.

E. The epineurium.

6. Which of the following best correlates with the rate of regeneration in peripheral nerves?

A. Nerve impulse velocity.

B. Slow axoplasmic flow.

C. Retrograde axoplasmic flow.

D. Fast axoplasmic flow.

E. None of the above.

7. Regeneration in the central nervous system:

A. Is likely to be impeded by mechanical problems such as proliferation of astrocytes and hemorrhage.

B. May take the form of collateral sprouting, where an intact neuron sends out processes to denervated areas.

C. Both A and B above are correct.

D. Neither A nor B above is correct.

In each of the following questions, answer:

A. If only (1), (2), and (3) are correct

B. If only (1) and (3) are correct

C. If only (2) and (4) are correct

D. If only (4) is correct

E. If all are correct

8. Which of the following statements is (are) correct concerning wallerian degeneration?

(1) The axon dissolves and disappears.

(2) The Schwann cells multiply.

(3) In peripheral nerves the endoneurium disappears.

(4) In the central nervous system the debris is removed by the microglial cells.

9. Which of the following explanations may be correct concerning the failure of regeneration in the central nervous system?

(1) The absence of sprouting of filaments from the proximal end of the cut axon.

(2) The absence of endoneurial tubes.

(3) The absence of lymph drainage to the central nervous system.

(4) The failure of the oligodendrocytes to form a band fiber.

10. The following factor(s) may explain the partial return of function following injury to the central nervous system:
    (1) The damaged nerve fiber proximal to the lesion may form new synapses with neighboring normal neurons.
    (2) Intense physiotherapy may enable the patient to use other muscles to compensate for the loss of paralyzed muscles.
    (3) The subsiding of edema at the site of injury.
    (4) Following a lesion of an afferent neuron an increased number of receptor sites may develop on a postsynaptic membrane.

In each of the following questions, answer:
A. If only (1) is correct
B. If only (2) is correct
C. If both (1) and (2) are correct
D. If neither (1) nor (2) is correct

11. (1) In a cut peripheral axon, degeneration extends proximally as far as the first node of Ranvier.
    (2) In a damaged peripheral axon, the axonal and myelin debris is phagocytosed by Schwann cells and tissue macrophages.
12. (1) Following section of a motor nerve, the synaptic contacts with the nerve cell body may retract and lose contact.
    (2) In the peripheral nervous system, following the death of a neuron, the space previously occupied by the cell body is left empty.
13. (1) In the central nervous system, following injury, chromatolysis is rarely seen.
    (2) Any small gap that exists between the proximal and distal stump of a sectioned peripheral nerve is filled by proliferating tissue macrophages.
14. (1) During regeneration in a peripheral nerve, the new axon only reaches about 10 percent of the original diameter.
    (2) The conduction velocity of a regenerated axon is identical to that of the original axon.
15. (1) Regeneration in a mixed peripheral nerve is more successful than in a pure sensory or motor nerve.
    (2) A regenerated motor fiber on reaching a sensory ending quickly adapts to its new function.
16. (1) A completely sectioned peripheral nerve has a better functional recovery than a crushed nerve.
    (2) In the central nervous system the process of regeneration, although not complete, continues for at least 18 months.
17. (1) The absence of nerve growth factors in the central nervous system may inhibit the process of regeneration.
    (2) When the proximal neuron degenerates, the distal neuron continues to function without structural changes.
18. (1) In old age a person loses up to 20 percent of the original number of neurons in the central nervous system.
    (2) For practical purposes the overall regeneration rate in a peripheral nerve is 1.5 mm daily.
19. (1) During the regeneration of a peripheral nerve, the nodes of Ranvier are not reformed.
    (2) Schmidt-Lanterman incisures are formed during the process of nerve regeneration.

20. (1) Following a lesion of the spinal cord, the microglial cells remain inactive.
(2) Following a brain lesion, monocytes do not enter the neuropile.

ANSWERS AND EXPLANATIONS

1. D
2. B
3. E
4. E: The Nissl substance is formed of rough endoplasmic reticulum, and in chromatolysis the Nissl substance is dispersed throughout the cell cytoplasm.
5. E
6. E
7. C
8. C: (1) The axon does not dissolve; it breaks up into fragments that are phagocytosed by Schwann cells and local macrophages. (3) The endoneurium does not disappear and it plays a vital role in the regeneration process.
9. C: (1) The proximal stump of an axon does send out large numbers of filaments, but the process ceases after about 2 weeks. (3) There are no lymph vessels in the central nervous system.
10. E
11. C
12. A: (2) The space previously occupied by a nerve cell body in the peripheral nervous system is filled with new connective tissue laid down by local fibroblasts.
13. A: (2) The small gap between the proximal and distal stumps of a cleanly sectioned peripheral nerve is filled in with proliferating Schwann cells.
14. D: (1) Under ideal conditions the new axon in a regenerating peripheral nerve reaches about 80 percent of the diameter of the original axon. (2) Because the diameter of the new axon is less than that of the original, the conduction velocity of the new axon is less than that of the original axon.
15. D: (1) The degree of recovery in a sectioned pure motor or a pure sensory nerve is greater than in a mixed nerve. The reason for this is that in a mixed nerve there is a good chance that regenerating motor and sensory axons may enter the wrong distal endoneurial tubes, ie., a motor axon may enter a sensory tube and vice versa. (2) A regenerating motor axon on reaching a distal sensory ending does not assume the function of a sensory nerve.
16. D: (1) In a simple nerve crush, the endoneurial tubes remain intact so that each regenerating axon enters the correct distal endoneurial tube. (2) In the central nervous system the attempted process of regeneration ceases after about 2 weeks.
17. A: (2) In many instances the second neuron undergoes some transneuronal degeneration when the proximal neuron in a functional pathway degenerates.
18. C
19. B: (1) In a regenerating peripheral nerve, the nodes of Ranvier are reformed.
20. D: (1) Following a lesion of the spinal cord, the resident microglial cells become active. (2) The microglial cells in the neuropile are joined by monocytes that have migrated from the blood and become new microglial cells.

4   Peripheral Nerves

SUGGESTED PLAN FOR REVIEW OF CHAPTER 4

1. Clearly understand the structure of a peripheral nerve and know how peripheral nerve fibers may be classified. Do nerve fibers of different diameters have different physiological properties?
2. Learn the composition of the 12 cranial nerves. Which cranial nerves are purely motor, which are purely sensory, and which are mixed nerves?
3. Be able to define what is a spinal nerve. How does it arise from the spinal cord? What is an anterior nerve root, a posterior nerve root, an anterior ramus, and a posterior ramus?
4. Understand how the cauda equina is formed during development. Does it consist of anterior or posterior roots or both of these roots? Are the spinal nerves included in the definition of the cauda equina? Which segments of the spinal cord contribute to the cauda equina?
5. Learn the structure of a sensory ganglion of a spinal or a cranial nerve and be able to compare it with the structure of an autonomic ganglion.
6. Understand how a nerve plexus is formed and appreciate the advantages of having nerve plexuses in different parts of the body.

INTRODUCTION

The peripheral nerves are the cranial and spinal nerves. Each peripheral nerve trunk consists of parallel bundles of nerve fibers, which may be myelinated or nonmyelinated, surrounded by connective tissue sheaths. The afferent nerve fibers connect the receptors to the central nervous system, while the efferent fibers connect the central nervous system to the muscles, glands, and blood vessels. There are 12 pairs of cranial nerves and 31 pairs of spinal nerves.

STRUCTURE OF PERIPHERAL NERVES

A nerve fiber is the name given to an axon (or dendrite) of a nerve cell. The structure of axons and dendrites is described on page 7. Each nerve trunk is surrounded by the following connective tissue sheaths.

Epineurium. The epineurium is the dense connective tissue sheath that surrounds the nerve trunk (Fig. 4-1).

Fig. 4-1   *The structure of a peripheral nerve.*

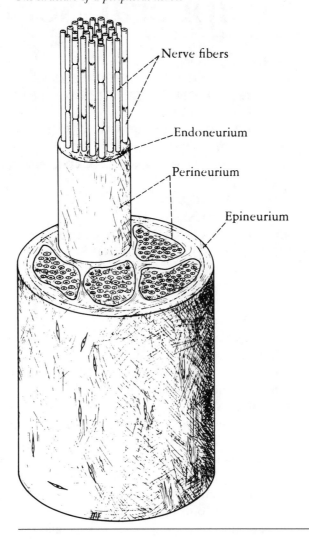

Nerve fibers

Endoneurium

Perineurium

Epineurium

Perineurium. The perineurium is the connective tissue sheath that surrounds the bundles of nerve fibers within the epineurium (Fig. 4-1).

Endoneurium. The endoneurium is a delicate connective tissue that lies between the individual nerve fibers (Fig. 4-1).

The function of the sheaths is to support the nerve fibers and their blood vessels and lymph vessels.

CLASSIFICATION OF PERIPHERAL NERVE FIBERS

Peripheral nerve fibers may be classified into three groups, depending on their size and speed of conduction:

Group A. These fibers are 1 to 20 μm in diameter and they conduct nerve impulses at the rate of 5 to 120 meters per second. They are myelinated somatic afferent and efferent fibers.

Group B. These fibers are 1 to 3 μm in diameter and they conduct nerve impulses at the rate of 3 to 15 meters per second. They are myelinated preganglionic autonomic fibers.

Group C. These fibers are 0.5 to 2.0 μm in diameter and they conduct nerve impulses at the rate of 0.5 to 2.0 meters per second. They are nonmyelinated postganglionic autonomic fibers.

CRANIAL NERVES

There are 12 pairs of cranial nerves, which leave the brain and pass through foramina in the skull. Some of these nerves are composed entirely of afferent nerve fibers bringing sensations to the brain (olfactory I, optic II, vestibulocochlear VIII), others are composed entirely of efferent fibers (oculomotor III, trochlear IV, abducent VI, accessory XI, hypoglossal XII), while the remainder possess both afferent and efferent fibers (trigeminal V, facial VII, glossopharyngeal IX, vagus X). The cranial nerves are described in Chapters 18, 19, and 20.

SPINAL NERVES AND SPINAL NERVE ROOTS

There are 31 pairs of spinal nerves, which leave the spinal cord and pass through intervertebral foramina in the vertebral column. The spinal nerves are named according to the regions of the vertebral column with which they are associated: 8 cervical, 12 thoracic, 5 lumbar, 5 sacral, and 1 coccygeal. Note that there are 8 cervical nerves and only 7 cervical vertebrae and that there is 1 coccygeal nerve and there are 4 coccygeal vertebrae.

Two spinal roots connect each spinal nerve to the spinal cord, an anterior root and a posterior root (Fig. 4-2). The **anterior root** consists of bundles of nerve fibers carrying nerve impulses away from the spinal cord; these nerve fibers are called efferent nerve fibers. The efferent fibers that pass to skeletal muscles and cause them to contract are called motor fibers. Their cells of origin lie in the anterior gray horn of the spinal cord. At certain levels the anterior roots also contain preganglionic nerve fibers of the autonomic system.

The **posterior root** consists of bundles of nerve fibers, called afferent fibers, that carry nervous impulses to the spinal cord. Since these fibers convey nerve impulses concerned with general sensations, they are called **sensory fibers.** The cell bodies of those nerve fibers are located in a swelling on the posterior root called the **posterior root ganglion** (Fig. 4-2).

The spinal nerve roots pass from the spinal cord to the level of their respective intervertebral foramina, where they unite to form a spinal nerve. Here the motor and sensory fibers mix so that a spinal nerve is made up of a mixture of motor and sensory fibers.

After emerging from the intervertebral foramen, each spinal nerve divides into a large **anterior ramus** and a smaller **posterior ramus,** each containing both motor and sensory fibers (Fig. 4-2). The posterior ramus runs posteriorly around the vertebral column to supply the muscles and skin of the back. The anterior ramus runs anteriorly to supply the muscles and skin over the anterolateral body wall and all the muscles and skin of the limbs.

CAUDA EQUINA

Because of the disproportionate growth in length of the vertebral column during fetal development, compared with that of the spinal cord, the length of the spinal nerve roots increases progressively from above downward (Fig. 4-3). In the upper cervical region the spinal nerve roots are short and run almost horizontally, but the roots of the lumbar and sacral nerves below the level of the termination of the cord (lower border of the first lumbar vertebra in the adult) form

Fig. 4-2

Cross section of the thoracic region of the spinal cord, showing roots, spinal nerve, and anterior and posterior rami and their branches. Note that an intercostal nerve is formed from the anterior rami of T1–11 spinal nerves.

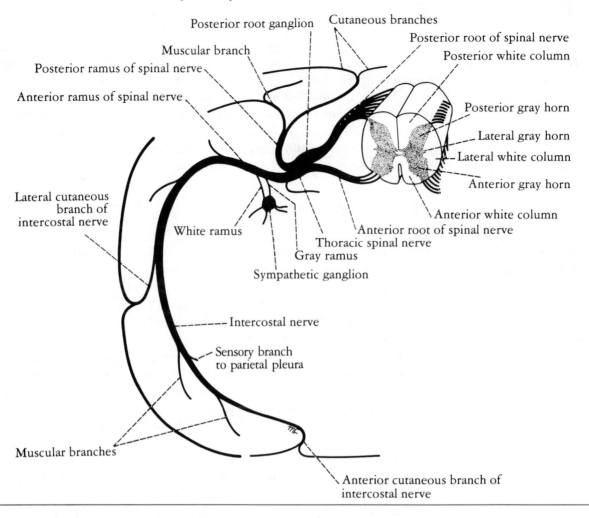

a vertical leash of nerves around the **filum terminale** (see p. 57). Together these lower nerve roots are called the **cauda equina** (Fig. 4-4).

POSTERIOR ROOT GANGLIA AND SENSORY GANGLIA OF CRANIAL NERVES

The sensory ganglia of the posterior spinal nerve roots (Fig. 4-2) and of the trunks of the trigeminal, facial, vestibulocochlear, glossopharyngeal, and vagal cranial nerves have the same structure. Each ganglion is covered by a layer of connective tissue that is continuous with the epineurium and perineurium of the peripheral nerve. The neurons are unipolar, possessing cell bodies that are rounded or oval in shape. The sensory ganglia of the vestibulocochlear nerves differ in that the cells are bipolar. The peripheral axon terminates in a series of dendrites in a peripheral sensory ending, and the central axon enters the central nervous system.

Each nerve cell body is closely surrounded by a layer of flattened cells called **capsular cells** or **satellite cells.** The capsule cells are similar in structure to Schwann cells and are continuous with these cells as they envelop the peripheral and central processes of each neuron.

Fig. 4-3

Posterior view of spinal cord, showing the origins of the roots of the spinal nerves and their relationship to the different vertebrae. On the right, the laminae have been removed to expose the right half of the spinal cord and the nerve roots.

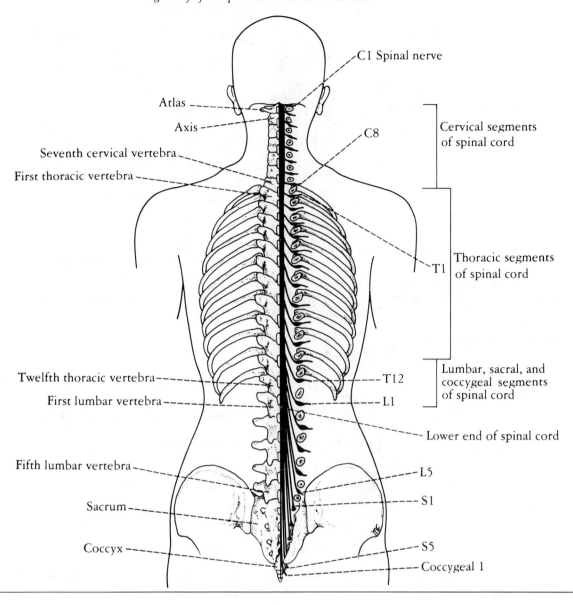

AUTONOMIC GANGLIA

The autonomic ganglia (sympathetic and parasympathetic ganglia) are situated at a distance from the brain and spinal cord (Fig. 4-2). They are located in the sympathetic trunks, in prevertebral plexuses (e.g., the celiac and mesenteric plexuses), and as ganglia in or close to viscera. Each ganglion is covered by a layer of connective tissue that is continuous with the epineurium and perineurium of the peripheral nerve. The neurons are multipolar and possess cell bodies that are irregular in shape. The dendrites of the neurons make synaptic connections with the myelinated axons of preganglionic neurons. The axons of the neurons are of small diameter (C fibers) and unmyelinated, and they pass to viscera, blood vessels, and sweat glands.

Each nerve cell body is closely surrounded by a layer of flattened cells called **capsular cells** or **satellite cells.** The capsular cells, like those of sensory ganglia, are similar in structure to Schwann cells and are continuous with them as they cover the peripheral and central processes of each neuron.

Fig. 4-4

Oblique posterior view of the lower end of the spinal cord and the cauda equina. On the right, the laminae have been removed to expose the right half of the spinal cord and the nerve roots.

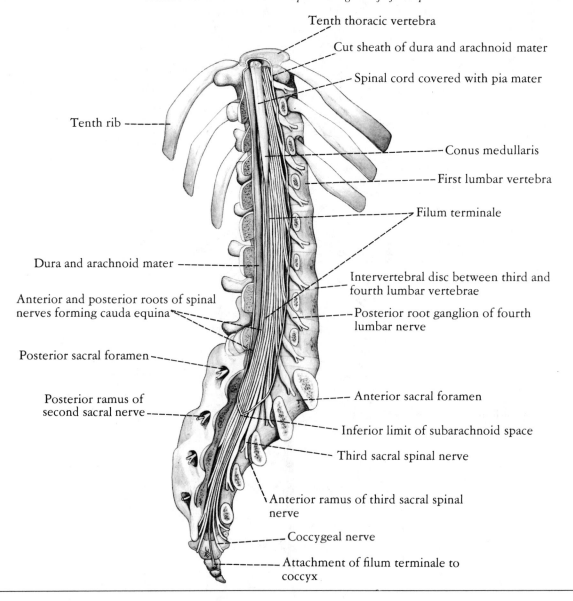

Tenth thoracic vertebra

Cut sheath of dura and arachnoid mater

Spinal cord covered with pia mater

Tenth rib

Conus medullaris

First lumbar vertebra

Filum terminale

Dura and arachnoid mater

Intervertebral disc between third and fourth lumbar vertebrae

Anterior and posterior roots of spinal nerves forming cauda equina

Posterior root ganglion of fourth lumbar nerve

Posterior sacral foramen

Posterior ramus of second sacral nerve

Anterior sacral foramen

Inferior limit of subarachnoid space

Third sacral spinal nerve

Anterior ramus of third sacral spinal nerve

Coccygeal nerve

Attachment of filum terminale to coccyx

NERVE PLEXUSES

In many parts of the body peripheral nerves divide into branches that join neighboring peripheral nerves. If this should occur frequently, a network of nerves is formed called a **nerve plexus.** Since a peripheral nerve is composed of bundles of nerve fibers, a nerve plexus permits individual nerve fibers to pass from one peripheral nerve to another and in most instances branching of nerve fibers does not take place. A nerve plexus thus permits a redistribution of the nerve fibers within the different peripheral nerves.

At the root of the limbs the anterior rami of the spinal nerves form the following plexuses—cervical, brachial, lumbar, and sacral. This allows the nerve fibers, derived from different segments of the spinal cord, to be arranged and distributed efficiently in different nerve trunks to the various parts of the upper and lower limbs.

Cutaneous nerves, as they approach their final destination, commonly form fine plexuses, which again permit a rearrangement of nerve fibers before they reach their terminal sensory endings.

The autonomic nervous system also possesses numerous nerve plexuses, which consist of pre- and postganglionic nerve fibers and ganglia.

In each of the following questions, answer:

A. If only (1) is correct
B. If only (2) is correct
C. If both (1) and (2) are correct
D. If neither (1) nor (2) is correct

1. (1) A peripheral nerve is composed entirely of axons.
   (2) Only myelinated nerve fibers are present in a peripheral nerve.
2. (1) The connective tissue sheaths that surround a peripheral nerve are devoid of blood and lymph vessels.
   (2) The epineurium is the outermost of the connective tissue sheaths that surround a peripheral nerve.
3. (1) The endoneurium supports individual nerve fibers and plays a vital role in regeneration of peripheral nerves.
   (2) Group A fibers are myelinated somatic afferent and efferent fibers.
4. (1) Group C fibers measure 1 to 20 μm in diameter, are nonmyelinated, and are postganglionic autonomic fibers.
   (2) The conduction velocity in group A fibers may be as high as 120 meters per second.

In each of the following questions, answer:

A. If only (1), (2), and (3) are correct
B. If only (1) and (3) are correct
C. If only (2) and (4) are correct
D. If only (4) is correct
E. If all are correct

5. The cranial nerves:
   (1) Are twelve in number and are paired.
   (2) Exit from the brain only.
   (3) Exit through formina in the skull.
   (4) Are entirely motor in function.
6. The spinal nerves:
   (1) Are 33 in number and are paired.
   (2) Leave the vertebral column through intervertebral foramina.
   (3) Include seven in the cervical region.
   (4) Include one coccygeal nerve in the coccygeal region.
7. Concerning the spinal nerve roots:
   (1) The anterior root contains motor fibers to skeletal muscle.
   (2) The posterior root contains sensory fibers.
   (3) The anterior root may contain autonomic nerve fibers.
   (4) The cells of origin of the posterior root nerve fibers are located in the posterior root ganglion.
8. (1) A spinal nerve is connected to the spinal cord by an anterior and a posterior ramus.
   (2) The posterior ramus of a spinal nerve is larger than the anterior ramus.
   (3) The anterior ramus contains only motor fibers.
   (4) A spinal nerve is formed as it passes through an intervertebral foramen.
9. (1) The nerve cells in the posterior root ganglion are devoid of capsular cells.

(2) The cells in the sensory ganglia of the vestibulocochlear nerve are bipolar.

(3) Autonomic ganglia are always situated close to the spinal cord.

(4) The cells situated in an autonomic ganglion are of the multipolar type.

10. Concerning the cauda equina:

(1) It is formed from the roots of the lumbar and sacral nerves below the level of the lower border of the first lumbar vertebra.

(2) It is made up of both anterior and posterior nerve roots.

(3) The nerve roots form a leash of nerves around the filum terminale.

(4) It lies below the lower end of the spinal cord.

11. Concerning large nerve plexuses:

(1) They permit nerve fibers to pass from one peripheral nerve to another.

(2) They are commonly found at the root of a limb.

(3) They permit nerve fibers from different segments of the spinal cord to enter a peripheral nerve.

(4) In most instances individual nerve fibers do not branch at large nerve plexuses.

12. Concerning autonomic ganglia:

(1) They are covered with connective tissue that is continuous with the epineurium and perineurium of the nerves.

(2) They are located, for example, in the celiac and mesenteric plexuses.

(3) The axons of the neurons are of the type C.

(4) The dendrites of the nerve cells synapse with myelinated axons.

ANSWERS AND EXPLANATIONS

1. D: (1) A peripheral nerve is composed of axons and dendrites. (2) A peripheral nerve contains both myelinated motor and sensory fibers and nonmyelinated postganglionic sympathetic fibers.

2. B: (1) Blood and lymph vessels are present in the connective tissue sheaths of peripheral nerves.

3. C

4. B: (1) Group C fibers measure about 0.5 to 2.0 μm in diameter.

5. B: (2) All the cranial nerves exit from the brain except the spinal part of the accessory nerve (XI), which exits from the upper five cervical segments of the spinal cord and joins the cranial part of the nerve within the skull; they then both exit through the jugular foramen. (4) Some cranial nerves are purely sensory (olfactory, optic, vestibulocochlear) and some are mixed (trigeminal, facial, glossopharyngeal, and vagus).

6. C: (1) There are 31 pairs of spinal nerves. (3) There are eight spinal nerves in the cervical region.

7. E

8. D: (1) A spinal nerve is connected to the spinal cord by anterior and posterior nerve roots. (2) The posterior ramus of a spinal nerve is smaller than an anterior ramus. (3) The anterior ramus contains motor, sensory, and autonomic nerve fibers.

9. C: (1) The nerve cells in a posterior root ganglion are surrounded with capsular or satellite cells (3) Autonomic ganglia are situated some distance from the spinal cord in plexuses, in ganglionated trunks, or suspended from nerves.

10. E

11. E

12. E

5 Peripheral Nerve Endings

SUGGESTED PLAN FOR REVIEW OF CHAPTER 5

1. Understand and be able to classify the different types of receptors.
2. Learn the detailed structure of hair follicle receptors, the Meissner's corpuscle, and the pacinian corpuscle.
3. Understand the function of cutaneous receptors.
4. What is meant by transduction of sensory stimuli into nerve impulses?
5. What are the different types of joint receptors?
6. The structure and function of neuromuscular and neurotendinous spindles must be learned. These structures are basic to the understanding of skeletal muscle tone, muscle movements, and posture.
7. Learn the anatomy and physiology of a stretch reflex. What is reciprocal inhibition?
8. What are gamma efferent nerve fibers?
9. Be able to define a motor unit.
10. Learn in detail the structure and function of a neuromuscular junction in skeletal muscle.

11. Understand how nerves end on smooth muscle, cardiac muscle, and secretory cells.

<table>
<tr><td>

INTRODUCTION

</td><td>

Special sensory nerve endings or **receptors** allow the individual to receive information from the environment and from within the body. **Exteroreceptors** are those that respond to stimuli from the external environment and include those of the eye, ear, nose, and taste buds in the mouth. The skin receptors are sensitive to touch, pressure, and temperature changes. **Interoreceptors** respond to stimuli from within the body and include **stretch receptors** within muscles, **visceroreceptors** in the walls of viscera, and **chemoreceptors,** such as the carotid and aortic bodies, and **baroreceptors,** such as the carotid sinus.

</td></tr>
<tr><td>

CLASSIFICATION OF RECEPTORS

</td><td>

From a functional standpoint, sensory receptors can be classified into five basic types:

1. **Mechanoreceptors.** These respond to mechanical deformation.
2. **Thermoreceptors.** These respond to changes in temperature; some receptors respond to cold and others to heat.
3. **Nocioreceptors.** These respond to any stimuli that bring about damage to the tissue.
4. **Electromagnetic receptors.** The rods and cones of the eyes are sensitive to changes in light intensity and wavelength.
5. **Chemoreceptors.** These respond to chemical changes associated with taste and smell and oxygen and carbon dioxide concentrations in the blood.

Until more is known about the genesis of subjective sensations, the sensory receptors will be classified in this text, on a structural basis, into nonencapsulated and encapsulated receptors. The eyes, ears, nose, and taste buds will be considered with the cranial nerves.

Nonencapsulated Receptors

FREE NERVE ENDINGS. Free nerve endings are found throughout the body, including the epithelia of the skin, cornea, and alimentary tract, and in connective tissues, including the dermis, ligaments, joint capsules, tendons, perichondrium, periosteum, and dental pulp. The afferent nerve fibers from the free nerve endings are of small diameter and are either myelinated or nonmyelinated. The terminal endings are devoid of a myelin sheath and there are no Schwann cells covering their tips.

The majority of these endings detect pain, while others detect crude touch, pressure, and tickle sensations, and possibly cold and heat.

MERKEL'S DISCS. Merkel's discs are found in hairless skin, for example the fingertips, and also in hair follicles. The nerve fiber passes into the epidermis and terminates as a disc-shaped expansion that is applied closely to a dark-staining epithelial cell in the deeper part of the epidermis, called the **Merkel cell.** In hairy skin, clusters of Merkel's discs known as **tactile domes** are found in the epidermis between the hair follicles. They measure about 0.2 mm in diameter and are supplied by branches of a single myelinated axon. Merkel's discs are slowly adapting touch receptors that transmit information about the degree of pressure exerted on the skin, as for example when holding a pen.

</td></tr>
</table>

HAIR FOLLICLE RECEPTORS. Nerve fibers wind around the follicle in its outer connective tissue sheath below the sebaceous gland (Fig. 5-1). Some branches surround the follicle while others run parallel to its long axis. Many naked axon filaments terminate among the cells of the outer root sheath. Bending of the hair stimulates the follicle receptor, which belongs to the rapidly adapting group of mechanoreceptors. While the hair remains bent the receptor is silent, but when the hair is released, a further burst of nerve impulses is initiated.

Encapsulated Receptors. These receptors vary in size and shape, and the termination of the nerve is covered by a capsule.

MEISSNER'S CORPUSCLES. Meissner's corpuscles are located in the dermal papillae of the skin, especially the skin of the hand and the foot (Fig. 5-1). Each corpuscle is ovoid in shape and consists of a stack of modified flattened Schwann cells arranged transversely across the long axis of the corpuscle. The corpuscle is

---

Fig. 5-1

A. Nerve endings around hair follicle. B. Meissner's corpuscle in skin. C. Pacinian corpuscle in skin.

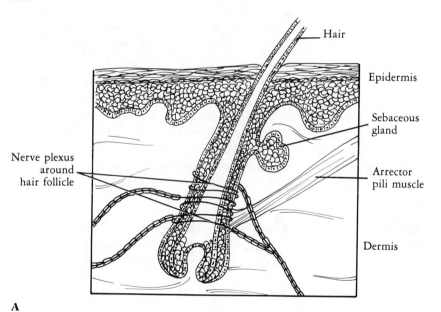

Hair

Epidermis

Sebaceous gland

Nerve plexus around hair follicle

Arrector pili muscle

Dermis

A

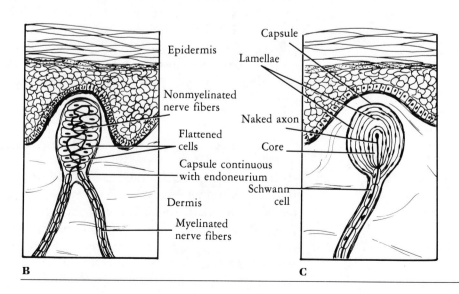

Epidermis

Nonmyelinated nerve fibers

Flattened cells

Capsule continuous with endoneurium

Dermis

Myelinated nerve fibers

Capsule

Lamellae

Naked axon

Core

Schwann cell

B

C

enclosed by a capsule of connective tissue that is continuous with the endoneurium of the nerves that enter it. A few myelinated nerve fibers enter the deep end of the corpuscle; myelinated and unmyelinated branches decrease in size and ramify among the Schwann cells. There is a considerable reduction in the number of Meissner's corpuscles between birth and old age.

Meissner's corpuscles are extremely sensitive to touch and are rapidly adapting mechanoreceptors. They enable an individual to distinguish between two pointed structures when they are placed close together on the skin (two-point tactile discrimination).

PACINIAN CORPUSCLES. Pacinian corpuscles are widely distributed throughout the body and they are present in large numbers in the dermis and subcutaneous tissue of the hands and feet (Fig. 5-1). Each corpuscle is ovoid in shape, measuring about 2 mm long and about 100 to 500 μm across. It consists of a capsule and a central core containing the nerve ending. The capsule consists of numerous concentric lamellae of flattened cells.

A large myelinated nerve fiber enters the corpuscle and loses its myelin sheath and then its Schwann cell covering. The naked axon, surrounded by lamellae formed of flattened cells, passes through the center of the core and terminates in an expanded end.

Pacinian corpuscles are rapidly developing mechanoreceptors and particularly sensitive to vibration. They can respond to up to 600 stimuli per second.

RUFFINI'S CORPUSCLES. Ruffini's corpuscles are located in the dermis of hairy skin. Each corpuscle consists of several unmyelinated nerve endings lying within a bundle of collagen fibers and surrounded by a cellular capsule. They are stretch receptors and respond when the skin is stretched. They are slowly adapting mechanoreceptors.

FUNCTION OF CUTANEOUS RECEPTORS

The main types of sensation that can be experienced by the skin are pain, temperature (heat and cold), touch, pressure, and vibration. Each receptor that has been described can be stimulated by a variety of stimuli such as mechanical deformation, application of chemicals, or change in the temperature. For a long time it was believed that the different histological types of receptors corresponded to specific sensations. However, it was soon pointed out that there are areas of the body that have only one or two histological types of receptors and yet they are sensitive to a variety of different stimuli. Moreover, in spite of the fact that we have these different receptors, all nerves only transmit nerve impulses. The type of sensation felt is determined by the specific area of the central nervous system to which the afferent nerve fiber passes. For example, if a pain nerve fiber is stimulated by heat, cold touch, or pressure, the individual will experience only pain.

TRANSDUCTION OF SENSORY STIMULI INTO NERVE IMPULSES

Transduction is the process by which one form of energy (the stimulus) is changed into another form of energy (electrochemical energy of the nerve impulse). The stimulus when applied to the receptor brings about a change in potential of the plasma membrane of the nerve ending. Since this process takes place in the receptor it is referred to as the **receptor potential.** The receptor potential, if large enough, will generate an action potential at the first node of Ranvier. This sets in motion the saltatory conduction of an action potential that travels along the afferent nerve fiber to the central nervous system.

JOINT RECEPTORS	Four types of sensory endings can be located in the capsule and ligaments of synovial joints. Three of these endings are encapsulated and resemble pacinian, Ruffini's, and tendon stretch receptors. They provide the central nervous system with information regarding the position and movements of the joint. A fourth type of ending is nonencapsulated and is thought to be sensitive to excessive movements and to transmit pain sensations.
MUSCLE RECEPTORS	**Neuromuscular Spindles.** Neuromuscular spindles, or muscular spindles (Fig. 5-2), are found in skeletal muscles and are most numerous toward the tendinous attachment of the muscle. They provide sensory information that is used by the central nervous system in the control of muscle activity.

Each spindle measures about 1 to 4 mm in length and is surrounded by a fusiform capsule of connective tissue. Within the capsule are 6 to 14 slender **intrafusal muscle fibers;** the ordinary muscle fibers situated outside the spindles are referred to as **extrafusal fibers.** The intrafusal fibers of the spindles are of two types: the **nuclear bag** and **nuclear chain** fibers. The nuclear bag fibers are recognized by the presence of numerous nuclei in the equatorial region, which consequently is expanded; also, cross-striations are absent in this region. In the nuclear chain fibers, the nuclei form a single longitudinal row or chain in the center of each fiber at the equatorial region. The nuclear bag fibers are larger in diameter than the nuclear chain fibers, and they extend beyond the capsule at each end to be attached to the endomysium of the extrafusal fibers.

Two types of sensory innervation of the muscle spindles exists, the annulospiral and the flower spray (Fig. 5-2). The **annulospiral endings** are located at the equator of the intrafusal fibers. The large myelinated nerve fiber pierces the capsule and loses its myelin sheath, and the naked axon winds spirally around the intrafusal fiber.

The **flower spray endings** are located chiefly on the nuclear chain fibers away from the equatorial region. A large myelinated nerve fiber pierces the capsule and loses its myelin sheath, and the naked axon breaks up into small branches with terminal expansions that resemble a spray of flowers.

Stretching (elongation) of the intrafusal muscle fibers causes stimulation of the annulospiral and flower spray endings and the passage of nerve impulses to the spinal cord in the afferent neurons.

Motor innervation of the intrafusal fibers is from small gamma efferent fibers (Fig. 5-2). The nerves terminate in small motor end-plates situated away from the equatorial region of the intrafusal fibers. Stimulation of the motor nerves causes both ends of the intrafusal fibers to contract and activates the sensory endings. The equatorial region, which is without cross-striations, is noncontractile.

The extrafusal muscle fibers receive their innervation from large alpha-size axons.

FUNCTION OF THE NEUROMUSCULAR SPINDLE. Under resting conditions, the muscle spindles give rise to afferent nerve impulses all the time, and most of this information is not consciously perceived. When muscle activity occurs, either actively or passively, the intrafusal fibers are stretched and there is an increase in the rate of passage of nerve impulses to the spinal cord in the afferent neurons. Similarly, if the intrafusal fibers are now relaxed due to the cessation of muscle activity, the result is a decrease in the rate of passage of nerve impulses to the spinal cord. The neuromuscular spindle thus plays a very important role in keeping the central nervous system informed about muscle activity, thereby indirectly influencing the control of voluntary muscle.

Fig. 5-2

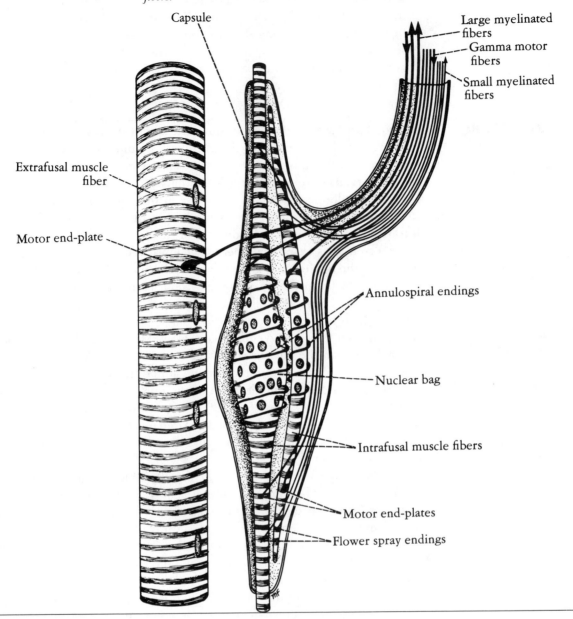

Capsule

Large myelinated fibers

Gamma motor fibers

Small myelinated fibers

Extrafusal muscle fiber

Motor end-plate

Annulospiral endings

Nuclear bag

Intrafusal muscle fibers

Motor end-plates

Flower spray endings

STRETCH REFLEX. The neurons involved in the simple stretch reflex are as follows: Stretching a muscle results in the elongation of the intrafusal fibers and stimulation of the annulospiral and the flower spray endings. The nerve impulses reach the spinal cord in the afferent neurons and synapse with the large alpha motor neurons situated in the anterior gray horns of the spinal cord. Nerve impulses now pass via the efferent motor nerves and stimulate the extrafusal muscle fibers and the muscle contracts. This simple stretch reflex depends on a two-neuron arc, an afferent neuron and an efferent neuron. It is interesting to note that the muscle spindle afferent impulses inhibit the alpha motor neurons supplying the antagonist muscles. This effect is called **reciprocal inhibition.**

Control of the Gamma Efferent Nerves. In the brain and spinal cord there are centers that give rise to tracts that synapse with gamma motor neurons in the spinal cord. Included in these centers are the reticular formation, the basal ganglia, and the cerebellum. By this means these centers can greatly influence voluntary muscle activity. The gamma efferent motor fibers cause shortening of the intrafusal fibers, stretching of the equatorial regions, and stimulation of the annulospiral and flower spray endings. This in turn will initiate the reflex contraction of the extrafusal fibers described previously. It is estimated that about one-third of all the motor fibers passing to a muscle are gamma efferents; the remaining two-thirds are the large alpha motor fibers. It is believed that the nuclear bag fibers are concerned with dynamic responses and are associated more with position and velocity of contraction, whereas the nuclear chain fibers are associated with slow static contractions of voluntary muscle.

Neurotendinous Spindles (Golgi Tendon Organs). Neurotendinous spindles are present in tendons at each end of muscles and they are located near the junctions of tendons with muscles. Each spindle consists of a fibrous capsule that surrounds a small bundle of loosely arranged tendon (collagen) fibers (intrafusal fibers). The tendon cells are larger and more numerous than those found elsewhere in the tendon. One or more myelinated sensory nerve fibers pierce the capsule, lose their myelin sheath, branch, and terminate in expanded endings. The nerve endings are activated by being squeezed by the adjacent tendon fibers within the spindle when tension develops in the tendon. Unlike the neuromuscular spindle, which is sensitive to changes in muscle length, the neurotendinous organ detects changes in muscle tension.

FUNCTION OF THE NEUROTENDINOUS SPINDLE. Increased muscle tension stimulates the neurotendinous spindles and an increased number of nerve impulses reach the spinal cord through the afferent nerve fibers. These fibers synapse with the large alpha motor neurons situated in the anterior gray horns of the spinal cord. Unlike the muscle spindle reflex, this reflex is inhibitory and inhibits muscle contraction. In this manner the tendon reflex prevents the development of too much tension in the muscle. Although this tendon reflex is probably important in protecting the muscle from developing too much tension and thus tearing or being avulsed from its bony attachments, its main function is to provide the central nervous system with information that can influence voluntary muscle activity.

EFFECTOR ENDINGS

Innervation of Skeletal Muscle. Skeletal muscle is innervated by one or more nerves. In the limbs and head and neck the innervation is usually single, but in the large muscles of the abdominal wall the innervation is multiple, the latter muscles having retained their embryonic segmental nerve supply.

The nerve supply to a muscle contains motor and sensory fibers. The motor fibers are of three types: (1) large alpha myelinated fibers, (2) small gamma myelinated fibers, and (3) fine unmyelinated fibers. The large myelinated axons of the alpha anterior horn cells supply the extrafusal fibers that form the main mass of the muscle. The small gamma myelinated fibers supply the intrafusal fibers of the neuromuscular spindles. The fine unmyelinated fibres are postganglionic autonomic efferents that supply the smooth muscle in the walls of blood vessels.

The sensory fibers are of three main types: (1) the myelinated fibers, which originate in the annulospiral and flower spray endings of the neuromuscular spindles, (2) the myelinated fibers, which originate in the neurotendinous spindles, and (3) the myelinated and nonmyelinated fibers, which originate from a variety of sensory endings in the connective tissue of the muscle.

MOTOR UNIT. The motor unit may be defined as the single alpha motor neuron and the muscle fibers that it innervates. The muscle fibers of a single motor unit are widely scattered throughout the muscle. Where fine, precise muscle control is required, such as in the extraocular muscles or the small muscles of the hand, the motor units possess only a few muscle fibers. However, in a large limb muscle, such as the gluteus maximus, where precise control is not necessary, a single motor nerve may innervate many hundreds of muscle fibers.

NEUROMUSCULAR JUNCTIONS IN SKELETAL MUSCLE. As each large alpha myelinated fiber enters a skeletal muscle it branches many times. The number of branches depends on the size of the motor unit. A single branch then terminates on a muscle fiber at a site referred to as a **neuromuscular junction** or **motor end-plate** (Fig. 5-3). The great majority of muscle fibers are innervated by just one motor end-plate. On reaching the muscle fiber, the nerve loses its myelin sheath and breaks up into a number of subsidiary branches. Each branch ends as a naked axon and constitutes the **neural element** of the motor end-plate (Fig. 5-3). The axon is expanded slightly and contains numerous mitochondria and vesicles (approximately 45 nm in diameter). At the site of the motor end-plate the surface of the muscle fiber is elevated slightly to form the **muscular element** of the plate, often referred to as the **sole plate.** The elevation is due to the local accumulation of granular sarcoplasm beneath the sarcolemma and the presence of numerous nuclei and mitochondria.

The expanded naked axon lies in a groove on the surface of the muscle fiber. Each groove is formed by the infolding of the sarcolemma. The groove may branch many times, each branch containing a division of the axon. It is important to realize that the axons are truly naked; the Schwann cells merely serve as a cap or roof to the groove and never project into it. The floor of the groove is formed of sarcolemma, which is thrown into numerous folds, called **junctional folds;** these serve to increase the surface area of the sarcolemma that lies close to the naked axon (Fig. 5-3). The plasma membrane of the axon (the axolemma or presynaptic membrane) is separated, by a space about 20 to 50 nm wide, from the plasma membrane of the muscle fiber (the sarcolemma or postsynaptic membrane). This space constitutes the **synaptic cleft.** The synaptic cleft is filled with the basement membranes of the axon and the muscle fiber. The motor end-plate is strengthened by the connective tissue sheath of the nerve fiber, the endoneurium, which becomes continuous with the connective tissue sheath of the muscle fiber, the endomysium.

A nerve impulse, on reaching a motor end-plate, causes the release of acetylcholine from some of the axonal vesicles. The acetylcholine is discharged into the synaptic cleft by a process of exocytosis and diffuses through the basement membranes to reach the receptors on the postsynaptic membrane. This makes the postsynaptic membrane more permeable to Na^+ ions, and a local potential is created called the **end-plate potential.** If the end-plate potential is large enough, an action potential will be initiated that will spread along the surface of the sarcolemma. The wave of depolarization is carried into the muscle fiber to the contractile myofibrils through the system of T tubules. This leads to the release of Ca^+ ions from the sarcoplasmic reticulum, which in turn causes the muscle to contract.

The amount of acetylcholine released at the motor end-plate will depend on the number of nerve impulses arriving at the nerve terminal. Once the acetylcholine crosses the synaptic cleft, it immediately undergoes hydrolysis due to the presence of **acetylcholinesterase** (AChE) in the basement membranes and the postsynaptic membrane or sarcolemma. The acetylcholine remains for about 1 millisecond in contact with the postsynaptic membrane, and it is rapidly destroyed to prevent reexcitation of the muscle fiber.

Skeletal muscle fiber contraction is thus controlled by the frequency of the

Fig. 5-3

A. A skeletal neuromuscular junction. B. Enlarged view of muscle fiber showing terminal naked axon lying in surface groove of muscle fiber.

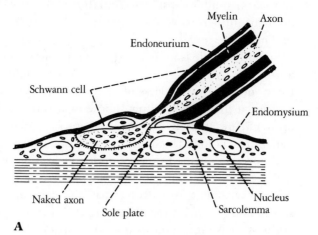

A

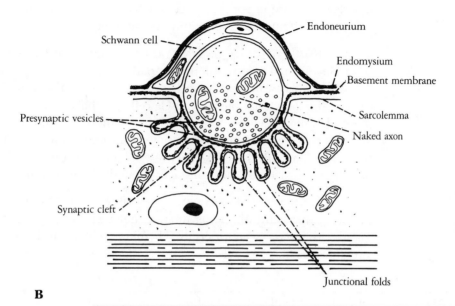

B

nerve impulses that arrive at the motor nerve terminal. A resting muscle fiber shows small occasional depolarizations (end-plate potentials) at the motor end-plate, which are insufficient to cause an action potential and make the fiber contract. These are believed to be due to the sporadic release of acetylcholine into the synaptic cleft from a single presynaptic vesicle.

NEUROMUSCULAR JUNCTIONS IN SMOOTH MUSCLE. In smooth muscle, where the action is slow and widespread, such as within the wall of the intestine, the autonomic nerve fibers branch extensively, so that a single neuron exerts control over a large number of muscle fibers. In some areas, for example, the longitudinal layer of smooth muscle in the intestine, only a few muscle fibers are associated with autonomic endings, the wave of contraction passing from one muscle cell to another by means of gap junctions.

In smooth muscle, in which the action is fast and precision is required, such as in the iris, the branching of the nerve fibers is less extensive, so that a single neuron exerts control over only a few muscle fibers.

The autonomic nerve fibers, which are postganglionic, are nonmyelinated and terminate as a series of varicosed branches. An interval of from 10 to 100 nm may exist between the axon and the muscle fiber. At the site where transmission is to occur, the Schwann cell is retracted so that the axon lies within a shallow groove on its surface. Part of the axon thus is naked, permitting free diffusion of the transmitter substance from the axon to the muscle cell. Here the axoplasm contains numerous vesicles similar to those seen at the motor end-plate of skeletal muscle.

Smooth muscle is innervated by sympathetic and parasympathetic parts of the autonomic system. Those nerves that are cholinergic liberate acetylcholine at their endings by a process of exocytosis, the acetylcholine being present in the vesicles at the nerve ending. Those nerves that are noradrenergic liberate **norepinephrine** at their endings by a process of exocytosis, the norepinephrine being present in dark-cored vesicles at the nerve endings. Both the acetylcholine and norepinephrine bring about depolarization of the muscle fibers innervated, which thereupon contract. The fate of these neurotransmitter substances differs. The acetylcholine is hydrolyzed in the presence of acetylcholinesterase in the sarcolemma of the muscle fiber and the norepinephrine is taken up by the nerve endings. It is important to note that in some areas of the body (e.g., bronchial muscle) the norepinephrine liberated from postganglionic sympathetic fibers causes smooth muscle to relax and not contract.

NEUROMUSCULAR JUNCTIONS IN CARDIAC MUSCLE. Cardiac muscle is innervated by nonmyelinated postganglionic sympathetic and parasympathetic nerve fibers. These nerves run in the connective tissue between the muscle fibers and end close to the individual cardiac muscle cells. At the site where transmission takes place, the axon becomes naked because of the retraction of the Schwann cell. This permits free diffusion of the neurotransmitter substance from the axon to the muscle cell. Because of the presence of gap junctions between adjacent muscle cells, excitation and contraction rapidly spread from fiber to fiber.

NERVE ENDINGS ON SECRETORY CELLS OF GLANDS. Nonmyelinated postganglionic sympathetic and parasympathetic nerves run in the connective tissue of glands close to the secretory cells. The nerve fibers entering some glands innervate only the blood vessels.

NATIONAL BOARD TYPE QUESTIONS

In each of the following questions, answer:
A. If only (1) is correct
B. If only (2) is correct
C. If both (1) and (2) are correct
D. If neither (1) nor (2) is correct

1. (1) The carotid and aortic bodies are examples of chemoreceptors.
   (2) The carotid sinus is an example of a baroreceptor.
2. (1) A mechanoreceptor is one that brings about damage to the tissue.
   (2) Free nerve endings are confined to the deep tissues of the body.
3. (1) Merkel's discs are slowly adapting touch receptors.
   (2) Merkel's discs are found only in hair follicles.
4. (1) The hair follicle receptors remain active once the hair has been bent out of shape.
   (2) Meissner's corpuscles become reduced in number with age.
5. (1) Meissner's corpuscles are located in the dermal papillae of the skin.
   (2) Meissner's corpuscles are sensitive to heat changes.
6. (1) Annulospiral endings are located at the ends of the intrafusal fibers in a neuromuscular spindle.
   (2) Nuclear bag and nuclear chain fibers are the names given to the intrafusal muscle fibers in a neuromuscular spindle.

Select the **best** response.

7. The following facts are correct concerning the pacinian corpuscle **except:**
   A. It is present in large numbers in the dermis and subcutaneous tissues.
   B. It measures about 2 mm long.
   C. The expanded end of the axon is covered by Schwann cells.
   D. It is particularly sensitive to vibration.
   E. The capsule consists of numerous concentric lamellae of flattened cells.

8. Concerning the neuromuscular spindles, all the following facts are correct **except:**
   A. They are most numerous toward the tendinous attachment of skeletal muscle.
   B. If the intrafusal fibers are relaxed there is an increase in the rate of passage of nerve impulses to the spinal cord.
   C. The intrafusal fibers receive their motor innervation from gamma nerve fibers.
   D. Flower spray endings are located on the nuclear chain fibers away from the equatorial region.
   E. The extrafusal fibers receive their nerve supply from alpha-size axons.

9. The following facts are **incorrect** concerning the neurotendinous spindles **except:**
   A. They are present in the tendon at only one end of a skeletal muscle.
   B. They have no fibrous capsule.
   C. They are innervated by nonmyelinated nerve fibers.
   D. Their main function is to detect changes in muscle tension.
   E. The nerve endings are activated by being elongated.

In each of the following questions, answer:
A. If only (1), (2), and (3) are correct
B. If only (1) and (3) are correct
C. If only (2) and (4) are correct
D. If only (4) is correct
E. If all are correct

10. Concerning the innervation of skeletal muscle:
    (1) Each muscle of the abdominal wall receives multiple innervations.
    (2) The motor nerve supply to a muscle contains motor and sensory fibers.
    (3) The motor fibers consist of alpha myelinated fibers, gamma myelinated fibers, and fine unmyelinated fibers.
    (4) A motor unit is a single muscle fiber and its nerve supply.

11. Concerning a neuromuscular junction in skeletal muscle:
    (1) The motor nerve loses its myelin sheath on reaching the muscle fiber.
    (2) The axon breaks up into a number of branches.
    (3) The expanded part of the terminal axon lies in a groove on the surface of the muscle fiber.
    (4) The terminal axon contains mitochondria and vesicles in its cytoplasm.

12. Concerning the muscular element of the motor end-plate:
    (1) The endomysium lines the grooves on the surface of the muscle fibers.
    (2) The surface area of the sarcolemma is increased by the presence of junctional folds.
    (3) The space between the presynaptic membrane and the postsynaptic membrane measures about 2 mm.
    (4) The neurotransmitter is acetylcholine.

13. Concerning the events that take place at a motor end-plate:
    (1) The neurotransmitter is released from the presynaptic vesicles.
    (2) The end-plate potential is created by the acetylcholine reaching the receptors on the postsynaptic membrane, resulting in an increased permeability to Na^+ ions.
    (3) The T tubules serve to conduct the wave of depolarization to the myofibrils.
    (4) Acetylcholinesterase limits the action of acetylcholine by the process of hydrolysis, which takes place inside the sarcoplasmic reticulum.

14. Concerning the innervation of smooth muscle:
    (1) Each smooth muscle fiber is innervated by several autonomic neurons.
    (2) The wave of contraction of smooth muscle travels from one muscle fiber to another by means of gap junctions.
    (3) The postganglionic autonomic fiber on reaching the muscle fiber retains its covering of myelin and Schwann cells.
    (4) Smooth muscle is innervated by sympathetic and parasympathetic parts of the autonomic system.

15. Neuromuscular junctions in cardiac muscle:
    (1) The nerves run in the connective tissue between the cardiac muscle fibers.
    (2) The nerve fibers are nonmyelinated.
    (3) The terminal axon is naked and devoid of Schwann cells.
    (4) Gap junctions on the cardiac muscle fibers permit the excitation and contraction to spread rapidly from fiber to fiber.

ANSWERS AND EXPLANATIONS

1. C
2. D: (1) A nocioreceptor is one that brings about damage to the tissue. (2) Free nerve endings are widely distributed throughout the body.
3. A: (2) Merkel's discs are found in the epidermis of hairless skin and in hair follicles.
4. B: (1) The hair follicle receptors are only activated by movement of the hair; once movement ceases (although the hair may be bent), the receptors are inactive.
5. A: (2) Meissner's corpuscles are sensitive to touch.
6. B: (1) Annulospiral endings are located at the equator of the intrafusal fibers.
7. C: The expanded end of the axon is naked.
8. B: If the intrafusal fibers are relaxed there is a decrease in the rate of passage of nerve impulses to the spinal cord.
9. D: (A) They are present in the tendons at both ends of a skeletal muscle. (B) They have a fibrous capsule. (C) They are innervated by myelinated nerve fibers. (E) The nerve endings are activated by being compressed.
10. A: (4) A motor unit is a single motor nerve cell and all the muscle fibers that it supplies.
11. E
12. C: (1) The endomysium does not line the grooves in the sarcolemma at a motor end-plate. (3) The synaptic cleft measures about 20 to 50 nm wide.
13. A: (4) Acetylcholinesterase is located in the basement membranes of the synaptic cleft and on the postsynaptic membrane.
14. C: (1) Each smooth muscle fiber is innervated by a single autonomic neuron. (2) The postganglionic autonomic fiber on reaching the muscle fiber loses its covering of myelin and Schwann cells.
15. E

6 Spinal Cord

SUGGESTED PLAN FOR REVIEW OF CHAPTER 6

1. Spend a long time absorbing the contents of this chapter. The information is repeatedly used in describing the various nerve pathways as they ascend and descend in the spinal cord.

2. Understand the general shape and arrangement of the spinal cord. Know the vertebral level of the lower end of the spinal cord in the adult and young child. What is a spinal segment?

3. Learn the arrangement of the gray and white matter at different segmental levels of the spinal cord. Be able to draw a representative cross section taken from the cervical, thoracic, lumbar, and sacral levels of the cord.

4. Be able to define the phrenic nucleus and the accessory nucleus.

5. Learn the location and function of the substantia gelatinosa, the nucleus proprius, the nucleus dorsalis (Clark's column), the visceral nucleus, and the lateral gray column cells.

6. Define the gray commissures and the central canal.

7. Learn the approximate position of the nerve fiber tracts in the white matter. You will need this knowledge when you learn about the various pathways in the central nervous system. Be able to draw a cross section of the spinal cord with the different tracts in position.

8. Understand the three meninges and learn the extent of the subarachnoid space, especially its lower extent in the vertebral column.

9. Have a good understanding of the formation and circulation of the cerebrospinal fluid (CSF).

10. Know the main blood supply to the spinal cord. Appreciate the seriousness of the situation should the blood supply be compromised.

The spinal cord is an elongated cylindrical part of the central nervous system (Fig. 6-1). It is situated in the upper two-thirds of the vertebral column and is continuous above with the brain. Like the vertebral column, the spinal cord is segmented, though the segments are not visible externally. Left and right spinal nerves, one pair per segment, connect the spinal cord to the tissues of the trunk, appendages, and the viscera.

The spinal cord contains large numbers of ascending and descending pathways, which serve as conduits for nervous information passing to and from different parts of the body to the brain. The spinal cord is also an important center for reflex activity, which is closely supervised by the brain.

Fig. 6-1

(A) Brain and spinal cord posterior view. (B) Transverse section of spinal cord in thoracic region, showing anterior and posterior roots of a spinal nerve and the meninges. (C) Posterior view of lower end of spinal cord and cauda equina.

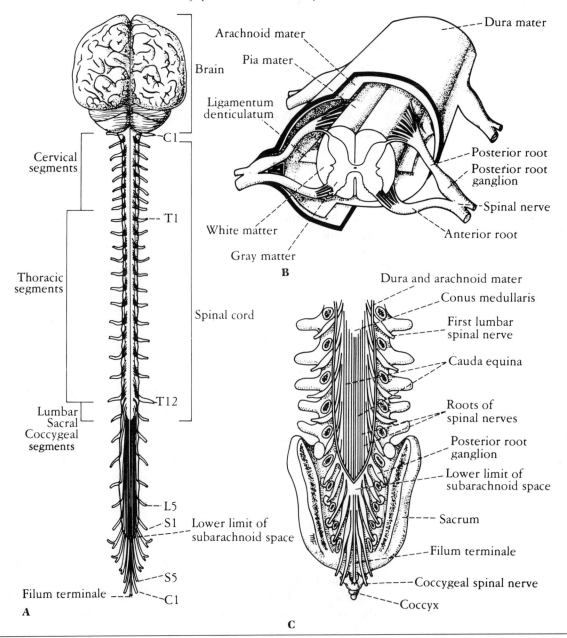

ORGANIZATION OF SPINAL CORD

The spinal cord begins superiorly at the foramen magnum in the skull, where it is continuous with the medulla oblongata of the brain. It terminates inferiorly in the adult at the level of the **lower border of the first lumbar vertebra.** In the young child it is relatively longer and ends at the upper border of the third lumbar vertebra. The spinal cord is situated within the vertebral canal of the vertebral column and is surrounded by three meninges, the **dura mater,** the **arachnoid mater,** and the **pia mater.** (Fig. 6-1). Further protection is provided by the cerebrospinal fluid, which surrounds the spinal cord in the subarachnoid space.

The spinal cord is roughly cylindrical in shape (Fig. 6-1). However, in the cervical region, where it gives origin to the brachial plexus, and in the lower thoracic and lumbar regions, where it gives origin to the lumbosacral plexus, there are fusiform enlargements, called the **cervical and lumbar enlargements** (Fig. 6-2). Inferiorly, the spinal cord tapers off into the **conus medullaris,** from the apex of which a prolongation of the pia mater, the **filum terminale,** descends to be attached to the back of the coccyx (Fig. 6-1). The cord possesses, in the

---

Fig. 6-2   *A. Transverse sections of the spinal cord at different levels. B. Posterior view of the spinal cord, showing cervical and lumbar enlargements.*

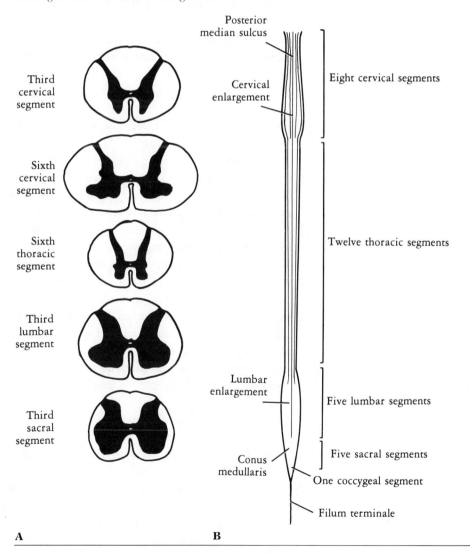

midline anteriorly, a deep longitudinal fissure, the **anterior median fissure,** and on the posterior surface, a shallow furrow, the **posterior median sulcus** (Fig. 6-2).

Along the entire length of the spinal cord are attached 31 pairs of spinal nerves by the **anterior or motor roots** and the **posterior or sensory roots** (Fig. 6-1). Each root is attached to the cord by a series of rootlets, which extend the whole length of the corresponding **root ganglion,** the cells of which give rise to peripheral and central nerve fibers.

STRUCTURE OF SPINAL CORD

The spinal cord is composed of an inner core of **gray matter,** which is surrounded by an outer covering of **white matter** (Fig. 6-1).

Gray Matter. The gray matter, on cross section, is seen as an H-shaped pillar with **anterior and posterior gray columns, or horns,** united by a thin **gray commissure** containing the small **central canal** (Fig. 6-3). A small **lateral gray column or horn** is present in the thoracic and upper lumbar segments of the cord.

STRUCTURE OF GRAY MATTER. As in other regions of the central nervous system, the gray matter of the spinal cord consists of a mixture of nerve cells and their processes, neuroglia, and blood vessels. The nerve cells are multipolar and the neuroglia forms an intricate network around the nerve cell bodies and their neurites.

Nerve Cell Groups in the Anterior Gray Columns. The majority of the nerve cells are large and multipolar and their axons pass out in the anterior roots of the spinal nerves as **alpha efferents,** which innervate skeletal muscles. The smaller nerve cells are also multipolar and the axons of many of these pass out in the anterior roots of the spinal nerves as **gamma efferents,** which innervate the intrafusal muscle fibers of neuromuscular spindles.

The nerve cells of the anterior gray column may be divided into three basic groups: medial, central, and lateral.

The medial group is present in most segments of the spinal cord and is responsible for innervating the skeletal muscles of the neck and trunk (Fig. 6-3). The central group is present in some cervical and lumbosacral segments. In the cervical part of the cord some of these nerve cells (segments C3, 4, and 5) specifically innervate the diaphragm and are collectively referred to as **phrenic nucleus.** In the upper five or six cervical segments, some of the nerve cells innervate the sternocleidomastoid and trapezius muscles and are referred to as the **accessory nucleus.** The axons of these cells form the spinal part of the accessory nerve. The **lumbosacral nucleus** present in the second lumbar down to the first sacral segments of the cord is made up of nerve cells whose axons have an unknown distribution.

The lateral group is present in the cervical and lumbosacral segments of the cord and is responsible for innervating the skeletal muscles of the limbs.

Nerve Cell Groups in the Posterior Gray Columns. There are four nerve cell groups of the posterior gray column.

The **substantia gelatinosa group** is situated at the apex of the posterior gray column throughout the length of the spinal cord (Fig. 6-3). It is largely composed of Golgi type II neurons and receives afferent fibers concerned with pain, temperature, and touch from the posterior root.

The **nucleus proprius** is a group of large nerve cells situated anterior to the

Fig. 6-3

A. Transverse section of the sixth thoracic segment of the spinal cord showing the arrangement of the gray matter. B. Transverse section of the spinal cord at the midcervical level, showing the general arrangement of the ascending tracts on the right and the descending tracts on the left.

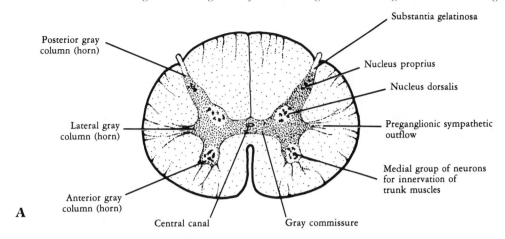

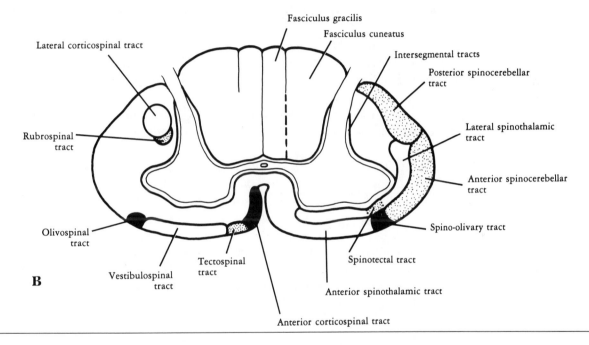

substantia gelatinosa throughout the spinal cord (Fig. 6-3). This nucleus constitutes the main bulk of cells present in the posterior gray column and receives fibers from the posterior white column that are associated with the senses of position and movement (proprioception), two-point discrimination, and vibration.

The **nucleus dorsalis (Clark's column)** is a group of nerve cells situated at the base of the posterior gray column and extending from the eighth cervical segment caudally to the third or fourth lumbar segment (Fig. 6-3). The majority of the cells are comparatively large and are associated with proprioceptive endings (neuromuscular spindles and tendon spindles).

The **visceral afferent nucleus** is a group of nerve cells of medium size situated lateral to the nucleus dorsalis; it extends from the first thoracic to the third lumbar segment of the spinal cord. It is believed to be associated with receiving visceral afferent information.

Nerve Cell Groups in the Lateral Gray Columns. The intermediolateral group of cells form the small lateral gray column, which extends from the first thoracic to the second or third lumbar segments of the spinal cord (Fig. 6-3). The cells are relatively small and give rise to preganglionic sympathetic fibers.

A similar group of cells found in the second, third, and fourth sacral segments of the spinal cord give rise to preganglionic parasympathetic fibers.

THE GRAY COMMISSURE AND CENTRAL CANAL. In transverse sections of the spinal cord, the anterior and posterior gray columns on each side are seen to be connected by a transverse **gray commissure,** so that the gray matter resembles the letter H (Fig. 6-3). In the center of the gray commissure is situated the **central canal.** The part of the gray commissure that is situated posterior to the central canal is often referred to as the **posterior gray commissure;** similarly, the part that lies anterior to the canal is called the **anterior gray commissure.**

The central canal is present throughout the spinal cord (Fig. 6-2). Superiorly, it is continuous with the central canal of the caudal half of the medulla oblongata, and above this it opens into the cavity of the fourth ventricle. Inferiorly in the conus medullaris, it expands into the fusiform **terminal ventricle** and terminates below within the root of the filum terminale. It is filled with cerebrospinal fluid and is lined with ciliated columnar epithelium, the **ependyma.**

White Matter. The white matter, for purposes of description, may be divided into **anterior, lateral, and posterior white columns.** The anterior column on each side lies between the midline and the point of emergence of the anterior nerve roots; the lateral column lies between the emergence of the anterior nerve roots and the entry of the posterior nerve roots; the posterior column lies between the entry of the posterior nerve roots and the midline.

STRUCTURE OF WHITE MATTER. As in other regions of the central nervous system, the white matter of the spinal cord consists of a mixture of nerve fibers, neuroglia, and blood vessels. It surrounds the gray matter and its white color is due to the high proportion of myelinated nerve fibers.

ARRANGEMENT OF NERVE FIBER TRACTS. The spinal tracts are divided into ascending, descending, and intersegmental tracts, and their relative positions in the white matter are shown in Figure 6-3). The connections and functions of the various tracts are given in Chapter 7.

MENINGES OF THE SPINAL CORD

The spinal cord, like the brain, is surrounded by three meninges: the dura mater, the arachnoid mater, and the pia mater.

Dura Mater of the Spinal Cord. The dura mater is a dense, fibrous membrane that encloses the spinal cord and cauda equina (Fig. 6-1). It is continuous above through the foramen magnum with the meningeal layer of dura covering the brain. Inferiorly, it ends on the filum terminale at the level of the lower border of the second sacral vertebra. The dural sheath lies loosely in the vertebral canal and is separated from the walls of the canal by the **extradural space.** This contains loose areolar tissue and the **internal vertebral venous plexus.** The dura mater extends along each nerve root and becomes continuous with the connective tissue surrounding each spinal nerve (epineurium). The inner surface of the dura mater is in contact with the arachnoid mater.

Arachnoid Mater of the Spinal Cord. The arachnoid mater is a delicate impermeable membrane that covers the spinal cord and lies between the pia mater internally and the dura mater externally (Fig. 6-1). It is separated from the pia mater by a wide space, the **subarachnoid space,** which is filled with **cerebrospinal fluid.** The arachnoid mater is continuous above through the foramen magnum with the arachnoid covering the brain. Inferiorly, it ends on the filum terminale at the level of the lower border of the second sacral vertebra (Fig. 6-1). The arachnoid mater continues along the spinal nerve roots, forming small lateral extensions of the subarachnoid space.

Pia Mater of the Spinal Cord. The pia mater, a vascular membrane that closely invests the spinal cord, is thickened on either side between the nerve roots to form the **ligamentum denticulatum,** which passes laterally to adhere to the arachnoid and dura (Fig. 6-1). It is by this means that the spinal cord is suspended in the middle of the dural sheath. The pia mater extends along each nerve root and becomes continuous with the connective tissue surrounding each spinal nerve.

CEREBROSPINAL FLUID	The cerebrospinal fluid is present in the subarachnoid space and in the central canal of the spinal cord. It is produced by the **choroid plexuses** within the lateral, third, and fourth ventricles of the brain. It escapes from the ventricular system of the brain through the three foramina in the roof of the fourth ventricle and so enters the subarachnoid space. The fluid now circulates both superiorly over the surface of the cerebral hemispheres and inferiorly around the spinal cord. The spinal part of the subarachnoid space extends down as far as the lower border of the second sacral vertebra. Eventually, the fluid enters the bloodstream by passing into the **arachnoid villi** of the intracranial venous sinuses and diffusing through their walls.

In addition to removing waste products associated with neuronal activity, the cerebrospinal fluid provides a medium that surrounds the spinal cord. This fluid, together with the bony and ligamentous walls of the vertebral canal, effectively protects the spinal cord from trauma.

BLOOD SUPPLY OF THE SPINAL CORD	The **posterior spinal arteries,** which arise either directly or indirectly from the vertebral arteries, run inferiorly along the side of the spinal cord, close to the attachments of the posterior spinal nerve roots (Fig. 6-4). The anterior spinal arteries, which arise from the vertebral arteries, unite to form a single artery, which runs down within the anterior median fissure. Both the posterior and anterior spinal arteries are small and are not sufficient to supply the entire length of the spinal cord.

The posterior and anterior spinal arteries are reinforced by **radicular arteries** (Fig. 6-4), which are branches of local arteries (deep cervical, intercostal, and lumbar arteries). Radicular arteries enter the vertebral canal through the intervertebral foramina. Commonly, one of the anterior radicular arteries is larger than the remainder and is referred to as the **arteria radicularis magna** (artery of Adamkiewicz). It usually arises from an intersegmental branch of the descending aorta in the lower thoracic or upper lumbar vertebral levels. Usually it arises on the left-hand side. The importance of this artery lies in the fact that it may be the major source of blood to the lower two-thirds of the spinal cord.

The branches of the anterior spinal artery supply approximately the anterior

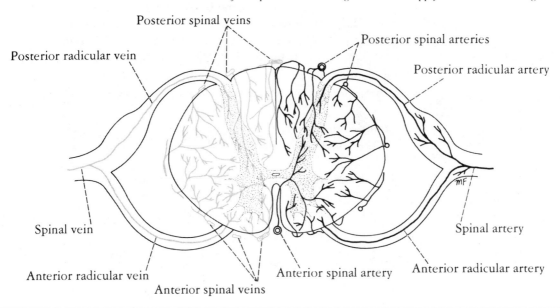

two-thirds of the spinal cord, while the remaining posterior third is supplied by branches from the posterior spinal arteries. A small area on the periphery of the spinal cord is supplied by small arteries from a plexus in the pia mater.

The veins of the spinal cord drain into six tortuous longitudinal channels that communicate superiorly within the skull with the veins of the brain and the venous sinuses. They drain mainly into the internal vertebral venous plexus.

NATIONAL BOARD TYPE QUESTIONS

In each of the following questions, answer:

A. If only (1), (2), and (3) are correct
B. If only (1) and (3) are correct
C. If only (2) and (4) are correct
D. If only (4) is correct
E. If all are correct

1. Concerning the spinal cord:
   (1) The spinal cord is segmented though the segments are not visible on the surface.
   (2) Each segment of the spinal cord has a pair of spinal nerves.
   (3) The spinal cord is an important reflex center.
   (4) The spinal cord terminates inferiorly in the adult at the level of the lower border of the first lumbar vertebra.
2. Concerning the protection of the spinal cord from external injury:
   (1) The spinal cord is located within the vertebral canal of the vertebral column.
   (2) The spinal cord is surrounded by the pia, arachnoid, and dura mater.
   (3) The spinal cord is floating in cerebrospinal fluid.
   (4) The spinal cord is protected by fatty areolar tissue in the vertebral canal.
3. Concerning the shape of the spinal cord:
   (1) The cervical enlargement is caused by the presence of the cervical and brachial plexuses.
   (2) The lumbar enlargement is caused by the parasympathetic outflow.
   (3) The conus medullaris contains the terminal ventricle.
   (4) The filum terminale attaches the lower end of the spinal cord to the back of the sacrum.

4. The gray matter of the spinal cord has the following features:
   (1) Lateral gray columns in the lower cervical region.
   (2) Anterior and posterior gray columns throughout the length of the spinal cord.
   (3) The gray commissure connects the tips of the posterior gray columns.
   (4) The central canal contains cerebrospinal fluid.
5. Concerning the gray matter of the spinal cord:
   (1) The phrenic nucleus is present in the third, fourth, and fifth cervical segments.
   (2) The accessory nucleus lies at the level of the fifth and sixth cervical segments.
   (3) The substantia gelatinosa occupies the tip of the posterior gray column throughout the length of the spinal cord.
   (4) The nucleus dorsalis (Clark's column) is situated at the level of the sacral segments of the spinal cord.
6. Concerning the efferent outflows of the autonomic system in the spinal cord:
   (1) The sympathetic outflow occurs at segmental levels T1–L2.
   (2) The sympathetic outflow occupies the lateral gray column.
   (3) The parasympathetic outflow occurs at segmental levels S2, S3, and S4.
   (4) The cells of origin give rise to axons that are called preganglionic nerve fibers.

In Figure 6-5, match the numbers listed on the left with the appropriate structure listed on the right.

7. Number 1   A. Nucleus dorsalis
8. Number 2   B. Central canal
9. Number 3   C. Lateral gray horn
10. Number 4   D. Anterior median fissure

In Figure 6-6, match the numbers listed on the left with the appropriate ascending or descending tract listed on the right.

11. Number 1   A. Posterior spinocerebellar tract
12. Number 2   B. Lateral corticospinal tract
13. Number 3   C. Fasciculus cuneatus
14. Number 4   D. Rubrospinal tract

In each of the following questions, answer:
A. If only (1) is correct
B. If only (2) is correct
C. If both (1) and (2) are correct
D. If neither (1) nor (2) is correct

15. (1) The dura mater covering the spinal cord is continuous above through the foramen magnum with the periosteal layer of dura of the brain.
    (2) The dura mater of the spinal cord ends below at the level of the second sacral vertebra.
16. (1) The arachnoid mater covering the spinal cord ends below at the level of the second sacral vertebra.
    (2) The subarachnoid space is filled with cerebrospinal fluid.
17. (1) The pia mater surrounds the spinal cord but does not extend along the spinal nerve roots.

Fig. 6-5

Transverse section of a thoracic segment of the spinal cord.

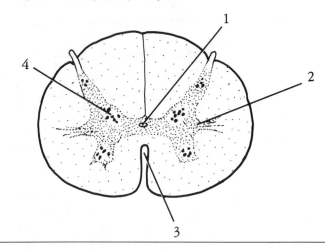

Fig. 6-6

Transverse section of a cervical segment of the spinal cord.

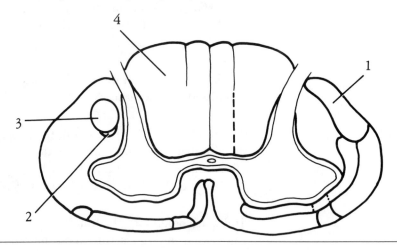

(2) The ligamentum denticulatum attaches the arachnoid mater to the dura between the nerve roots.

18. (1) The posterior spinal arteries supply the posterior third of the spinal cord.
    (2) The radicular arteries reinforce only the anterior spinal artery.
19. (1) Each spinal nerve is attached to the spinal cord by an anterior and a posterior nerve root.
    (2) Each root of the spinal nerve is attached to the spinal cord by a series of rootlets that extend the whole length of each segment of the spinal cord.
20. (1) The neurons in a posterior root ganglion are unipolar and give rise to peripheral and central sensory nerve fibers.
    (2) At each segment of the spinal cord, the subarachnoid space extends laterally as a diverticulum around the nerve roots as far as the spinal nerve.

ANSWERS AND EXPLANATIONS

1. E
2. E
3. B: (2) The lumbar enlargement is caused by the lumbosacral plexus. (4) The

filum terminale connects the lower end of the spinal cord to the back of the coccyx.

4. C: (1) The lateral gray columns of the spinal cord are associated with the sympathetic outflow and are located from T1–L2 segments. (3) The gray commissure connects the anterior and posterior gray columns on each side so that the gray matter resembles the letter H.

5. B: (2) The accessory nucleus occupies the upper five cervical segments of the spinal cord. (4) The nucleus dorsalis (Clark's column) is present from the eighth cervical segment to the third or fourth lumbar segment of the spinal cord.

6. E

7. B

8. C

9. D

10. A

11. A

12. D

13. B

14. C

15. B: (1) The dura mater covering the spinal cord is continuous above through the foramen magnum with the meningeal layer of the dura of the brain.

16. C

17. D: (1) The pia mater extends laterally around each nerve root as far as the beginning of the spinal nerve. (2) The ligamentum denticulatum connects the pia of the spinal cord to the arachnoid and dura mater; it thus assists in anchoring the spinal cord in the subarachnoid space.

18. A: (2) The radicular arteries reinforce both the anterior and the posterior spinal arteries.

19. C

20. C

7 Ascending and Descending Tracts and Reflex Activity

SUGGESTED PLAN FOR REVIEW OF CHAPTER 7

1. Each of the ascending and descending tracts listed in this chapter must be memorized. The function of each pathway must be committed to memory.
2. Distinguish between light touch and discriminative touch.

3. Understand the analgesia system and the gating theory.
4. What are enkephalins and endorphins?
5. Be able to define a reflex arc. Know what is meant by the law of reciprocal innervation and the crossed extensor reflex.
6. What is a Renshaw cell?

By the time that you have finished this chapter, it should be possible for you to make simple line drawings of each of the ascending and descending pathways showing their cells of origin, their course through the central nervous system, and their destination. Particular attention should be paid to whether a particular tract crosses the midline to the opposite side of the central nervous system or remains on the same side. If the tract does cross the midline, the level of cross-over is important.

INTRODUCTION

The ascending and descending tracts of the spinal cord are embedded in neuroglia and are situated in the white matter. They are the axons of nerve cells that carry nerve impulses up to the brain and down from the brain to the different segments of the spinal cord.

The position of the tracts has been determined by clinical and pathological studies and by animal experimentation. It must be emphasized that the positions of the tracts are only approximate and considerable overlap and mixing occurs. Nevertheless, from a practical standpoint, the arrangement of the tracts outlined below can be of considerable clinical value in making neurological diagnoses.

ASCENDING TRACTS

On entering the spinal cord, the sensory nerve fibers of different functions are sorted out and segregated into bundles of nerves or tracts (Fig. 7-1). Some of the nerve fibers serve to link different segments of the spinal cord, while others ascend from the spinal cord to higher centers and thus connect the spinal cord with the brain. The bundles of the ascending fibers are referred to as the **ascending tracts.**

In its simplest form, the ascending pathway to consciousness consists of three neurons. The first neuron, the **first-order neuron,** has its cell body in the **posterior root ganglion** of the spinal nerve. A peripheral process connects with a sensory receptor ending, whereas a central process enters the spinal cord through the posterior root to synapse on the **second-order neuron.** The second-order neuron gives rise to an axon that crosses to the opposite side and ascends to a higher level of the central nervous system, where it synapses with the **third-order neuron.** The third-order neuron is usually in the thalamus and gives rise to a projection fiber that passes to a sensory region of the cerebral cortex. The three-neuron chain described is the most common arrangement, but some afferent pathways use more or fewer neurons. Many of the neurons branch and participate in reflex activity.

Functions of the Ascending Tracts. Painful and thermal sensations ascend in the lateral spinothalamic tract; light touch and pressure ascend in the anterior spinothalamic tract. Discriminative touch—that is, the ability to localize accurately the area of the body touched and also to be aware that two points are touched simultaneously, even though they are close together (two-point discrimination)—ascends in the posterior white columns. Also ascending in the posterior white columns is information from muscles and joints pertaining to move-

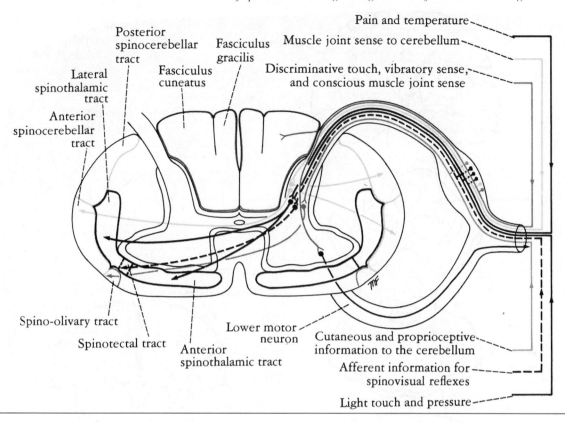

Posterior
spinocerebellar
tract

Lateral
spinothalamic
tract

Anterior
spinocerebellar
tract

Fasciculus
cuneatus

Fasciculus
gracilis

Pain and temperature

Muscle joint sense to cerebellum

Discriminative touch, vibratory sense,
and conscious muscle joint sense

Spino-olivary tract

Spinotectal tract

Anterior
spinothalamic tract

Lower motor
neuron

Cutaneous and proprioceptive
information to the cerebellum

Afferent information for
spinovisual reflexes

Light touch and pressure

ment and position of different parts of the body. In addition, vibratory sensations ascend in the posterior white column. Unconscious information from muscles, joints, the skin, and subcutaneous tissue reaches the cerebellum by way of the anterior and posterior spinocerebellar tracts and by the cuneocerebellar tract. Pain, thermal, and tactile information is passed to the superior colliculus of the midbrain through the spinotectal tract for the purpose of spinovisual reflexes. The spinoreticular tract provides a pathway from the muscles, joints, and skin to the reticular formation, while the spino-olivary tract provides an indirect pathway for further afferent information to reach the cerebellum.

Pain and Temperature Pathways

LATERAL SPINOTHALAMIC TRACT. The pain and thermal receptors in the skin and other tissues are free nerve endings. The pain impulses are transmitted to the spinal cord in fast-conducting delta A type fibers and slow-conducting C type fibers. The fast-conducting fibers alert the individual to the initial sharp pain and the slow-conducting fibers are responsible for the prolonged burning aching pain. The sensations of heat and cold also travel by delta A and C fibers.

The axons entering the spinal cord from the posterior root ganglion proceed to the tip of the posterior gray column and divide into ascending and descending branches (Fig. 7-2). These branches travel for a distance of one or two segments of the spinal cord and form the **posterolateral tract of Lissauer.** These fibers of the first-order neuron terminate by synapsing with cells in the posterior gray column, including cells in the substantia gelatinosa. Substance P, a peptide, is thought to be the neurotransmitter at these synapses.

The axons of the second-order neurons now cross obliquely to the opposite side in the anterior gray and white commissures within one spinal segment of

Fig. 7-2 *Pain and temperature pathways—lateral spinothalamic tract.*

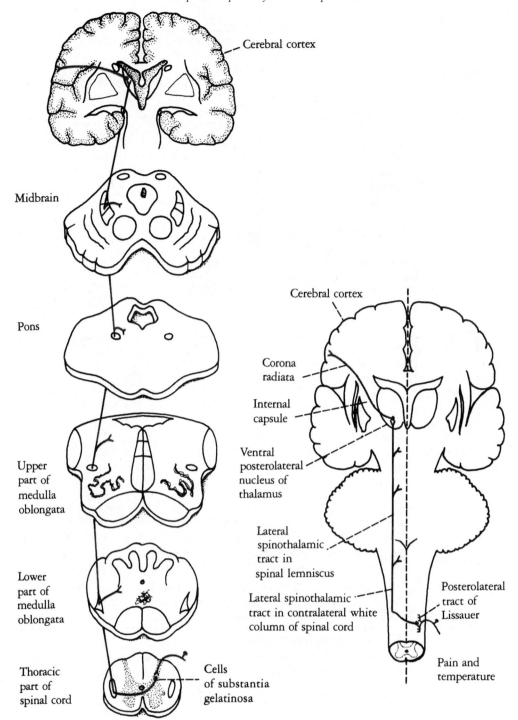

the cord and ascend in the contralateral white column as the lateral spinothalamic tract (Fig. 7-2). As the lateral spinothalamic tract ascends through the spinal cord, new fibers are added to the anteromedial aspect of the tract, so that in the upper cervical segments of the cord the sacral fibers are posterolateral and the cervical segments are anteromedial.

As the lateral spinothalamic tract ascends through the medulla oblongata, it is accompanied by the anterior spinothalamic tract and the spinotectal tract, which all together form the **spinal lemniscus** (Fig. 7-2).

The spinal lemniscus continues to ascend through the posterior part of the pons (Fig. 7-2). In the midbrain it lies in the tegmentum lateral to the medial lemniscus. Many of the fibers of the lateral spinothalamic tract end by synapsing with the third-order neuron in the ventral posterolateral nucleus of the thalamus (Fig. 7-2). It is believed that here crude pain and temperature sensations are appreciated and emotional reactions are initiated.

The axons of the third-order neurons in the ventral posterolateral nucleus of the thalamus now pass through the posterior limb of the internal capsule and the corona radiata to reach the somesthetic area in the postcentral gyrus of the cerebral cortex (Fig. 7-2). The contralateral half of the body is represented as inverted, with the hand and mouth situated inferiorly and the leg situated superiorly, and with the foot and anogenital region on the medial surface of the hemisphere. The role of the cerebral cortex is the interpretation of the sensory information at the level of consciousness.

Other Terminations of the Lateral Spinothalamic Tract. Pain impulses ascending through the lateral spinothalamic tract travel in two pathways. The initial sharp, pricking pain terminates in the ventral posterolateral nucleus of the thalamus and is then relayed to the cerebral cortex.

The burning pain terminates in the reticular formation, which then activates the entire nervous system. It is these impulses that alert the individual to an injury, and although the site of the injury is poorly localized, nevertheless they arouse the nervous system and create a sense of urgency.

THE ANALGESIA SYSTEM. Experimental stimulation of certain areas of the brainstem can reduce or block sensations of pain. These areas include the periventricular area of the diencephalon, the periaqueductal gray matter of the midbrain, and midline nuclei of the brainstem. It is believed that fibers of the reticulospinal tract pass down to the spinal cord and synapse on cells concerned with pain sensation in the posterior gray column. The analgesic system can suppress both sharp pricking pain and burning pain sensations.

Recently two compounds with morphinelike actions, called the **enkephalins** and the **endorphins,** have been isolated in the central nervous system. It has been suggested that these compounds serve as neurotransmitter substances in the analgesic system of the brain and that they may inhibit the release of substance P in the posterior gray column.

THE GATING THEORY. It has long been known that massage and the application of liniments to painful areas in the body can be very effective in relieving pain. Although the precise mechanism for these phenomena is not understood, the gating theory was proposed some years ago. It was suggested that at the site where the pain fiber enters the central nervous system, inhibition could occur by means of connector neurons excited by large, myelinated afferent fibers carrying nonpainful information of touch and pressure. The excess tactile stimulation, produced by massage for example, "closed the gate" for pain. Once the nonpainful tactile stimulation ceased, however, "the gate was opened" and the painful stimuli ascended the lateral spinothalamic tract. While the gate theory may partially explain the phenomena, it is probable that the analgesia system, noted above, is also involved with the liberation of enkephalins and endorphins in the posterior gray columns.

Light Touch and Pressure Pathways

ANTERIOR SPINOTHALAMIC TRACT. The axons enter the spinal cord from the posterior root ganglion and proceed to the tip of the posterior gray column, where they divide into ascending and descending branches (Fig. 7-3). These

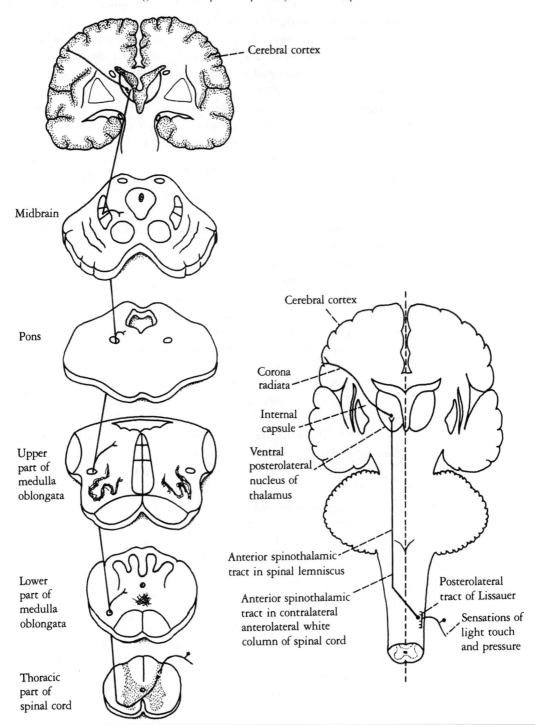

branches travel for a distance of one or two segments of the spinal cord, contributing to the **posterolateral tract of Lissauer.** It is believed that these fibers of the first-order neuron terminate by synapsing with cells in the substantia gelatinosa group in the posterior gray column.

The axons of the second-order neuron now cross very obliquely to the opposite side in the anterior gray and white commissures and ascend in the opposite anterolateral white column as the anterior spinothalamic tract (Fig. 7-3). As the anterior spinothalamic tract ascends through the spinal cord, new fibers are added to the medial aspect of the tract, so that in the upper cervical segments of the cord the sacral fibers are mostly lateral and the cervical segments are mostly medial.

As the anterior spinothalamic tract ascends through the medulla oblongata, it accompanies the lateral spinothalamic tract and the spinotectal tract, all of which form the **spinal lemniscus** (Fig. 7-3).

The spinal lemniscus continues to ascend through the posterior part of the pons, and the tegmentum of the midbrain and the fibers of the anterior spino-thalamic tract terminate by synapsing with the third-order neuron in the ventral posterolateral nucleus of the thalamus (Fig. 7-3). Crude awareness of touch and pressure is believed to be appreciated here.

The axons of the third-order neurons in the ventral posterolateral nucleus of the thalamus pass through the posterior limb of the **internal capsule** and the **corona radiata** to reach the somesthetic area in the postcentral gyrus of the cerebral cortex. The contralateral half of the body is represented inverted, with the hand and mouth situated inferiorly. The conscious appreciation of touch and pressure depends on the activity of the cerebral cortex. The sensations can only be crudely localized and very little discrimination of intensity is possible.

Discriminative Touch, Vibratory Sense, and Conscious Muscle Joint Sense

POSTERIOR WHITE COLUMN: FASCICULUS GRACILIS AND FASCICULUS CUNEATUS. The axons enter the spinal cord from the posterior root ganglion and pass directly to the posterior white column of the same side (Fig. 7-4). Here the fibers divide into long ascending and short descending branches. The descending branches pass down a variable number of segments, giving off collateral branches that synapse with cells in the posterior gray horn, with internuncial neurons, and with anterior horn cells. It is clear that these short descending fibers are involved with intersegmental reflexes.

The long ascending fibers may also end by synapsing with cells in the posterior gray horn, with internuncial neurons, and with anterior horn cells. This distribution may extend over many segments of the spinal cord. As in the case of the short descending fibers, they are involved with intersegmental reflexes.

Many of the long ascending fibers travel upward in the posterior white column as the **fasciculus gracilis and fasciculus cuneatus** (Fig. 7-4). The fasciculus gracilis is present throughout the length of the spinal cord and contains the long ascending fibers from the sacral, lumbar, and lower six thoracic spinal nerves. The fasciculus cuneatus is situated laterally in the upper thoracic and cervical segments of the spinal cord and is separated from the fasciculus gracilis by a septum. The fasciculus cuneatus contains the long ascending fibers from the upper six thoracic and all the cervical spinal nerves.

The fibers of the fasciculus gracilis and cuneatus ascend ipsilaterally and terminate by synapsing on the second-order neurons in the **nuclei gracilis and cuneatus** of the medulla oblongata (Fig. 7-4). The axons of the second-order neurons, called the **internal arcuate fibers,** sweep anteromedially around the central gray matter and cross the median plane decussating with the corresponding fibers of the opposite side in the **sensory decussation** (Fig. 7-4). The fibers then ascend as a single compact bundle, the **medial lemniscus,** through the medulla oblongata, the pons, and the midbrain (Fig. 7-4). The fibers terminate by synapsing on the third-order neurons in the ventral posterolateral nucleus of the thalamus.

The axons of the third-order neuron leave and pass through the posterior limb of the **internal capsule and corona radiata** to reach the somesthetic area in the postcentral gyrus of the cerebral cortex. The contralateral half of the body

Fig. 7-4

Discriminative touch, vibratory sense, and conscious muscle joint sense pathways—fasciculus gracilis and cuneatus.

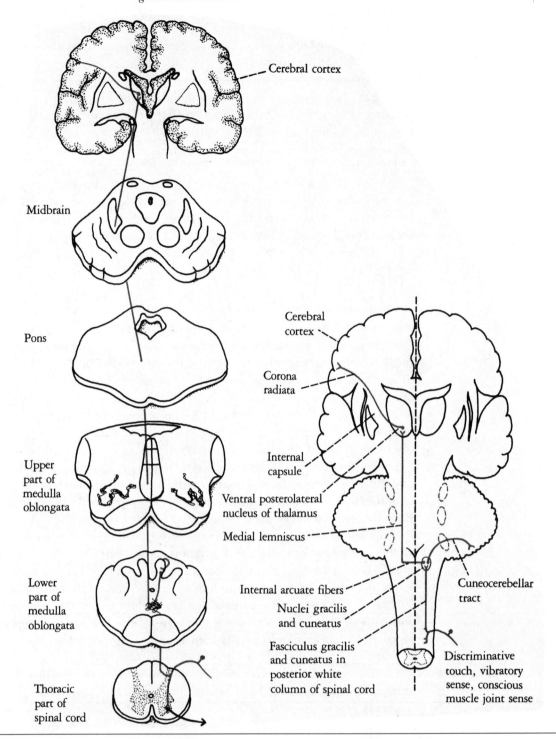

Cerebral cortex

Midbrain

Pons

Upper part of medulla oblongata

Lower part of medulla oblongata

Thoracic part of spinal cord

Cerebral cortex

Corona radiata

Internal capsule

Ventral posterolateral nucleus of thalamus

Medial lemniscus

Internal arcuate fibers

Nuclei gracilis and cuneatus

Fasciculus gracilis and cuneatus in posterior white column of spinal cord

Cuneocerebellar tract

Discriminative touch, vibratory sense, conscious muscle joint sense

is represented inverted, with the hand and mouth situated inferiorly. In this manner, the impressions of touch with fine gradations of intensity, exact localization, and two-point discrimination can be appreciated. Vibratory sense and the position of the different parts of the body can be consciously recognized.

A number of fibers in the fasciculus cuneatus from the cervical and upper thoracic segments, having terminated on the second-order neuron of the nucleus cuneatus, are relayed and travel as the axons of the second-order neurons to enter the cerebellum through the inferior cerebellar peduncle of the same side (Fig. 7-4). The pathway is referred to as the **cuneocerebellar tract** and the fibers are known as the **posterior external arcuate fibers.** The function of these fibers is to convey information of muscle joint sense to the cerebellum.

Muscle Joint Sense Pathways to the Cerebellum

POSTERIOR SPINOCEREBELLAR TRACT. The axons entering the spinal cord from the posterior root ganglion enter the posterior gray column and terminate by synapsing on the second-order neurons at the base of the posterior gray column (Fig. 7-5). These neurons are known collectively as the **nucleus dorsalis (Clark's column).** The axons of the second-order neurons enter the posterolateral part of the lateral white column on the same side and ascend as the posterior spinocerebellar tract to the medulla oblongata. Here the tract joins the inferior cerebellar peduncle and terminates in the cerebellar cortex (Fig. 7-5). Note that it does not ascend to the cerebral cortex. Since the nucleus dorsalis (Clark's col-

---

Fig. 7-5 *Muscle joint sense pathways to cerebellum—anterior and posterior spinocerebellar tracts.*

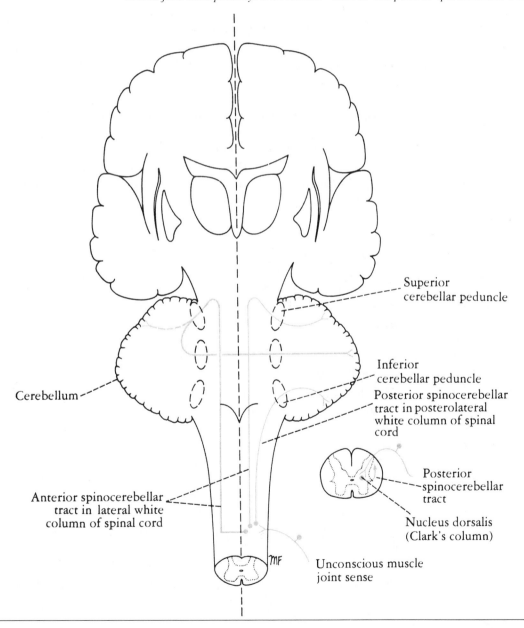

Superior cerebellar peduncle

Inferior cerebellar peduncle

Posterior spinocerebellar tract in posterolateral white column of spinal cord

Cerebellum

Posterior spinocerebellar tract

Anterior spinocerebellar tract in lateral white column of spinal cord

Nucleus dorsalis (Clark's column)

Unconscious muscle joint sense

---

umn) extends only from the eighth cervical segment caudally to the third or fourth lumbar segments, axons entering the spinal cord from the posterior roots of the lower lumbar and sacral segments ascend in the posterior white column until they reach the third or fourth lumbar segments, where they enter the nucleus dorsalis.

The posterior spinocerebellar fibers receive muscle joint information from the muscle spindles, tendon organs, and joint receptors of the trunk and lower limbs. This information concerning tension of muscle tendons and the movements of muscles and joints is used by the cerebellum in the coordination of limb movements and the maintenance of posture.

ANTERIOR SPINOCEREBELLAR TRACT. The axons entering the spinal cord from the posterior root ganglion terminate by synapsing with the second-order neurons in the nucleus dorsalis at the base of the anterior gray column (Fig. 7-5). The majority of the axons of the second-order neurons cross to the opposite side and ascend as the anterior spinocerebellar tract in the contralateral white column; the minority of the axons ascend as the anterior spinocerebellar tract in the lateral white column of the same side (Fig. 7-5). The fibers, having ascended through the medulla oblongata and pons, enter the cerebellum through the superior cerebellar peduncle and terminate in the cerebellar cortex. It is believed that those fibers that crossed over to the opposite side in the spinal cord cross back within the cerebellum (Fig. 7-5). The anterior spinocerebellar tract conveys muscle joint information from the muscle spindles, tendon organs, and joint receptors of the trunk and the upper and lower limbs. It is also believed that the cerebellum receives information from the skin and superficial fascia by this tract.

CUNEOCEREBELLAR TRACT. These fibers have already been described on page 75. They originate in the nucleus cuneatus and enter the cerebellum through the inferior cerebellar peduncle of the same side (Fig. 7-4). The fibers are known as the **posterior external arcuate fibers** and their function is to convey information of muscle joint sense to the cerebellum.

Other Ascending Pathways

SPINOTECTAL TRACT. The axons enter the spinal cord from the posterior root ganglion and travel to the gray matter where they synapse on unknown second-order neurons (Fig. 7-6). The axons of the second-order neurons cross the median plane and ascend as the spinotectal tract in the anterolateral white column lying close to the lateral spinothalamic tract. After they pass through the medulla oblongata and pons, they terminate by synapsing with neurons in the superior colliculus of the midbrain (Fig. 7-6). This pathway provides afferent information for spinovisual reflexes and brings about movements of the eyes and head toward the source of the stimulation.

SPINORETICULAR TRACT. The axons enter the spinal cord from the posterior root ganglion and terminate on unknown second-order neurons in the gray matter (Fig. 7-6). The axons from these second-order neurons ascend the spinal cord as the spinoreticular tract in the lateral white column mixed with the lateral spinothalamic tract. The majority of the fibers are uncrossed and terminate by synapsing with neurons of the reticular formation in the medulla oblongata, pons, and midbrain (Fig. 7-6). The spinoreticular tract provides an afferent pathway for the reticular formation, which plays an important role in influencing levels of consciousness. (For details, see p. 129.)

Fig. 7-6   *Spinotectal, spinorecticular, and spino-olivary tracts.*

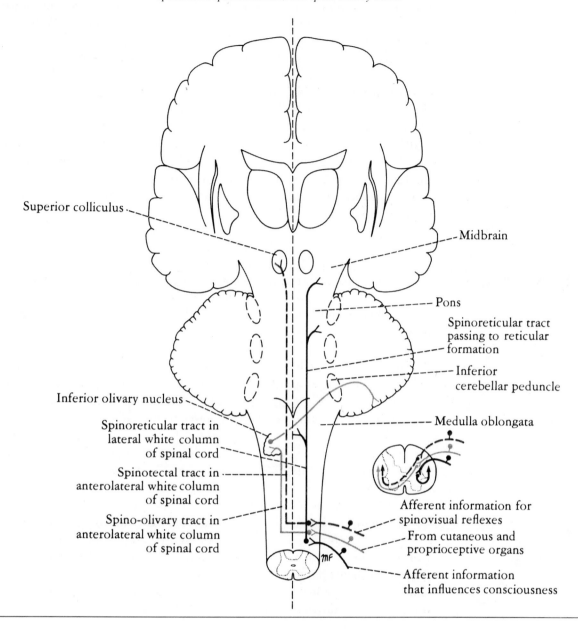

Superior colliculus

Midbrain

Pons

Spinoreticular tract passing to reticular formation

Inferior cerebellar peduncle

Inferior olivary nucleus

Spinoreticular tract in lateral white column of spinal cord

Spinotectal tract in anterolateral white column of spinal cord

Spino-olivary tract in anterolateral white column of spinal cord

Medulla oblongata

Afferent information for spinovisual reflexes

From cutaneous and proprioceptive organs

Afferent information that influences consciousness

SPINO-OLIVARY TRACT. The axons enter the spinal cord from the posterior root ganglion and terminate on unknown second-order neurons in the posterior gray column (Fig. 7-6). The axons from the second-order neurons cross the midline and ascend as the spino-olivary tract in the white matter at the junction of the anterior and lateral columns. The axons end by synapsing on third-order neurons in the inferior olivary nuclei in the medulla oblongata (Fig. 7-6). The axons of the third-order neurons cross the midline and enter the cerebellum through the inferior cerebellar peduncle. The spino-olivary tract conveys information to the cerebellum from cutaneous and proprioceptive organs.

VISCERAL SENSORY TRACTS. Sensations that arise in viscera located in the thorax and abdomen enter the spinal cord through the posterior roots. The cell bodies of the first-order neuron are situated in the posterior root ganglia. The peripheral processes of these cells receive nerve impulses from pain* and stretch receptor endings in the viscera. The central processes, having entered the spinal cord, synapse with second-order neurons in the gray matter, probably in the posterior or lateral gray columns.

The axons of the second-order neurons are believed to join the spinothalamic tracts and ascend and terminate on the third-order neurons in the ventral posterolateral nucleus of the thalamus. The final destination of the axons of the third-order neurons has not been established, but it may well be in the postcentral gyrus of the cerebral cortex.

It has been reported that sensations from a full rectum and a full urinary bladder experienced prior to defecation and micturition are carried by ascending tracts located in the posterior white columns of the spinal cord.

Many of the visceral afferent fibers that enter the spinal cord branch and participate in reflex activity.

DESCENDING TRACTS

The motor neurons situated in the anterior gray columns of the spinal cord send axons to innervate skeletal muscle through the anterior roots of the spinal nerves. These motor neurons are sometimes referred to as the **lower motor neurons.**

The lower motor neurons are constantly bombarded by nervous impulses that descend from the medulla, pons, midbrain, and cerebral cortex, as well as those that enter along sensory fibers from the posterior roots. The nerve fibers that descend in the white matter from different supraspinal nerve centers are segregated into nerve bundles called the **descending tracts.** These supraspinal neurons and their tracts sometimes are referred to as the **upper motor neurons** and they provide numerous separate pathways that can influence motor activity.

The descending pathway from the cerebral cortex is often made up of three neurons. The first neuron, the **first-order neuron,** has its cell body in the cerebral cortex. Its axon descends to synapse on the **second-order neuron,** an internuncial neuron, situated in the anterior gray column of the spinal cord. The axon of the second-order neuron is short and synapses with the **third-order neuron,** the lower motor neuron, in the anterior gray column. The axon of the third-order neuron innervates the skeletal muscle through the anterior root and spinal nerve. In some instances, the axon of the first-order neuron terminates directly on the third-order neuron (as in reflex arcs).

Functions of the Descending Tracts. The **corticospinal tracts** (Fig. 7-7) are the pathways concerned with voluntary, discrete, skilled movements, especially those of the distal parts of the limbs. The **reticulospinal tracts** (Fig. 7-7) may facilitate or inhibit the activity of the alpha and gamma motor neurons in the anterior gray columns and may therefore facilitate or inhibit voluntary movement or reflex activity. The **tectospinal tract** (Fig. 7-7) is concerned with reflex postural movements in response to visual stimuli. Those fibers that are associated with the sympathetic neurons in the lateral gray column are concerned with the pupillodilation reflex in response to darkness. The **rubrospinal tract** (Fig. 7-7) acts on both the alpha and gamma motor neurons in the anterior gray columns and facilitates the activity of flexor muscles and inhibits the activity of extensor or antigravity muscles. The **vestibulospinal tract** (Fig. 7-7), by acting on the motor neurons in the anterior gray columns, facilitates the activity of the extensor

*The causes of visceral pain include ischemia, chemical damage,
spasm of smooth muscle, and distention.

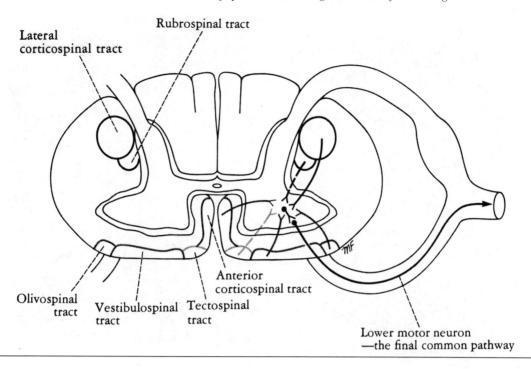

muscles, inhibits the activity of the flexor muscles, and is concerned with the postural activity associated with balance. The **olivospinal tract** (Fig. 7-7) may play a role in muscular activity, but its precise function is unknown. The **descending autonomic fibers** are concerned with the control of visceral activity.

Corticospinal Tracts. Fibers of the corticospinal tract arise as axons of pyramidal cells situated in the fifth layer of the cerebral cortex (Fig. 7-8). About one-third of the fibers originate from the primary motor cortex (area 4), one-third from the parietal lobe (areas 3, 1, and 2); thus, two-thirds of the fibers arise from the precentral gyrus and one-third from the postcentral gyrus.* Since electrical stimulation of different parts of the precentral gyrus produces movements of different parts of the opposite side of the body, we can represent the parts of the body in this area of the cortex. Such a homunculus is shown in Figure 7-8. Note that the region controlling the face is situated inferiorly and the lower limb is situated superiorly and on the medial surface of the hemisphere. The homunculus is a distorted picture of the body, with the various parts having a size proportional to the area of the cerebral cortex devoted to their control. It is interesting to find that the majority of the corticospinal fibers are myelinated and are relatively slow-conducting, small fibers.

The descending fibers converge in the **corona radiata** and then pass through the posterior limb of the **internal capsule** (Fig. 7-8). Here the fibers are organized so that those closest to the genu are concerned with cervical portions of the body, while those situated more posteriorly are concerned with the lower extremity. The tract then continues through the middle three-fifths of the **basis pedunculi of the midbrain** (Fig. 7-8). Here, the fibers concerned with cervical portions of the body are situated medially, while those concerned with the leg are placed laterally.

On entering the pons, the tract is broken into many bundles by the **transverse**

*These fibers do not control motor activity but influence sensory input to the nervous system.

Fig. 7-8   *Corticospinal tracts.*

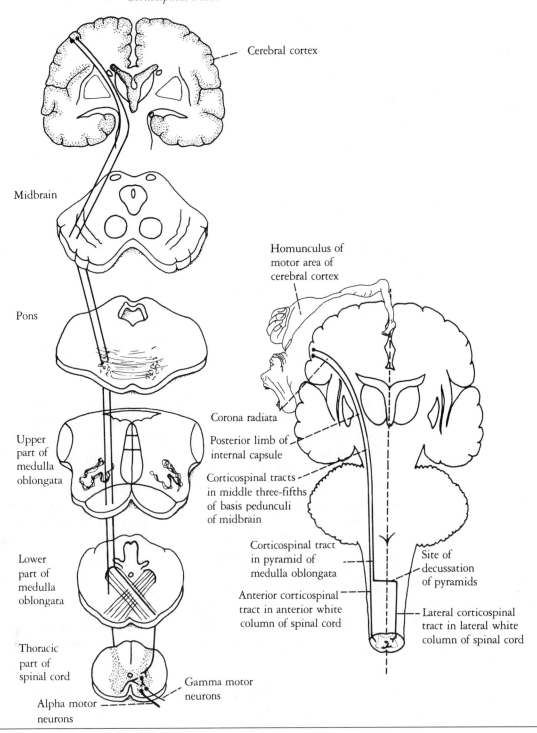

Cerebral cortex

Midbrain

Pons

Homunculus of motor area of cerebral cortex

Corona radiata

Posterior limb of internal capsule

Corticospinal tracts in middle three-fifths of basis pedunculi of midbrain

Corticospinal tract in pyramid of medulla oblongata

Anterior corticospinal tract in anterior white column of spinal cord

Site of decussation of pyramids

Lateral corticospinal tract in lateral white column of spinal cord

Upper part of medulla oblongata

Lower part of medulla oblongata

Thoracic part of spinal cord

Gamma motor neurons

Alpha motor neurons

pontocerebellar fibers. In the medulla oblongata, the bundles become grouped together along the anterior border to form a swelling known as the **pyramid** (hence the alternative name, **pyramidal tract;** see Fig. 8-1). At the junction of the medulla oblongata and the spinal cord, the majority of the fibers cross the midline at the **decussation of the pyramids** (Fig. 7-8) and enter the lateral white column of the spinal cord to form the **lateral corticospinal tract.** The remaining fibers do not cross in the decussation but descend in the anterior white column of the spinal cord as the **anterior corticospinal tract** (Fig. 7-8). These fibers eventually cross the midline and terminate in the anterior gray column of the spinal cord segments in the cervical and upper thoracic regions.

The lateral corticospinal tract descends the length of the spinal cord and its fibers terminate in the anterior gray column of all the spinal cord segments.

The majority of the corticospinal fibers synapse with internuncial neurons, which in turn synapse with alpha motor neurons and some gamma motor neurons. Only the largest corticospinal fibers synapse directly with the motor neurons.

The corticospinal tracts form the pathway that confers speed and agility to voluntary movements and are thus used in performing rapid skilled movements. Many of the simple, basic voluntary movements are believed to be mediated by other descending tracts.

BRANCHES OF CORTICOSPINAL TRACTS
1. Branches are given off early in their descent and return to the cerebral cortex to inhibit activity in adjacent regions of the cortex.
2. Branches pass to the caudate and lentiform nuclei, the red nuclei, and the olivary nuclei and the reticular formation. These branches keep the subcortical regions informed about the cortical motor activity. Once alerted, the subcortical regions may react and send their own nervous impulses to the alpha and gamma motor neurons by other descending pathways.

Reticulospinal Tracts. Throughout the midbrain, pons, and medulla oblongata, groups of scattered nerve cells and nerve fibers exist that are collectively known as the **reticular formation** (see p. 127). From the pons, these neurons send axons, which are mostly uncrossed, down into the spinal cord and form the **pontine reticulospinal tract** (Fig. 7-9). From the medulla, similar neurons send axons, which are crossed and uncrossed, to the spinal cord and form the **medullary reticulospinal tract.**

The reticulospinal fibers from the pons descend through the anterior white column, while those from the medulla oblongata descend in the lateral white column (Fig. 7-9). Both sets of fibers enter the anterior gray columns of the spinal cord and may facilitate or inhibit the activity of the alpha and gamma motor neurons. By this means the reticulospinal tracts influence voluntary movements and reflex activity. The reticulospinal fibers are also now thought to include the descending autonomic fibers. The reticulospinal tracts thus provide a pathway by which the hypothalamus can control the sympathetic outflow and the sacral parasympathetic outflow.

Tectospinal Tract. Fibers of this tract arise from nerve cells in the **superior colliculus** of the midbrain (Fig. 7-10). The majority of the fibers cross the midline soon after their origin and descend through the brainstem close to the **medial longitudinal fasciculus.** The tectospinal tract descends through the anterior white column of the spinal cord close to the anterior median fissure. The majority of the fibers terminate in the anterior gray column in the upper cervical segments of the spinal cord by synapsing with internuncial neurons. These fibers are believed to be concerned with reflex postural movements in response to visual stimuli.

Rubrospinal Tract. The **red nucleus** is situated in the tegmentum of the midbrain at the level of the superior colliculus (Fig. 7-11). The axons of neurons in this nucleus cross the midline at the level of the nucleus and descend as the rubrospinal tract through the pons and medulla oblongata to enter the lateral

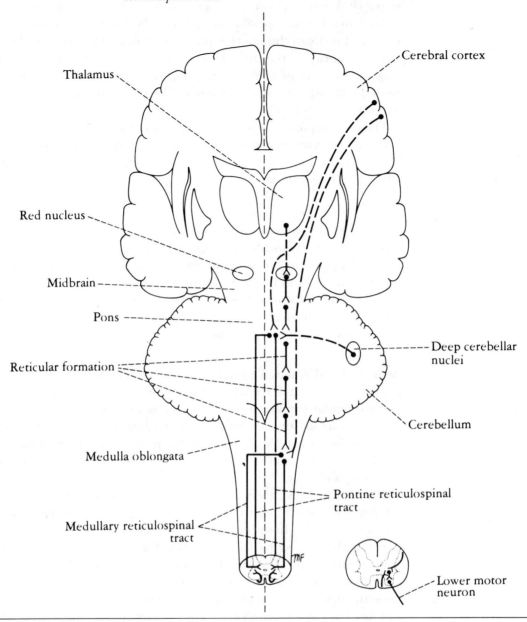

white column of the spinal cord. The fibers terminate by synapsing with internuncial neurons in the anterior gray column of the cord.

The neurons of the red nucleus receive afferent impulses through connections with the cerebral cortex and the cerebellum. This is believed to be an important indirect pathway by which the cerebral cortex and the cerebellum can influence the activity of the alpha and gamma motor neurons of the spinal cord. The tract facilitates the activity of the flexor muscles and inhibits the activity of the extensor or antigravity muscles.

Vestibulospinal Tract. The **vestibular nuclei** are situated in the pons and medulla oblongata beneath the floor of the fourth ventricle (Fig. 7-12). The vestibular nuclei receive afferent fibers from the inner ear through the vestibular nerve and from the cerebellum. The neurons of the lateral vestibular nucleus give rise to the axons that form the vestibulospinal tract. The tract descends uncrossed through the medulla and through the length of the spinal cord in the

Fig. 7-10   *Tectospinal tract.*

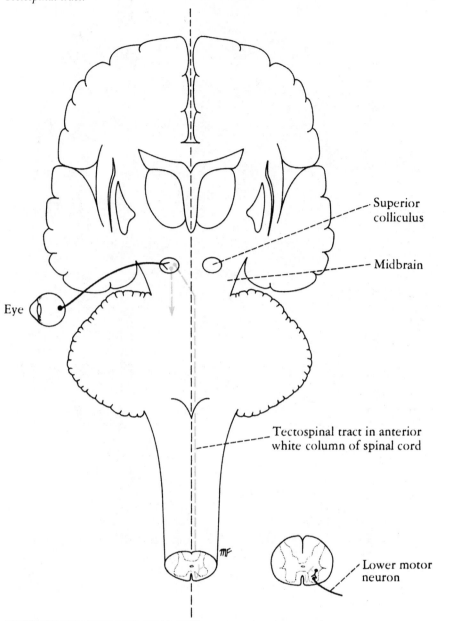

Superior
colliculus

Midbrain

Eye

Tectospinal tract in anterior
white column of spinal cord

Lower motor
neuron

anterior white column. The fibers terminate by synapsing with internuncial neurons of the anterior gray column of the spinal cord.

The inner ear and the cerebellum, by means of this tract, facilitate the activity of the extensor muscles and inhibit the activity of the flexor muscles in association with the maintenance of balance.

Olivospinal Tract. The olivospinal tract was thought to arise from the inferior olivary nucleus and to descend in the lateral white column of the spinal cord to influence the activity of the motor neurons in the anterior gray column. There is now considerable doubt that it exists.

Descending Autonomic Fibers. The higher centers of the central nervous system associated with the control of autonomic activity are situated in the cerebral cortex, hypothalamus, amygdaloid complex, and reticular formation. Although distinct tracts have not been recognized, it is known, as the result of study of

Fig. 7-11   *Rubrospinal tract.*

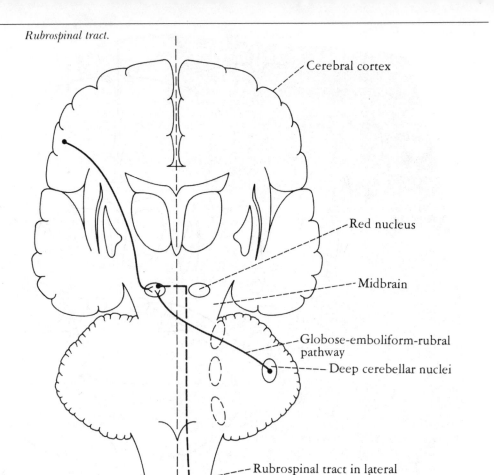

Cerebral cortex

Red nucleus

Midbrain

Globose-emboliform-rubral pathway

Deep cerebellar nuclei

Rubrospinal tract in lateral white column of spinal cord

Lower motor neuron

spinal cord lesions, that descending autonomic tracts do exist and probably form part of the reticulospinal tract.

The fibers arise from neurons in the higher centers and cross the midline in the brainstem. They are believed to descend in the lateral white column of the spinal cord and to terminate by synapsing on the autonomic motor cells in the lateral gray columns in the thoracic and upper lumbar (sympathetic outflow) and midsacral (parasympathetic) levels of the spinal cord.

INTERSEGMENTAL TRACTS

Short ascending and descending tracts, which originate and end within the spinal cord, exist in the anterior, lateral, and posterior white columns. The function of these pathways is to interconnect the neurons of different segmental levels, and they are particularly important in intersegmental spinal reflexes.

Fig. 7-12   *Vestibulospinal tract.*

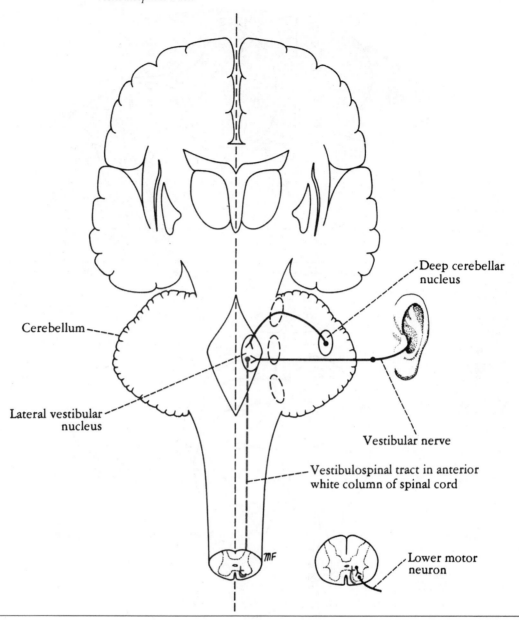

Deep cerebellar nucleus

Cerebellum

Lateral vestibular nucleus

Vestibular nerve

Vestibulospinal tract in anterior white column of spinal cord

Lower motor neuron

REFLEX ARC

A **reflex** may be defined as an involuntary response to a stimulus. It depends on the integrity of the reflex arc (Fig. 7-13). In its simplest form, a reflex arc consists of the following anatomical structures: (1) a receptor organ, (2) an afferent neuron, (3) an effector neuron, and (4) an effector organ. Such a reflex arc involving only one synapse is referred to as a **monosynaptic reflex arc.** Interruption of the reflex arc at any point along its course would abolish the response.

In the spinal cord, reflex arcs play an important role in maintaining muscle tone, which is the basis for body posture. The receptor organ is situated in the skin, muscle, or tendon. The cell body of the afferent neuron is located in the posterior root ganglion, and the central axon of this first-order neuron terminates by synapsing on the effector neuron. Since the afferent fibers are of large diameter and are rapidly conducting, and because of the presence of only one synapse, a very quick response is possible.

Fig. 7-13

A monosynaptic reflex arc.

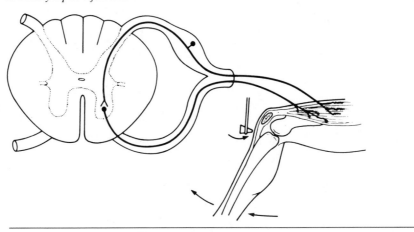

Fig. 7-14

Law of reciprocal innervation and the crossed extensor reflex.

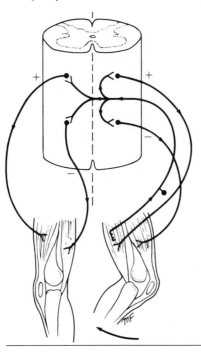

Law of Reciprocal Innervation. In considering reflex skeletal muscle activity it is important to understand the law of reciprocal innervation (Fig. 7-14). Simply stated, it means that the flexor and extensor reflexes of the same limb cannot be made to contract simultaneously. For this law to work, the afferent nerve fibers responsible for flexor reflex muscle action must have branches that synapse with the extensor motor neurons of the same limb, causing them to be inhibited.

Crossed Extensor Reflex. The evocation of a reflex on one side of the body causes opposite effects on the limb of the other side of the body. This crossed extensor reflex (Fig. 7-14) may be demonstrated as follows: Afferent stimulation of the reflex arc that causes the ipsilateral limb to flex results in the contralateral limb being extended.

HIGHER NEURONAL CENTERS AND THE ACTIVITIES OF SPINAL REFLEXES

The spinal segmental reflex arc involving motor activity is greatly influenced by higher centers in the brain. These influences are mediated through the corticospinal, reticulospinal, tectospinal, rubrospinal, and vestibulospinal tracts. In the clinical condition known as spinal shock, which follows the sudden removal of these influences by severance of the spinal cord, the segmental spinal reflexes are depressed. When the so-called spinal shock disappears in a few weeks, the segmental spinal reflexes return and the muscle tone is increased. This so-called **decerebrate rigidity** is due to the overactivity of the gamma efferent nerve fibers to the muscle spindles, which results from the release of these neurons from the higher centers. The next stage may be **paraplegia in extension** with domination of the increased tone of the extensor muscles over the flexor muscles. Some neurologists believe that this condition is due to incomplete severance of all the descending tracts with persistence of the vestibulospinal tract. Should all the descending tracts be severed, the condition of **paraplegia in flexion** occurs. In this condition, the reflex responses are flexor in nature and the tone of the extensor muscles is diminished.

RENSHAW CELLS AND LOWER MOTOR NEURON INHIBITION

Lower motor neuron axons give off collateral branches as they pass through the white matter to reach the anterior roots of the spinal nerve. These collaterals synapse on neurons described by Renshaw, which in turn synapse on the lower motor neurons. These internuncial neurons are believed to provide feedback on the lower motor neurons, inhibiting their activity.

NATIONAL BOARD TYPE QUESTIONS

Match the tracts listed below on the left with their cell of origin listed below on the right. An answer may be used more than once.

1. Lateral spinothalamic tract.
2. Fasciculus gracilis.
3. Anterior spinothalamic tract.
4. Fasciculus cuneatus.
5. Posterior spinocerebellar tract.

A. Posterior root ganglion.
B. Substantia gelatinosa.
C. Nucleus proprius.
D. None of the above.

Match the tracts listed below on the left with the appropriate statement listed below on the right. An answer may be used more than once.

6. Anterior spinothalamic tract.

7. Lateral corticospinal tract.

8. Fasciculus gracilis.

9. Fasciculus cuneatus.

10. Anterior corticospinal tract.

A. Crosses the midline of the spinal cord.
B. Crosses the midline of the medulla oblongata.
C. Is uncrossed in the spinal cord or the medulla oblongata.

Match the cell columns listed below on the left with distribution in the spinal cord. An answer may be used more than once.

11. Nucleus dorsalis.
12. Spinal part of accessory.
13. Phrenic.
14. Parasympathetic outflow.

A. Entire length of the spinal cord.
B. T1–L3.
C. S2, S3, S4.
D. C8–L3 or L4.
E. None of the above.

Match the tracts listed below on the left with the nucleus of termination listed below on the right. An answer may be used more than once.

15. Lateral corticospinal tract.
16. Anterior spinothalamic tract.
17. Fasciculus gracilis.
18. Lissauer's tract.
19. Fasciculus cuneatus.
20. Lateral spinothalamic tract.

A. Substantia gelatinosa.
B. Ventroposterolateral nucleus of the thalamus.
C. Clarke's column.
D. Ventroposteromedial nucleus of the thalamus.
E. None of the above.

In each of the following questions, answer:

A. If only (1), (2), and (3) are correct
B. If only (1) and (3) are correct
C. If only (2) and (4) are correct
D. If only (4) is correct
E. If all are correct

21. Muscle tone is dependent on the integrity of the following:
    (1) Posterior root of the spinal nerve.
    (2) Afferent fibers from facial and other muscles of the head.
    (3) Spinal nerves.
    (4) Lower motor neurons in anterior roots of spinal nerves.
22. Following section of a motor nerve, an atonic muscle has the following characteristics:
    (1) Soft and flabby.
    (2) Atrophies.
    (3) Loss of reflexes.
    (4) Responds to faradic stimulation 2 weeks after nerve section.
23. The precentral gyrus receives inputs either directly or indirectly from the following areas of the nervous system when voluntary movements are performed:
    (1) Limbic system.
    (2) Ascending tracts concerned with pain and touch.
    (3) Eyes.
    (4) Cerebellum.
24. Lesions that are restricted to the corticospinal tracts produce the following clinical signs:
    (1) Presence of superficial abdominal reflexes.
    (2) Babinski sign is present.
    (3) Cremasteric reflex is present.
    (4) Loss of fine, skilled voluntary movements.

25. Lesions of the descending tracts (other than the corticospinal tracts) produce the following clinical signs:
    (1) Usually hypertonicity.
    (2) Paralysis.
    (3) Exaggerated knee jerk.
    (4) Finger or ankle clonus.
26. The knee jerk reflex:
    (1) Is a muscle stretch reflex.
    (2) Is a response to painful stimulation of the skin.
    (3) Has only a single synapse in the spinal cord between afferent nerve fibers and spinal motor neurons.
    (4) Is an inverse muscle stretch reflex.
27. Which of the following observations would be consistent with the "gate theory" of pain?
    (1) Stimulation of large myelinated nerve fibers increases pain sensitivity.
    (2) Stimulation of group IV fibers decreases pain sensitivity.
    (3) Degeneration of large myelinated fibers decreases pain sensitivity.
    (4) Vibratory stimulation to the skin could diminish pain sensitivity.
28. Which of the following regions of white matter would **not** contain corticospinal fibers?
    (1) Pyramid of medulla oblongata.
    (2) Anterior limb of internal capsule.
    (3) Lateral white column of spinal cord.
    (4) Superior cerebellar peduncle.
29. Are the following statements correct concerning the reception of pain?
    (1) The enkephalins and endorphins may serve to inhibit the release of substance P in the posterior gray column.
    (2) Substance P, a peptide, is thought to be the neurotransmitter at the synapses where first-order neurons terminate on the cells in the posterior gray column.
    (3) Slow-conducting C type fibers are responsible for prolonged, burning pain.
    (4) The anterior spinothalamic tracts conduct the initial sharp pain.
30. Following a traumatic hemisection of the spinal cord on the right at the level of C7 segment, the patient presents with the following signs and symptoms:
    (1) Left hemiplegia.
    (2) Right positive Babinski sign.
    (3) Loss of pain and temperature on the right below the level of the lesion.
    (4) Loss of position sense on the right below the level of the lesion.

ANSWERS AND EXPLANATIONS

1. B
2. A
3. B
4. A
5. D: Nucleus dorsalis (Clark's column).
6. A
7. B
8. C
9. C
10. A
11. D

12. E: The spinal part of the accessory nerve arises from the accessory nucleus situated in the upper five or six cervical segments of the spinal cord.
13. E: The phrenic nerve arises from the phrenic nucleus situated in segments C3, C4, and C5 of the spinal cord.
14. C
15. E: The motor anterior gray column (horn) cells of the spinal cord.
16. B
17. E: The fasciculus gracilis ends by synapsing with the second-order neurons in the nucleus gracilis.
18. A
19. E: The fasciculus cuneatus ends by synapsing with the second-order neurons in the nucleus cuneatus.
20. B
21. E
22. A: (4) A paralyzed muscle ceases to respond to faradic stimulation after 4 to 7 days.
23. E
24. C: (1) The superficial abdominal reflexes are absent. (3) The cremasteric reflex is absent.
25. E
26. B: (2) It responds to a sharp tap on the ligamentum patellae, which stimulates the stretch receptors. (4) There is no inverse muscle stretch reflex.
27. D
28. C
29. A: (4) The anterior spinothalamic tract conducts sensations of light touch and pressure and not pain.
30. C: (1) In the spinal cord, the anterior gray column motor cells on the left, which control the voluntary muscles on the left side of the body, receive lateral corticospinal fibers that have descended on the left from the decussation of the pyramids in the medulla. Right hemiplegia would be present, not left hemiplegia. (3) Sensations of pain and temperature from the lower right side of the body travel in the lateral spinothalamic tract, which crosses to the contralateral side of the spinal cord before ascending to the brain. Loss of the sensations of pain and temperature would be present on the left but not on the right side.

8 Brainstem

SUGGESTED PLAN FOR REVIEW OF CHAPTER 8

1. Learn the general shape and parts of the brainstem so that you can understand the position of the cranial nerve nuclei and how the cranial nerves exit from the brainstem. A three-dimensional picture of the region in your mind will assist you in the visualization of the pathways taken by the various ascending and descending tracts.

2. Be able to make rough drawings of cross sections of the brainstem at the following levels: the medulla at the levels of the decussation of the pyramids, the decussation of the lemnisci, and the olives; the caudal and cranial parts of pons; and the midbrain at the levels of the inferior colliculi and the superior colliculi. At each level insert the main structures, including the cranial nerve nuclei and other masses of gray matter, and the main tracts.

3. Understand the Arnold-Chiari phenomenon, the lateral medullary syndrome

of Wallenberg, the medial medullary syndrome, Weber's syndrome, and Benedikt's syndrome. Examiners like asking questions on these clinical problems.
4. Learn the significance of blockage of the cerebral aqueduct in the production of hydrocephalus.

INTRODUCTION

The brainstem is made up of the medulla oblongata, the pons, and the midbrain. It is stalklike in shape and connects the narrow spinal cord with the expanded forebrain.

The brainstem participates in three broad functions: (1) It serves as a conduit for the ascending and descending tracts connecting the spinal cord to the different parts of the brain. (2) It contains important reflex centers associated with the control of respiration and the cardiovascular system; it also is associated with the control of consciousness. (3) It contains the important nuclei of cranial nerves 3 through 12.

The purpose of this chapter is to review the structure of the different parts of the brainstem so that the student can understand the spatial relationships of these parts to one another; the various connections of these parts are dealt with elsewhere as indicated in the text.

MEDULLA OBLONGATA

External Appearance. The medulla oblongata connects the pons superiorly with the spinal cord inferiorly (Fig. 8-1). The junction of the medulla and spinal cord is at the level of the foramen magnum. The medulla oblongata is conical in shape, its broad extremity being directed superiorly. The **central canal** of the spinal cord continues upward into the lower half of the medulla; in the upper half of the medulla it expands as the **cavity of the fourth ventricle** (Fig. 8-1).

On the anterior surface of the medulla is the **anterior median fissure,** which is continuous inferiorly with the **anterior median fissure** of the spinal cord (Fig. 8-1). On each side of the median fissure there is a swelling called the **pyramid.** The pyramids are composed of bundles of corticospinal nerve fibers that originate in large nerve cells in the precentral gyrus of the cerebral cortex. The pyramids taper inferiorly, and it is here that the majority of the descending fibers cross over to the opposite side, forming the **decussation of the pyramids** (Fig. 8-1). The **anterior external arcuate fibers** are a few nerve fibers that emerge from the anterior median fissure above the decussation and pass laterally over the surface of the medulla oblongata. Posterolateral to the pyramids are the **olives,** which are oval elevations produced by the underlying **inferior olivary nuclei.** In the groove between the pyramid and the olive emerge the rootlets of the hypoglossal nerve. Posterior to the olives are the **inferior cerebellar peduncles** (Fig. 8-1), which connect the medulla to the cerebellum. In the groove between the olive and the inferior cerebellar peduncle emerge the roots of the glossopharyngeal and vagus nerves and the cranial roots of the accessory nerve (Fig. 8-1).

The posterior surface of the superior half of the medulla oblongata forms the lower part of the **floor of the fourth ventricle** (Fig. 8-1). The posterior surface of the inferior half of the medulla is continuous with the posterior aspect of the spinal cord and possesses a **posterior median sulcus.** On each side of the median sulcus there is an elongated swelling, the **gracile tubercle,** produced by the underlying **gracile nucleus** (Fig. 8-1). Lateral to the gracile tubercle is a similar swelling, the **cuneate tubercle,** produced by the underlying **cuneate nucleus.**

Fig. 8-1

The medulla oblongata. A. Anterior view. B. Posterior view. Note that the roof of the fourth ventricle and the cerebellum have been removed.

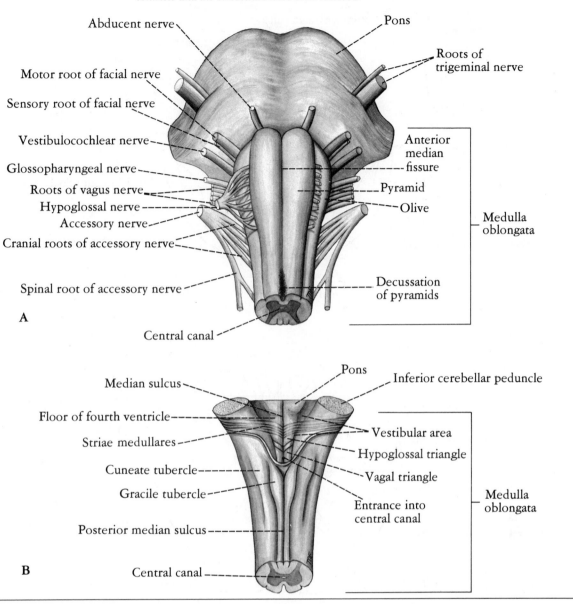

Internal Structure of the Medulla Oblongata. As in the spinal cord, the medulla oblongata consists of white matter and gray matter, but a study of transverse sections of this region shows that they have been extensively rearranged.

The internal structure of the medulla oblongata will be considered at four levels: (1) level of decussation of pyramids, (2) level of decussation of lemnisci, (3) level of the olives, and (4) level just inferior to the pons.

LEVEL OF DECUSSATION OF PYRAMIDS. A transverse section through the inferior half of the medulla oblongata (Fig. 8-2) passes through the **decussation of the pyramids,** the great motor decussation. In the superior part of the medulla the corticospinal fibers occupy and form the pyramid, but inferiorly about three-quarters of the fibers cross the median plane and continue down the spinal cord in the lateral white column as the **lateral corticospinal tract.** As these fibers cross

Fig. 8-2

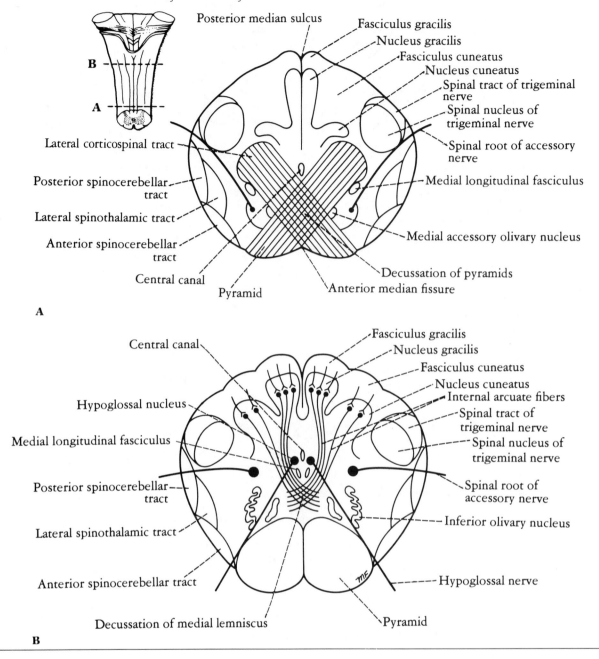

A

B

the midline, they sever the continuity between the anterior column of the gray matter of the spinal cord and the gray matter that surrounds the central canal.

The **fasciculus gracilis** and the **fasciculus cuneatus** continue to ascend superiorly posterior to the central gray matter (Fig. 8-2). The **nucleus gracilis** and the **nucleus cuneatus** appear as posterior extensions of the central gray matter.

The **substantia gelatinosa** in the posterior gray column of the spinal cord becomes continuous with the inferior end of the **nucleus of the spinal tract of the trigeminal nerve.** The fibers of the tract of the nucleus are situated between the nucleus and the surface of the medulla oblongata.

The lateral and anterior white columns of the spinal cord are easily identified in these sections and their fiber arrangement is unchanged (Fig. 8-2).

LEVEL OF DECUSSATION OF LEMNISCI. A transverse section through the inferior half of the medulla oblongata, a short distance above the level of the decussation of the pyramids, passes through the **decussation of lemnisci,** the great sensory decussation (Fig. 8-2). The decussation of the lemnisci takes place anterior to the central gray matter and posterior to the pyramids. It should be understood that the lemnisci have been formed from the **internal arcuate fibers,** which have emerged from the anterior aspects of the **nucleus gracilis and nucleus cuneatus.** The internal arcuate fibers first travel anteriorly and laterally round the central gray matter. They then curve medially toward the midline, where they decussate with the corresponding fibers of the opposite side (Fig. 8-2).

The **nucleus of the spinal tract of the trigeminal nerve** lies lateral to the internal arcuate fibers. The **spinal tract of the trigeminal nerve** lies lateral to the nucleus (Fig. 8-2).

The **lateral and anterior spinothalamic tracts and the spinotectal tracts** occupy an area lateral to the decussation of the lemnisci. They are very close to one another and collectively are known as the **spinal lemniscus.** The **spinocerebellar, vestibulospinal,** and the **rubrospinal tracts** are situated in the anterolateral region of the medulla oblongata.

LEVEL OF THE OLIVES. A transverse section through the olives passes across the inferior part of the fourth ventricle (Fig. 8-3). The amount of gray matter has increased at this level owing to the presence of the olivary nuclear complex, the nuclei of the vestibulocochlear, glossopharyngeal, vagus, accessory, and hypoglossal nerves, and the arcuate nuclei.

OLIVARY NUCLEAR COMPLEX. The largest nucleus of this complex is the **inferior olivary nucleus** (Fig. 8-3). The gray matter is shaped like a crumpled bag with its mouth directed medially; it is responsible for the elevation on the surface of the medulla called the **olive.** Smaller **dorsal and medial accessory olivary nuclei** also are present. The cells of the inferior olivary nucleus send fibers medially

---

Fig. 8-3   *Transverse section of the medulla oblongata at the level of the olivary nuclei.*

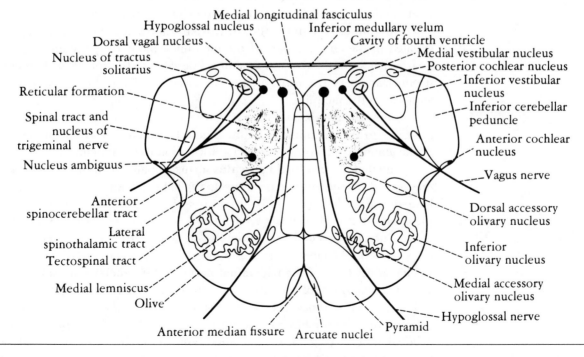

95

across the midline to enter the cerebellum through the inferior cerebellar peduncle. Afferent fibers reach the inferior olivary nuclei from the spinal cord (the **spino-olivary tracts**) and from the cerebellum and cerebral cortex. The function of the olivary nuclei is associated with voluntary muscle movement.

VESTIBULOCOCHLEAR NUCLEI. The **vestibular nuclear complex** is made up of the following nuclei: (1) **medial vestibular nucleus,** (2) **inferior vestibular nucleus,** (3) **lateral vestibular nucleus,** and (4) **superior vestibular nucleus.** For connections of these nuclei, see page 231. It should be noted that the medial and inferior vestibular nuclei can be seen on section at this level (Fig. 8-3).

The **cochlear nuclei** are two in number. The **anterior cochlear nucleus** is situated on the anterolateral aspect of the inferior cerebellar peduncle and the **posterior cochlear nucleus** is situated on the posterior aspect of the peduncle lateral to the floor of the fourth ventricle. The connections of these nuclei are described on page 232.

NUCLEUS AMBIGUUS. The nucleus ambiguus consists of large motor neurons and is situated deep within the reticular formation (Fig. 8-3). The emerging nerve fibers join the glossopharyngeal, vagus, and cranial part of the accessory nerve and are distributed to voluntary skeletal muscle.

CENTRAL GRAY MATTER. The central gray matter lies beneath the floor of the fourth ventricle at this level (Fig. 8-3). Passing from medial to lateral, the following important structures may be recognized: (1) the **hypoglossal nucleus,** (2) the **dorsal nucleus of the vagus,** (3) the **nucleus of the tractus solitarius,** and (4) the **medial and inferior vestibular nuclei** (see above). The nucleus ambiguus, referred to above, has become deeply placed within the reticular formation (Fig. 8-3). The connections and functional significance of these nuclei are described on pages 242 and 245.

ARCUATE NUCLEI. The arcuate nuclei are thought to be inferiorly displaced **pontine nuclei** (see p. 101) and are situated on the anterior surface of the pyramids (Fig. 8-3). They receive nerve fibers from the cerebral cortex and send efferent fibers to the cerebellum through the **anterior external arcuate fibers.**

The **pyramids** containing the corticospinal and some corticonuclear fibers are situated in the anterior part of the medulla separated by the anterior median fissure (Fig. 8-3); the corticospinal fibers descend to the spinal cord and the corticonuclear fibers are distributed to the motor nuclei of the cranial nerves situated within the medulla.

The **medial lemniscus** forms a flattened tract on each side of the midline posterior to the pyramid (Fig. 8-3). These fibers emerge from the decussation of the lemnisci and convey sensory information to the thalamus.

The **medial longitudinal fasciculus** forms a small tract of nerve fibers situated on each side of the midline posterior to the medial lemniscus and anterior to the hypoglossal nucleus (Fig. 8-3). It consists of ascending and descending fibers, the connections of which will be described on pages 214, 216, 228, and 232.

The **inferior cerebellar peduncle** is situated in the posterolateral corner of the section on the lateral side of the fourth ventricle (Fig. 8-3).

The **spinal tract of the trigeminal nerve and its nucleus** are situated on the anteromedial aspect of the inferior cerebellar peduncle (Fig. 8-3).

The **anterior spinocerebellar tract** is situated near the surface in the interval between the inferior olivary nucleus and the nucleus of the spinal tract of the trigeminal nerve (Fig. 8-3). The **spinal lemniscus,** consisting of the **lateral spinothalamic and spinotectal tracts** and the rubrospinal tract, are deeply placed.

The **reticular formation,** consisting of a diffuse mixture of nerve fibers and small groups of nerve cells, is deeply placed posterior to the olivary nucleus (Fig. 8-3). The reticular formation represents, at this level, only a small part of this system, which is also present in the pons and midbrain.

The **glossopharyngeal, vagus,** and **cranial part of the accessory nerves** can be seen running forward and laterally through the reticular formation (Fig. 8-3). The nerve fibers emerge between the olives and the inferior cerebellar peduncles. The **hypoglossal nerves** also run anteriorly and laterally through the reticular formation and emerge between the pyramids and the olives (Fig. 8-3).

LEVEL OF THE MEDULLA OBLONGATA JUST INFERIOR TO THE PONS. There are no major changes in the distribution of the gray and white matter. The lateral vestibular nucleus has replaced the inferior vestibular nucleus, and the cochlear nuclei now are visible on the anterior and posterior surfaces of the inferior cerebellar peduncle.

Blood Supply of the Medulla Oblongata. The vertebral, anterior and posterior spinal, posterior inferior cerebellar, and basilar arteries all send branches to the medulla oblongata.

Arnold-Chiari Phenomenon. The Arnold-Chiari malformation is a congenital anomaly in which there is a herniation of the tonsils of the cerebellum and the medulla oblongata through the foramen magnum into the vertebral canal. This results in the blockage of the exits in the roof of the fourth ventricle to the cerebrospinal fluid, causing internal hydrocephalus.

Vascular Disorders of the Medulla Oblongata

LATERAL MEDULLARY SYNDROME OF WALLENBERG. The lateral part of the medulla oblongata is supplied by the posterior inferior cerebellar artery, which is usually a branch of the vertebral artery. Thrombosis of either of these arteries (Fig. 8-4) produces the following signs and symptoms: dysphagia and dysarthria due to paralysis of the ipsilateral palatal and laryngeal muscles (innervated by the nucleus ambiguus); analgesia and thermoanesthesia on the ipsilateral side of the face (nucleus and spinal tract of the trigeminal nerve); vertigo, nausea, vomiting, and nystagmus (vestibular nuclei); ipsilateral Horner's syndrome (descending sympathetic fibers); ipsilateral cerebellar signs—gait and limb ataxia (cerebellum or inferior cerebellar peduncle); contralateral loss of sensations of pain and temperature (spinal lemniscus—spinothalamic tract).

MEDIAL MEDULLARY SYNDROME. The medial part of the medulla oblongata is supplied by the vertebral artery. Thrombosis of the medullary branch (Fig. 8-4) produces the following signs and symptoms: contralateral hemiparesis (pyramidal tract); contralateral impaired sensations of position and movement and tactile discrimination (medial lemniscus); ipsilateral paralysis of tongue muscles with deviation of paralyzed side when protruded (hypoglossal nerve).

PONS

External Appearance. The pons is anterior to the cerebellum (Fig. 8-5) and connects the medulla oblongata to the midbrain. It is about 1 inch (2.5 mm) long.

The anterior surface is convex from side to side and shows many transverse fibers that converge on each side to form the **middle cerebellar peduncle** (Fig. 8-5). There is a shallow groove in the midline, the **basilar groove,** which lodges the basilar artery. On the anterolateral surface of the pons the **trigeminal nerve**

Fig. 8-4

Transverse sections of the medulla oblongata. A. Shows the lesion that produces the lateral medullary syndrome. B. Shows the lesion that produces the medial medullary syndrome.

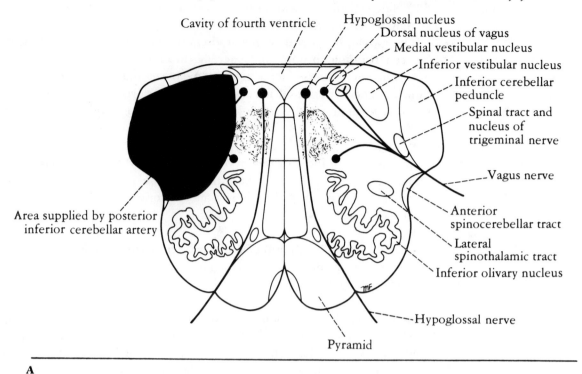

Cavity of fourth ventricle

Hypoglossal nucleus

Dorsal nucleus of vagus

Medial vestibular nucleus

Inferior vestibular nucleus

Inferior cerebellar peduncle

Spinal tract and nucleus of trigeminal nerve

Vagus nerve

Anterior spinocerebellar tract

Lateral spinothalamic tract

Inferior olivary nucleus

Area supplied by posterior inferior cerebellar artery

Hypoglossal nerve

Pyramid

A

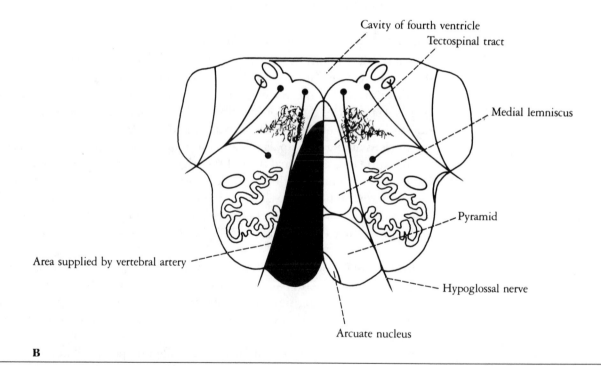

Cavity of fourth ventricle

Tectospinal tract

Medial lemniscus

Pyramid

Hypoglossal nerve

Area supplied by vertebral artery

Arcuate nucleus

B

emerges on each side. Each nerve consists of a smaller, medial **motor root** and a larger, lateral **sensory root.** In the groove between the pons and the medulla oblongata there emerge, from medial to lateral, the **abducent, facial,** and **vestibulocochlear nerves** (Fig. 8-5).

The posterior surface of the pons is hidden from view by the cerebellum. It forms the upper half of the floor of the fourth ventricle and is triangular in

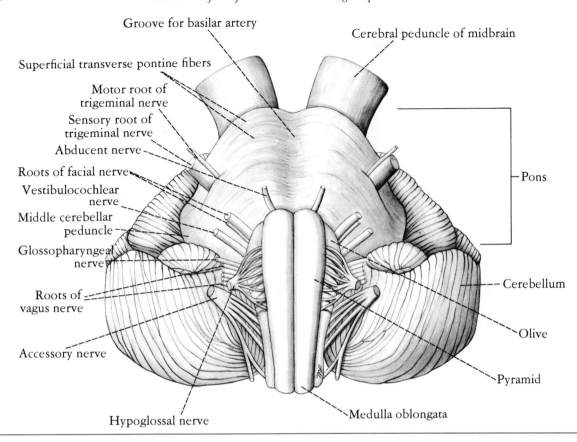

shape (Fig. 8-6). The posterior surface is limited laterally by the **superior cere-bellar peduncles** and is divided into symmetrical halves by a **median sulcus.** Lateral to this sulcus is an elongated elevation, the **medial eminence,** which is bounded laterally by a sulcus, the **sulcus limitans** (Fig. 8-6). The inferior end of the medial eminence is slightly expanded to form the **facial colliculus,** which is produced by the root of the facial nerve winding around the nucleus of the abducent nerve (Fig. 8-7). The floor of the superior part of the **sulcus limitans** is bluish-gray in color and is called the **substantia ferruginea;** it owes its color to a group of deeply pigmented nerve cells. Lateral to the sulcus limitans is the **area vestibuli** produced by the underlying vestibular nuclei (Fig. 8-6).

Internal Structure of Pons. For purposes of description, the pons is commonly divided into a posterior part, the **tegmentum,** and an anterior **basal part** by the transversely running fibers of the **trapezoid body** (Fig. 8-7).

The structure of the pons may be studied at two levels: (1) transverse section through the caudal part, passing through the facial colliculus, and (2) transverse section through the cranial part, passing through the trigeminal nuclei.

TRANSVERSE SECTION THROUGH THE CAUDAL PART OF THE PONS. The **medial lemniscus** rotates as it passes from the medulla into the pons. It is situated in the most anterior part of the tegmentum with its long axis running transversely (Fig. 8-7).

The **facial nucleus** lies posterior to the lateral part of the medial lemniscus. The fibers of the facial nerve wind round the **nucleus of the abducent nerve,** producing the **facial colliculus** (Fig. 8-7). The fibers of the facial nerve then

Fig. 8-6   *Posterior surface of the brainstem showing the pons. The cerebellum has been removed.*

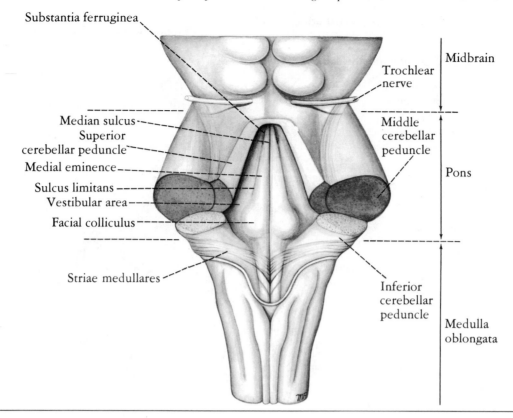

Substantia ferruginea

Trochlear nerve

Midbrain

Median sulcus
Superior cerebellar peduncle

Middle cerebellar peduncle

Medial eminence

Pons

Sulcus limitans
Vestibular area
Facial colliculus

Striae medullares

Inferior cerebellar peduncle

Medulla oblongata

Fig. 8-7   *Transverse section of the caudal part of the pons at the level of the facial colliculus.*

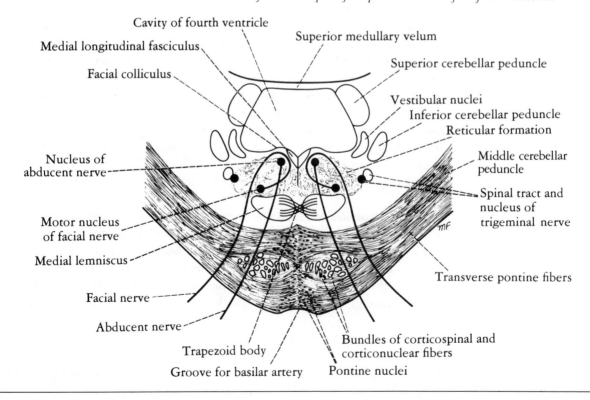

Cavity of fourth ventricle

Medial longitudinal fasciculus

Superior medullary velum

Facial colliculus

Superior cerebellar peduncle

Vestibular nuclei
Inferior cerebellar peduncle
Reticular formation

Nucleus of abducent nerve

Middle cerebellar peduncle

Spinal tract and nucleus of trigeminal nerve

Motor nucleus of facial nerve

Medial lemniscus

Transverse pontine fibers

Facial nerve

Abducent nerve

Trapezoid body

Groove for basilar artery

Bundles of corticospinal and corticonuclear fibers

Pontine nuclei

pass anteriorly between the facial nucleus and the superior end of the nucleus of the spinal tract of the trigeminal nerve.

The medial longitudinal fasciculus is situated beneath the floor of the fourth ventricle on either side of the midline (Fig. 8-7). The medial longitudinal fasciculus is the main pathway that connects the vestibular and cochlear nuclei with the nuclei controlling the extraocular muscles (oculomotor, trochlear, and abducent nuclei).

The **medial vestibular nucleus** is situated lateral to the abducent nucleus (Fig. 8-7) and is in close relationship to the inferior cerebellar peduncle. The superior part of the lateral and the inferior part of the superior vestibular nucleus are found at this level. The **posterior and anterior cochlear nuclei** are also found at this level (see p. 232).

The **spinal nucleus of the trigeminal nerve and its tract** lie on the anteromedial aspect of the inferior cerebellar peduncle (Fig. 8-7).

The **trapezoid body** is made up of fibers derived from the cochlear nuclei and the nuclei of the trapezoid body. They run transversely (Fig. 8-7) in the anterior part of the tegmentum (see p. 232).

The basilar part of the pons, at this level, contains small masses of nerve cells called **pontine nuclei** (Fig. 8-7). The **corticopontine fibers** of the crus cerebri of the midbrain terminate in the pontine nuclei. The axons of these cells give origin to the **transverse fibers** of the pons, which cross the midline and intersect the corticospinal and corticonuclear tracts, breaking them up into small bundles. The transverse fibers of the pons enter the middle cerebellar peduncle and are distributed to the cerebellar hemisphere. This connection forms the main pathway linking the cerebral cortex to the cerebellum.

TRANSVERSE SECTION THROUGH THE CRANIAL PART OF THE PONS. The internal structure of the pons is similar to that seen at the caudal level (Fig. 8-8), but it now contains the motor and principal sensory nuclei of the trigeminal nerve.

Fig. 8-8   *Transverse section of the pons at the level of the trigeminal nuclei.*

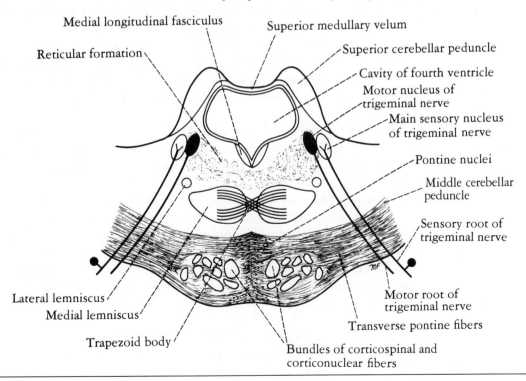

The **motor nucleus of the trigeminal nerve** is situated beneath the lateral part of the fourth ventricle within the reticular formation (Fig. 8-8). The emerging motor fibers travel anteriorly through the substance of the pons and exit on its anterior surface.

The **principal sensory nucleus of the trigeminal nerve** is situated on the lateral side of the motor nucleus (Fig. 8-8); it is continuous inferiorly with the nucleus of the spinal tract. The entering sensory fibers travel through the substance of the pons and lie lateral to the motor fibers (Fig. 8-8).

The **superior cerebellar peduncle** is situated posterolateral to the motor nucleus of the trigeminal nerve (Fig. 8-8). It is joined by the **anterior spinocerebellar tract.**

The **trapezoid body** and the **medial lemniscus** are situated in the same position as they were in the previous section (Fig. 8-8). The **lateral lemniscus** lies at the lateral extremity of the medial lemniscus (Fig. 8-8).

MIDBRAIN

External Appearance. The midbrain measures about 0.8 inch (2 cm) in length and connects the pons and cerebellum with the forebrain. The midbrain is traversed by a narrow channel, the **cerebral aqueduct,** which is filled with cerebrospinal fluid (Fig. 8-9).

On the posterior surface are four **colliculi** (corpora quadrigemina). These are rounded eminences that are divided into superior and inferior pairs by a vertical and a transverse groove. The superior colliculi are centers for visual reflexes (see p. 211), and the inferior are lower auditory centers. In the midline below the inferior colliculi, the **trochlear** nerves emerge (Fig. 8-9). These are delicate nerves that wind round the lateral aspect of the midbrain to enter the lateral wall of the cavernous sinus.

On the lateral aspect of the midbrain, the superior and inferior brachia ascend in an anterolateral direction. The **superior brachium** passes from the superior colliculus to the lateral geniculate body and the optic tract. The **inferior brachium** connects the inferior colliculus to the **medial geniculate body.**

On the anterior aspect of the midbrain (Fig. 8-9) there is a deep depression in the midline, the **interpeduncular fossa,** which is bounded on either side by the **crus cerebri.** Many small blood vessels perforate the floor of the interpeduncular fossa and this region is termed the **posterior perforated substance.** The **oculomotor** nerve emerges from a groove on the medial side of the crus cerebri and passes forward in the lateral wall of the cavernous sinus (Fig. 8-9).

Internal Structure of the Midbrain. The midbrain comprises two lateral halves, called the **cerebral peduncles;** each of these is divided into an anterior part, the **crus cerebri,** and a posterior part, the **tegmentum,** by a pigmented band of gray matter, the **substantia nigra** (Fig. 8-9). The narrow cavity of the midbrain is the **cerebral aqueduct,** which connects the third and fourth ventricles. The **tectum** is the part of the midbrain posterior to the cerebral aqueduct; it has four small surface swellings referred to previously: the **two superior** and **two inferior colliculi** (Fig. 8-9). The cerebral aqueduct is lined by ependyma and is surrounded by the **central gray matter.** On transverse sections of the midbrain, the interpeduncular fossa can be seen to separate the crura cerebri, whereas the tegmentum is continuous across the median plane (Fig. 8-9).

TRANSVERSE SECTION OF THE MIDBRAIN AT THE LEVEL OF THE INFERIOR COLLICULI. The **inferior colliculus,** consisting of a large nucleus of gray matter, lies beneath the corresponding surface elevation and forms part of the auditory

Fig. 8-9

Transverse sections of the midbrain. A. At the level of the inferior colliculus. B. At the level of the superior colliculus.

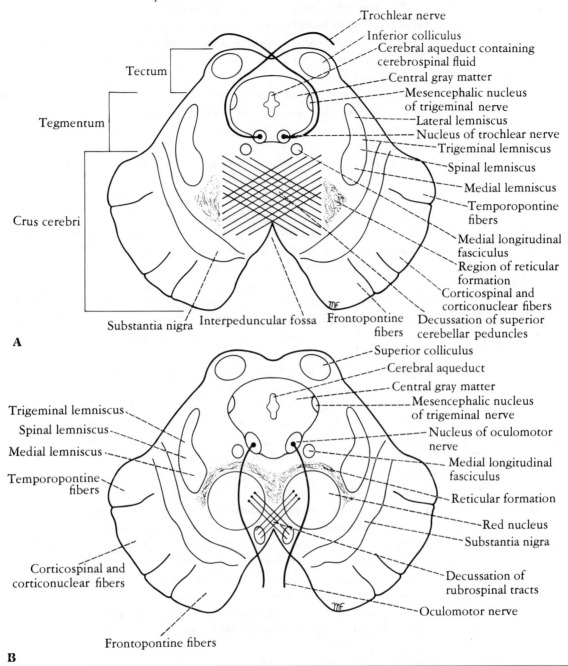

pathway (Fig. 8-9). It receives many of the terminal fibers of the lateral lemniscus. The pathway then continues (see p. 232) through the inferior brachium to the medial geniculate body.

The **trochlear nucleus** is situated in the central gray matter close to the median plane just posterior to the **medial longitudinal fasciculus.** The emerging fibers of the trochlear nucleus pass laterally and posteriorly round the central gray matter and leave the midbrain just below the inferior colliculi. The fibers of the trochlear nerve now decussate completely in the superior medullary velum. The **mesencephalic nuclei of the trigeminal nerve** are lateral to the cerebral aqueduct (Fig. 8-9). The **decussation of the superior cerebellar peduncles** occupies the central part of the tegmentum anterior to the cerebral aqueduct. The **reticular formation** is smaller than that of the pons and is situated lateral to the decussation.

The **medial lemniscus** ascends posterior to the substantia nigra; the **spinal** and **trigeminal lemnisci** are situated lateral to the medial lemniscus (Fig. 8-9). The **lateral lemniscus** is located posterior to the trigeminal lemniscus.

The **substantia nigra** (Fig. 8-9) is a large motor nucleus situated between the tegmentum and the crus cerebri and is found throughout the midbrain. The nucleus is composed of medium-size multipolar neurons that possess inclusion granules of melanin pigment within their cytoplasm. The substantia nigra is concerned with muscle tone and is connected to the cerebral cortex, spinal cord, hypothalamus, and basal nuclei.

The **crus cerebri** contains important descending tracts and is separated from the tegmentum by the substantia nigra (Fig. 8-9). The corticospinal and corticonuclear fibers occupy the middle two-thirds of the crus. The frontopontine fibers occupy the medial part of the crus and the temporopontine fibers occupy the lateral part of the crus (Fig. 8-9). These descending tracts connect the cerebral cortex to the anterior gray column cells of the spinal cord, the cranial nerve nuclei, the pons, and the cerebellum.

TRANSVERSE SECTION OF THE MIDBRAIN AT THE LEVEL OF THE SUPERIOR COLLICULI. The **superior colliculus** (Fig. 8-9), a large nucleus of gray matter that lies beneath the corresponding surface elevation, forms part of the visual reflexes (see p. 211). It is connected to the lateral geniculate body by the superior brachium. It receives afferent fibers from the optic nerve, the visual cortex, and the spinotectal tract. The efferent fibers form the tectospinal and tectobulbar tracts, which are probably responsible for the reflex movements of the eyes, head, and neck in response to visual stimuli. The afferent pathway for the **light reflex** ends in the **pretectal nucleus.** This is a small group of neurons situated close to the lateral part of the superior colliculus. After relaying in the pretectal nucleus, the fibers pass to the parasympathetic nucleus of the oculomotor nerve (Edinger-Westphal nucleus). The emerging fibers then pass to the oculomotor nerve. The **oculomotor nucleus** is situated in the central gray matter close to the median plane, just posterior to the **medial longitudinal fasciculus** (Fig. 8-9). The fibers of the oculomotor nucleus pass anteriorly through the red nucleus to emerge on the medial side of the crus cerebri in the interpeduncular fossa. The nucleus of the oculomotor nerve is divisible into a number of cell groups, the details of which are described on p. 214.

The **medial, spinal, and trigeminal lemnisci** form a curved band posterior to the substantia nigra but the **lateral lemniscus** does not extend superiorly to this level (Fig. 8-9).

The **red nucleus** (Fig. 8-9) is a rounded mass of gray matter situated between the cerebral aqueduct and the substantia nigra. Afferent fibers reach the red nucleus from: (1) the cerebral cortex through the corticospinal fibers, (2) the cerebellum through the superior cerebellar peduncle, and (3) the lentiform nucleus, subthalamic and hypothalamic nuclei, substantia nigra, and spinal cord. Efferent fibers leave the red nucleus and pass to (1) the spinal cord through the rubrospinal tract (as this tract descends it decussates), (2) the reticular formation through the rubroreticular tract, (3) the thalamus, and (4) the substantia nigra.

The **reticular formation** is situated in the tegmentum lateral and posterior to the red nucleus (Fig. 8-9).

The **crus cerebri** contains the identical important descending tracts, the **corticospinal, corticonuclear,** and **corticopontine** fibers, that are present at the level of the inferior colliculus.

Blockage of the Cerebral Aqueduct. The cavity of the midbrain, the cerebral aqueduct, is one of the narrower parts of the ventricular system. Normally, cerebrospinal fluid that has been produced in the lateral and third ventricles passes through this channel to enter the fourth ventricle and so escapes through the foramina in its roof to enter the subarachnoid space. In congenital hydrocephalus, the cerebral aqueduct may be blocked. A tumor of the midbrain or pressure on the midbrain from a tumor arising outside the midbrain may compress the aqueduct and produce hydrocephalus.

Vascular Disorders of the Midbrain

WEBER'S SYNDROME. Weber's syndrome (Fig. 8-10), which is commonly produced by occlusion of a branch of the posterior cerebral artery that supplies the midbrain, results in the necrosis of brain tissue involving the oculomotor nerve and the crus cerebri. There is ipsilateral ophthalmoplegia and contralateral paralysis of the lower part of the face, the tongue, and the arm and leg. The eyeball is deviated laterally because of the paralysis of the medial rectus muscle; there is drooping (ptosis) of the upper lid and the pupil is dilated and fixed to light and accommodation.

BENEDIKT'S SYNDROME. Benedikt's syndrome (Fig. 8-10) is similar to Weber's syndrome, but the necrosis involves the medial lemniscus and red nucleus, pro-

---

Fig. 8-10   *Vascular disorders of the midbrain. A. Weber's syndrome, involving the oculomotor nerve and the crus cerebri. B. Benedikt's syndrome, involving the red nucleus and the medial lemniscus.*

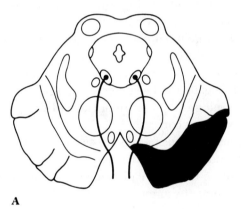

A

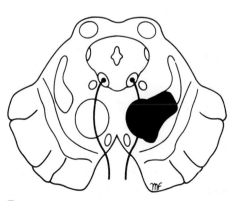

B

ducing contralateral hemianesthesia and involuntary movements of the limbs of the opposite side.

NATIONAL BOARD
TYPE QUESTIONS

In each of the following questions, answer:
A. If only (1) is correct
B. If only (2) is correct
C. If both (1) and (2) are correct
D. If neither (1) nor (2) is correct

1. Concerning the anterior surface of the medulla oblongata, which of the following statements is (are) correct?
   (1) On each side of the midline there is a swelling called the pyramid.
   (2) The corticospinal fibers take part in the decussation of the pyramids.
2. Concerning the posterior surface of the medulla oblongata, which of the following statements is (are) correct?
   (1) It forms the upper half of the floor of the fourth ventricle.
   (2) It has two small swellings produced by the underlying cuneate and gracile nuclei.
3. Concerning the emergence of the cranial nerves from the medulla oblongata, which of the following statements is (are) correct?
   (1) The glossopharyngeal nerve emerges between the olive and the inferior cerebellar peduncle.
   (2) The cranial part of the accessory nerve emerges between the pyramid and the olive.
4. Concerning the anterior surface of the pons, which of the following statements is (are) correct?
   (1) The trigeminal nerve emerges as a small medial motor root and a large lateral sensory root.
   (2) In the groove between the lower border of the pons and the medulla oblongata, the facial nerve emerges.
5. Concerning the posterior surface of the pons, which of the following statements is (are) correct?
   (1) The colliculus facialis is a swelling caused by the abducent nerve winding round the facial nucleus.
   (2) The vestibular area lies medial to the medial eminence.
6. Concerning the anterior surface of the midbrain, which of the following facts is (are) correct?
   (1) The oculomotor nerve emerges between the cerebral peduncles.
   (2) The space between the cerebral peduncles is called the interpeduncular fossa.
7. Concerning the posterior surface of the midbrain, which of the following facts is (are) correct?
   (1) The fibers of the trochlear nerve decussate completely on emerging on the posterior surface.
   (2) The superior colliculi are associated with visual reflexes.

Select the **best** response.

8. The following statements concerning the interior of the lower part of the medulla are correct **except:**
   A. It contains the central canal.
   B. About three-quarters of the corticospinal fibers cross the median plane.

C. The substantia gelatinosa of the spinal cord becomes continuous with the nucleus of the spinal tract of the trigeminal nerve.

D. The medial lemniscus is formed by nerve fibers entering the hypoglossal nucleus.

E. The nucleus gracilis lies lateral to the posterior median sulcus.

9. The following statements concerning the interior of the upper part of the medulla are true **except:**

A. The medial longitudinal fasciculus lies on either side of the midline.

B. The dorsal nucleus of the vagus nerve lies between the pyramid and the olive.

C. The hypoglossal nucleus lies just beneath the floor of the fourth ventricle.

D. The nucleus ambiguus is situated within the reticular formation.

E. The inferior cerebellar peduncle is located along the lateral border of this part of the medulla.

10. The following statements concerning a transverse section through the caudal part of the pons are correct **except:**

A. All the transverse pontine fibers cross the pons posterior to the cortico-spinal fibers.

B. The motor nucleus of the facial nerve lies posterior to the medial lemniscus.

C. The trapezoid body is present.

D. The cavity of the fourth ventricle is roofed over by the superior medullary velum.

E. The spinal tract and nucleus of the trigeminal nerve are present.

11. The following statements concerning a transverse section through the mid-brain at the level of the superior colliculus are true **except:**

A. The nucleus of the oculomotor nerve is present in the central gray matter.

B. The red nucleus is traversed by the emerging fibers of the third cranial nerve.

C. The medial lemniscus lies anterior to the substantia nigra.

D. The spinal lemniscus lies a short distance lateral to the medial longitudinal bundle.

E. The rubrospinal tracts decussate at this level of the brainstem.

12. The following statements concerning a transverse section of the midbrain at the level of the inferior colliculus are true **except:**

A. The frontopontine fibers are situated lateral to the temporopontine fibers.

B. The superior cerebellar peduncles decussate at this level.

C. The nucleus of the trochlear nerve lies in the central gray matter.

D. The reticular formation lies posterior to the substantia nigra.

E. The tectum lies posterior to the cerebral aqueduct.

In each of the following questions, answer:
A. If only (1), (2), and (3) are correct
B. If only (1) and (3) are correct
C. If only (2) and (4) are correct
D. If only (4) is correct
E. If all are correc'

13. Which of the following statement(s) concerning the medulla is (are) correct?

(1) The central canal is continuous below with the central canal of the spinal cord.

(2) The inferior medullary velum stretches between the inferior cerebellar peduncles.

(3) The blood supply is derived from the vertebral, anterior and posterior spinal, posterior inferior cerebellar, and basilar arteries.

(4) The tectospinal tract is formed from the external arcuate fibers.

14. Which of the following statements concerning the pons is (are) correct?

(1) The pons lies anterior to the cerebellum.

(2) The basilar artery lies on its anterior surface, producing a groove.

(3) The posterior surface of the pons forms part of the floor of the fourth ventricle.

(4) The posterior part of the pons is often referred to as the tegmentum.

15. Which of the following statements concerning the midbrain is (are) correct?

(1) It is surrounded by cerebrospinal fluid.

(2) The crus cerebri form the posterior part of the cerebral peduncles.

(3) The inferior colliculi are concerned with auditory reflexes.

(4) The inferior brachium connects the inferior colliculus with the lateral geniculate body.

16. Which of the following statements concerning the lateral medullary syndrome of Wallenberg is (are) correct?

(1) The syndrome can be caused by thrombosis of the posterior inferior cerebellar artery.

(2) There is analgesia and thermoanesthesia on the ipsilateral side of the face.

(3) There is ipsilateral Horner's syndrome.

(4) There is contralateral loss of sensations of pain and temperature.

17. Which of the following signs and symptoms is (are) correct concerning the medial medullary syndrome?

(1) Ipsilateral impaired sensations of position and movement.

(2) Contralateral hemiparesis.

(3) Ipsilateral loss of tactile descrimination.

(4) Ipsilateral paralysis of the tongue.

18. Which of the following facts is (are) true concerning the Arnold-Chiari phenomenon?

(1) It is a congenital anomaly.

Fig. 8-11   *Transverse section of the medulla oblongata.*

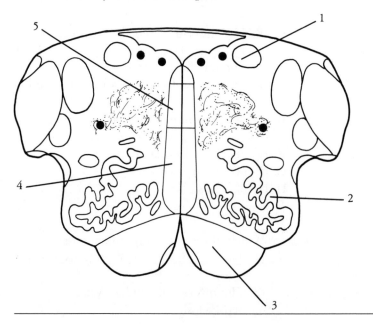

(2) There is a herniation of part of the cerebellum through the foramen magnum.

(3) The apertures in the roof of the fourth ventricle become blocked.

(4) Internal hydrocephalus occurs.

19. Which of the following statements concerning the cerebral aqueduct is (are) correct?

(1) It is lined by ependyma.

(2) It is continuous above with the third ventricle.

(3) It drains below into the fourth ventricle.

(4) It is one of the narrower parts of the ventricular system of the brain.

20. Which of the following statements concerning Weber's syndrome is (are) correct?

(1) It results in necrosis of the brain tissue involving the oculomotor nerve.

(2) There is ipsilateral ophthalmoplegia.

(3) There is contralateral paralysis of the upper and lower limbs.

(4) There is ptosis of the contralateral upper eyelid.

Match the numbers listed below on the left in Figure 8-11 with the appropriate structure listed below on the right.

21. Number 1	A. Inferior cerebellar peduncle.
22. Number 2	B. Inferior olivary nucleus.
23. Number 3	C. Pyramid.
24. Number 4	D. Medial lemniscus
25. Number 5	E. None of the above.

Match the numbers listed below on the left in Figure 8-12 with the appropriate structure listed below on the right.

26. Number 1	A. Middle cerebellar peduncle.
27. Number 2	B. Transverse pontine fibers.
28. Number 3	C. Medial lemniscus.
29. Number 4	D. Decussation of the superior cerebellar peduncles.
30. Number 5	E. None of the above.

Fig. 8-12   *Transverse section of the pons.*

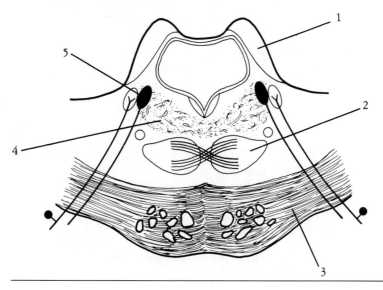

Fig. 8-13 *Transverse section of the midbrain.*

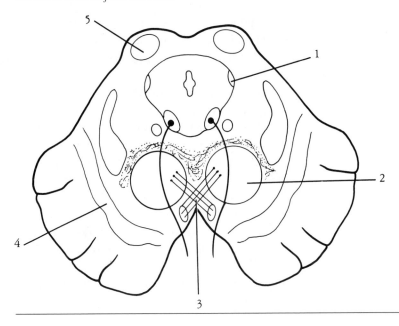

Match the numbers listed below on the left in Figure 8-13 with the appropriate structure listed below on the right.

31. Number 1   A. Superior colliculus.
32. Number 2   B. Mesencephalic nucleus.
33. Number 3   C. Reticular formation.
34. Number 4   D. Red nucleus.
35. Number 5   E. None of the above.

ANSWERS AND EXPLANATIONS

1. C
2. B: (1) The pons forms the upper part of the floor of the fourth ventricle.
3. A: (2) The cranial part of the accessory nerve emerges from the medulla in the groove between the olive and the inferior cerebellar peduncle.
4. C
5. D: (1) The colliculus facialis is produced by the motor root of the facial nerve winding round the nucleus of the abducent nerve. (2) The vestibular area on the floor of the fourth ventricle lies lateral to the medial eminence.
6. C
7. C
8. D: The medial lemniscus is formed from the internal arcuate fibers that have emerged from the nucleus gracilis and the nucleus cuneatus.
9. B: The dorsal nucleus of the vagus nerve lies beneath the floor of the fourth ventricle just lateral to the hypoglossal nucleus.
10. A: The corticospinal and corticonuclear fibers lie in amongst the transverse pontine fibers.
11. C: The medial lemniscus lies posterior to the substantia nigra.
12. A: The frontopontine fibers lie medial to the temporopontine fibers.
13. A: (4) The tectospinal tract is formed from nerve cells in the superior colliculus of the midbrain; the tract is concerned with the influence of visual stimuli on postural movements.
14. E

15. B: (2) The crus cerebri forms the anterior part of the cerebral peduncle. (4) The inferior brachium connects the inferior colliculus to the medial geniculate body.
16. E: The lateral medullary syndrome of Wallenberg is described on page 97.
17. C: (1) Contralateral impaired sensations of position and movement (involvement of the medial lemniscus). (3) Contralateral loss of tactile descrimination (involvement of the medial lemniscus). The medial medullary syndrome is described on page 97.
18. E
19. E
20. A: (4) Ptosis occurs on the same side of the lesion and is caused by paralysis of the levator palpebrae superioris due to the involvement of the oculomotor nerve.
21. E: Medial vestibular nucleus.
22. B
23. C
24. D
25. E: Tectospinal tract.
26. E: Superior cerebellar peduncle.
27. C
28. B
29. E: Reticular formation.
30. E: Motor nucleus of trigeminal nerve.
31. B
32. D
33. E: Decussation of rubrospinal tract.
34. E: Substantia nigra.
35. A

9 Cerebellum

SUGGESTED PLAN FOR REVIEW FOR CHAPTER 9

1. Learn the structure of the gray matter of the cerebellar cortex and the arrangement of the intracerebellar nuclei. Memorize the connections of the cells of the cerebellar cortex. Examiners are fond of asking questions about the Purkinje cells.
2. Understand the difference between the climbing and the mossy fibers. Where do these fibers terminate in the cerebellar cortex?
3. Learn the main connections between the cerebellum and the remainder of the nervous system. Do not just commit connections to memory but understand the functions of the various connections. You will find that this approach helps one to retain the material.
4. Know the functions of the cerebellum and understand what happens if the cerebellum fails to function because of disease. Remember that each cerebellar hemisphere controls muscular movement on the same side of the body. Also note that the cerebellum has no direct pathway to the lower motor neurons but exerts its control via the cerebral cortex and the brainstem.

INTRODUCTION

The cerebellum lies in the posterior cranial fossa of the skull and forms the roof of the fourth ventricle. It is joined to the brainstem by three pairs of peduncles: the superior, middle, and inferior peduncles.

The essential function of the cerebellum is to coordinate, by synergistic action, all reflex and voluntary muscular activity. It thus graduates and harmonizes muscle tone and maintains normal body posture. It permits voluntary movements to take place with precision and economy of effort.

EXTERNAL APPEARANCES

The cerebellum is somewhat ovoid in shape and constricted in its median part. It consists of two **cerebellar hemispheres** joined by a narrow median **vermis** (Figs. 9-1 and 9-2).

The cerebellum is divided into three main lobes: the **anterior lobe,** the **middle lobe,** and the **flocculonodular lobe.** The **anterior lobe** may be seen on the superior surface of the cerebellum and is separated from the middle lobe by a wide V-shaped fissure called the **primary fissure** (Fig. 9-2). The **middle lobe** (sometimes called the posterior lobe), which is the largest part of the cerebellum, is situated between the primary and **uvulonodular fissures.** The **flocculonodular lobe** is situated posterior to the uvulonodular fissure. A deep **horizontal fissure** that is found along the margin of the cerebellum separates the superior from the inferior surfaces; it is of no morphological or functional significance (Fig. 9-2).

The superior surface of the cerebellum shows the superior aspect of the vermis as a ridge that is not separated from the hemispheres by fissures (Fig. 9-2). The primary fissure, noted above, is visible on this surface.

The inferior surface of the cerebellum shows a deep groove, the **vallecula,** the floor of which is formed by the inferior aspect of the vermis (Fig. 9-2).

INTERNAL STRUCTURE

The cerebellum is made up of gray matter and white matter. The gray matter is found mainly covering the surface of the cerebellum as **cortex;** small aggrega-

Fig. 9-1   *Sagittal section through the brainstem and the cerebellum.*

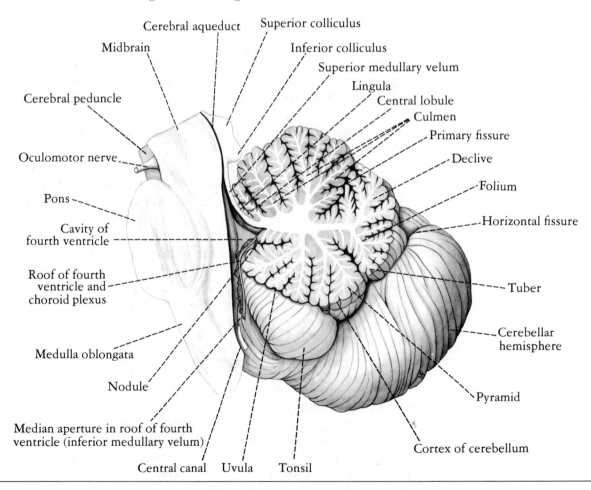

Fig. 9-2   *The cerebellum. (A) Superior view. (B) Inferior view.*

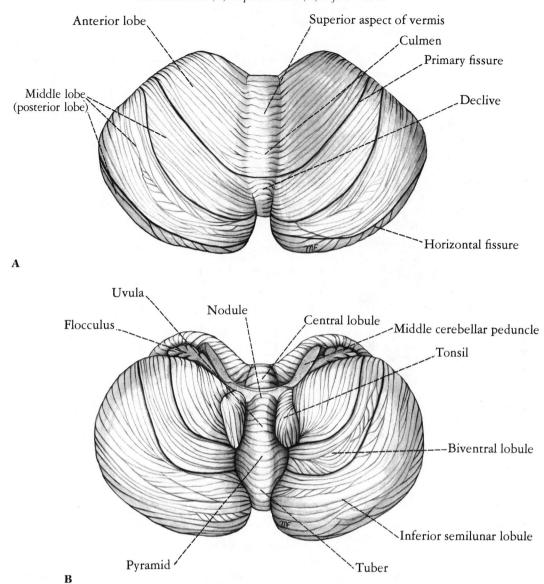

A

B

tions of gray matter, the **intracerebellar nuclei,** are also found in the interior of the cerebellum.

Gray Matter of the Cerebellum

CEREBELLAR CORTEX. The cortex of the cerebellum is folded by many parallel transverse fissures into the **cerebellar folia** (Fig. 9-1). Each folium contains a core of white matter covered superficially by gray matter. A section made through the cerebellum parallel with the median plane divides the folia at right angles, and the cut surface has a branched appearance, called the **arbor vitae** (Fig. 9-1).

The cerebellar cortex throughout its extent has a uniform structure. The cortex may be divided into three layers: (1) an external layer, the **molecular layer;** (2) a middle layer, the **Purkinje cell layer;** and (3) an internal layer, the **granular layer** (Fig. 9-3).

Molecular Layer. The molecular layer contains two types of neurons: the outer **stellate cell** and the inner **basket cell** (Fig. 9-3). These neurons are scattered

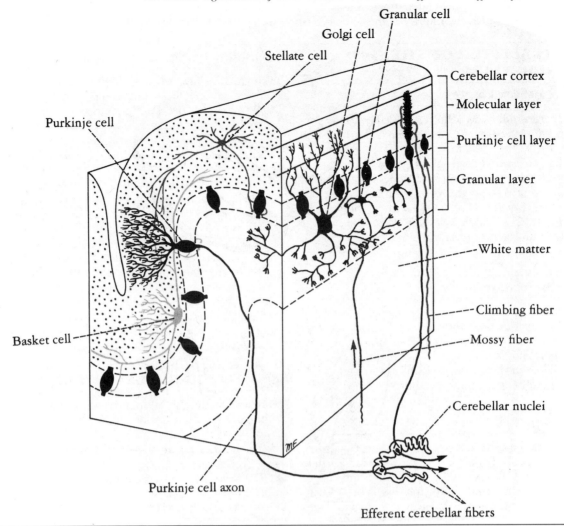

among dendritic arborizations and numerous thin axons that run parallel to the long axis of the folia. Neuroglial cells are found between these structures.

Purkinje Cell Layer. The Purkinje cells are large Golgi type I neurons. They are flask-shaped and are arranged in a single layer (Fig. 9-3). In a plane transverse to the folium, the dendrites of these cells are seen to pass into the molecular layer, where they undergo profuse branching. The primary and secondary branches are smooth and subsequent branches are covered by short, thick **dendritic spines.** It has been shown that the spines form synaptic contacts with the parallel fibers derived from the granule cell axons.

At the base of the Purkinje cell, the axon arises and passes through the granular layer to enter the white matter. On entering the white matter, the axon acquires a myelin sheath and it terminates by synapsing with cells of one of the intracerebellar nuclei. Collateral branches of the Purkinje axon make synaptic contacts with the dendrites of basket and stellate cells of the granular layer in the same area or in distant folia. A few of the Purkinje cell axons pass directly to end in the vestibular nuclei of the brainstem.

Granular Layer. The granular layer is packed with small cells with densely staining nuclei and scanty cytoplasm (Fig. 9-3). Each cell gives rise to four or five dendrites, which make clawlike endings and have synaptic contact with mossy fiber input. The axon of each granule cell passes into the molecular layer, where it bifurcates at a T junction, the branches running parallel to the long axis of the cerebellar folium. These fibers, known as **parallel fibers,** run at right angles to the dendritic processes of the Purkinje cells. The majority of the parallel fibers make synaptic contacts with the spinous processes of the dendrites of the Purkinje cells. Neuroglial cells are found throughout this layer. Scattered throughout the granular layer are Golgi cells (Fig. 9-3). Their dendrites ramify in the molecular layer and their axons terminate by splitting up into branches that synapse with the dendrites of the granular cells.

INTRACEREBELLAR NUCLEI. Four masses of gray matter are embedded in the white matter of the cerebellum on each side of the midline. From lateral to medial these nuclei are the **dentate,** the **emboliform,** the **globose,** and the **fastigial.**

The **dentate nucleus,** the largest of the cerebellar nuclei, is situated in the white matter of each cerebellar hemisphere (Fig. 9-4). It has the shape of a crumpled bag with the opening facing medially (Fig. 9-4). The interior of the bag is filled with white matter made up of efferent fibers that leave the nucleus through the opening to form a large part of the superior cerebellar peduncle.

The **emboliform nucleus** is oval-shaped and situated medial to the dentate nucleus, partially covering its hilus (Fig. 9-4).

The **globose nucleus** consists of one or more rounded cell groups that lie medial to the emboliform nucleus (Fig. 9-4).

The **fastigial nucleus** lies near the midline in the vermis and close to the roof of the fourth ventricle; it is larger than the globose nucleus (Fig. 9-4).

The intracerebellar nuclei are composed of large, multipolar neurons with simple branching dendrites. The axons form the cerebellar outflow in the superior and inferior cerebellar peduncles.

White Matter of the Cerebellum. The white matter is made up of three groups of fibers: (1) intrinsic, (2) afferent, and (3) efferent.

The **intrinsic fibers** do not leave the cerebellum but connect up different re-

---

Fig. 9-4   *Coronal section through the cerebellum and pons showing the intracerebellar nuclei.*

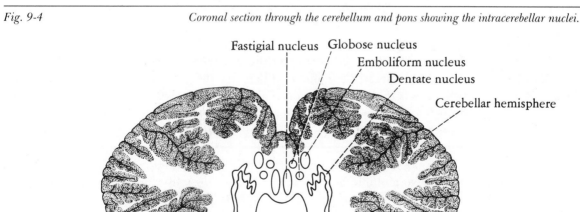

Fastigial nucleus   Globose nucleus
Emboliform nucleus
Dentate nucleus
Cerebellar hemisphere

Cavity of the fourth ventricle

Pons

gions of the organ. Some interconnect folia of the cerebellar cortex and vermis on the same side; others connect the two cerebellar hemispheres together.

The **afferent fibers** form the greater part of the white matter and proceed to the cerebellar cortex. Here, they lose their myelin sheath and end as either **climbing** or **mossy fibers** (Fig. 9-3). The afferent fibers enter the cerebellum mainly through the inferior and middle cerebellar peduncles.

The **efferent fibers** constitute the output of the cerebellum and commence as the axons of the Purkinje cells of the cerebellar cortex. The great majority of the Purkinje cell axons pass to and synapse with the neurons of the cerebellar nuclei (fastigial, globose, emboliform, and dentate). The axons of the neurons then leave the cerebellum. A few Purkinje cell axons in the flocculonodular lobe and in parts of the vermis bypass the cerebellar nuclei and leave the cerebellum without synapsing.

Fibers from the dentate, emboliform, and globose nuclei leave the cerebellum through the superior cerebellar peduncle. Fibers from the fastigial nucleus leave through the inferior cerebellar peduncle.

CEREBELLAR PEDUNCLES	The efferent and afferent fibers of the cerebellum are grouped together on each side into three large bundles, or peduncles. The superior cerebellar peduncles connect the cerebellum to the midbrain, the middle cerebellar peduncles connect the cerebellum to the pons, and the inferior cerebellar peduncles connect the cerebellum to the medulla oblongata.

The **inferior cerebellar peduncle** is formed on the posterolateral aspect of the superior half of the medulla oblongata. The two peduncles diverge as they ascend and pass into their respective cerebellar hemispheres.

The **middle cerebellar peduncle** is the largest of the three peduncles. It arises from the posterolateral region of the pons and becomes continuous with the white matter within the cerebellar hemisphere.

The **superior cerebellar peduncle** emerges from the superior part of the vallecula (anterior cerebellar notch) and runs superiorly, lateral to the upper half of the fourth ventricle, to enter the lower part of the midbrain.

INTERCONNECTIONS OF THE NEURONS OF THE CEREBELLAR CORTEX	Two types of afferent fibers enter the cerebellar cortex, the **climbing fibers** and the **mossy fibers.** The climbing fibers are the terminal fibers of the olivocerebellar tracts (Fig. 9-3). They enter the molecular layer of the cortex, where they branch and make multiple synaptic contacts with one Purkinje cell. A few side branches leave each climbing fiber and synapse with adjacent stellate and basket cells.

The mossy fibers are the terminal fibers of all other cerebellar afferent tracts. They have multiple branches, so a single mossy fiber may stimulate thousands of Purkinje cells through the granule cells (Fig. 9-3).

CEREBELLAR AFFERENT FIBERS FROM THE CEREBRAL CORTEX	The cerebral cortex sends information to the cerebellum by three pathways: (1) the corticopontocerebellar pathway, (2) the cerebro-olivocerebellar pathway, and (3) the cerebroreticulocerebellar pathway.

Corticopontocerebellar Pathway. The corticopontine fibers arise from nerve cells in the frontal, parietal, temporal, and occipital lobes of the cerebral cortex and descend through the corona radiata and internal capsule and terminate upon the pontine nuclei (Fig. 9-5). The pontine nuclei give rise to the **transverse fibers of the pons,** which cross the midline and enter the opposite cerebellar hemisphere as the middle cerebellar peduncle.

Cerebro-olivocerebellar Pathway. The cortico-olivary fibers arise from nerve cells in the frontal, parietal, temporal, and occipital lobes of the cerebral cortex and descend through the corona radiata and internal capsule to terminate bilaterally upon the inferior olivary nuclei (Fig. 9-5). The inferior olivary nuclei give rise to fibers that cross the midline and enter the opposite cerebellar hemisphere through the inferior cerebellar peduncle. These fibers terminate as the climbing fibers in the cerebellar cortex.

Cerebroreticulocerebellar Pathway. The corticoreticular fibers arise from nerve cells from many areas of the cerebral cortex, particularly the sensorimotor areas.

Fig. 9-5   *The main connections of the cerebellum; the cerebellar peduncles are shown as ovoid dashes.*

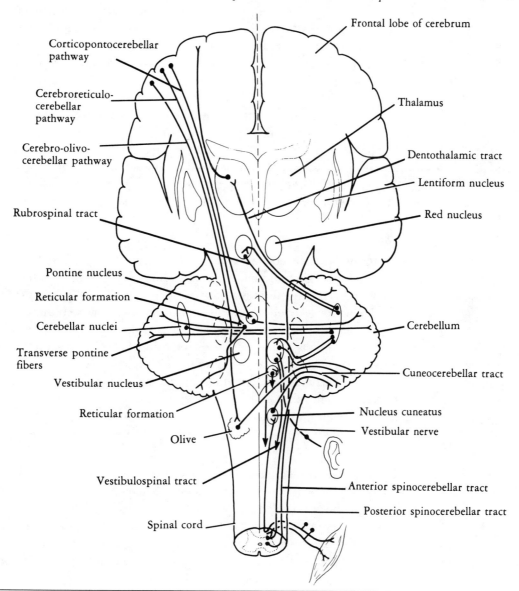

They descend to terminate in the reticular formation on the same side and on the opposite side in the pons and medulla (Fig. 9-5). The cells in the reticular formation give rise to the reticulocerebellar fibers that enter the cerebellar hemisphere on the same side through the inferior and middle cerebellar peduncles.

This connection between the cerebrum and the cerebellum is important in the control of voluntary movement. Information regarding the initiation of movement in the cerebral cortex is probably transmitted to the cerebellum so that the movement can be monitored and appropriate adjustments in the muscle activity can be made.

CEREBELLAR AFFERENT FIBERS FROM THE SPINAL CORD

The spinal cord sends information to the cerebellum by three pathways: (1) the anterior spinocerebellar tract, (2) the posterior spinocerebellar tract, and (3) the cuneocerebellar tract.

Anterior Spinocerebellar Tract. The axons entering the spinal cord from the posterior root ganglion terminate by synapsing with the neurons in the **nucleus dorsalis** (Clark's column) at the base of the posterior gray column. The majority of the axons of these neurons cross to the opposite side and ascend as the **anterior spinocerebellar tract** in the contralateral white column; the minority of the axons ascend as the anterior spinocerebellar tract in the lateral white column of the same side (Fig. 9-5). The fibers enter the cerebellum through the superior cerebellar peduncle and terminate as mossy fibers in the cerebellar cortex. Collateral branches that end in the deep cerebellar nuclei are also given off. It is believed that those fibers that crossed over to the opposite side in the spinal cord cross back within the cerebellum.

The anterior spinocerebellar tract is found at all segments of the spinal cord and its fibers convey muscle joint information from the muscle spindles, tendon organs, and joint receptors of the upper and lower limbs. It is also believed that the cerebellum receives information from the skin and superficial fascia by this tract.

Posterior Spinocerebellar Tract. The axons entering the spinal cord from the posterior root ganglion enter the posterior gray column and terminate by synapsing on the neurons at the base of the posterior gray column. These neurons are known collectively as the nucleus dorsalis (Clark's column). The axons of these neurons enter the posterolateral part of the lateral white column on the same side and ascend as the **posterior spinocerebellar tract** to the medulla oblongata (Fig. 9-5). Here the tract enters the cerebellum through the inferior cerebellar peduncle and terminates as mossy fibers in the cerebellar cortex. Collateral branches that end in the deep cerebellar nuclei are also given off. The posterior spinocerebellar tract receives muscle joint information from the muscle spindles, tendon organs, and joint receptors of the trunk and lower limbs.

Cuneocerebellar Tract. These fibers originate in the nucleus cuneatus of the medulla oblongata and enter the cerebellar hemisphere on the same side through the inferior cerebellar peduncle (Fig. 9-5). The fibers terminate as mossy fibers in the cerebellar cortex. Collateral branches that end in the deep cerebellar nuclei are also given off. The cuneocerebellar tract receives muscle joint information from the muscle spindles, tendon organs, and joint receptors of the upper limb and upper part of the thorax.

CEREBELLAR AFFERENT FIBERS FROM THE VESTIBULAR NERVE	The vestibular nerve sends many afferent fibers directly to the cerebellum through the inferior cerebellar peduncle on the same side. Other vestibular afferent fibers pass first to the vestibular nuclei in the brainstem, where they synapse and are relayed to the cerebellum (Fig. 9-5). They enter the cerebellum through the inferior cerebellar peduncle on the same side. All the afferent fibers from the inner ear terminate as mossy fibers in the flocculonodular lobe of the cerebellum.
OTHER AFFERENT FIBERS	In addition, the cerebellum receives small bundles of afferent fibers from the red nucleus and the tectum.
CEREBELLAR EFFERENT FIBERS	The entire output of the cerebellar cortex is through the axons of the Purkinje cells. The majority of the axons of the Purkinje cells end by synapsing on the neurons of the deep cerebellar nuclei (Fig. 9-3). The axons of the neurons that form the cerebellar nuclei constitute the efferent outflow from the cerebellum. A few Purkinje cell axons pass directly out of the cerebellum to the lateral vestibular nucleus. The efferent fibers from the cerebellum connect with the red nucleus, thalamus, vestibular complex, and reticular formation.

Globose-Emboliform-Rubral Pathway. Axons of neurons in the globose and emboliform nuclei travel through the superior cerebellar peduncle and cross the midline to the opposite side in the **decussation of the superior cerebellar peduncles** (Fig. 9-5). The fibers end by synapsing with cells of the contralateral red nucleus, which give rise to axons of the **rubrospinal tract** (Fig. 9-5). Thus it is seen that this pathway crosses twice, once in the decussation of the superior cerebellar peduncle, and again in the rubrospinal tract close to its origin. By this means, the globose and emboliform nuclei influence motor activity on the same side of the body.

Dentothalamic Pathway. Axons of neurons in the dentate nucleus travel through the superior cerebellar peduncle and cross the midline to the opposite side in the **decussation of the superior cerebellar peduncle** (Fig. 9-5). The fibers end by synapsing with cells in the contralateral **ventrolateral nucleus of the thalamus.** The axons of the thalamic neurons ascend through the internal capsule and corona radiata and terminate in the primary motor area of the cerebral cortex. By this pathway, the dentate nucleus can influence motor activity by acting upon the motor neurons of the opposite cerebral cortex; impulses from the motor cortex are transmitted to spinal segmental levels through the corticospinal tract. The majority of the fibers of the corticospinal tract cross to the opposite side in the decussation of the pyramids or later at the spinal segmental levels. The dentate nucleus thus is able to coordinate muscle activity on the same side of the body.

Fastigial Vestibular Pathway. The axons of neurons in the fastigial nucleus travel through the inferior cerebellar peduncle and end by projecting on the neurons of the **lateral vestibular nucleus** on both sides (Fig. 9-5). It will be remembered that some Purkinje cell axons project directly to the lateral vestibular nucleus. The neurons of the lateral vestibular nucleus form the **vestibulospinal**

tract. The fastigial nucleus exerts a facilitory influence mainly on the ipsilateral extensor muscle tone.

Fastigial Reticular Pathway. The axons of neurons in the fastigial nucleus travel through the inferior cerebellar peduncle and end by synapsing with neurons of the reticular formation (Fig. 9-5). Axons of these neurons influence spinal segmental motor activity through the reticulospinal tract.

CEREBELLAR CORTICAL MECHANISMS	Certain basic mechanisms have been attributed to the cerebellar cortex. The climbing and the mossy fibers constitute the two main lines of input to the cortex and are excitatory to the Purkinje cells. The climbing fibers pass through the granular layer of the cortex and terminate by dividing repeatedly. Each climbing fiber makes a large number of synaptic contacts with the dendrites of a single Purkinje cell. A few side branches leave each climbing fiber and synapse with the stellate cells and basket cells. The mossy fibers, on the other hand, exert a much more diffuse excitatory effect, so that a single mossy fiber may stimulate thousands of Purkinje cells through the granule cells. The Purkinje cells, by means of their axons, exert an inhibitory effect upon the intracerebellar and vestibular nuclei. The remaining cells of the cerebellar cortex, namely, the stellate, basket, and Golgi cells serve as inhibitory interneurons. It is believed that they not only limit the area of cortex excited but influence the degree of Purkinje cell excitation produced by the climbing and mossy fiber input. By this means, fluctuating inhibitory impulses are transmitted by the Purkinje cells to the intracerebellar nuclei, which in turn modify muscular activity through the motor control areas of the brainstem and cerebral cortex.
FUNCTIONS OF THE CEREBELLUM	The cerebellum receives afferent information concerning voluntary movement from the cerebral cortex and from the muscles, tendons, and joints. It also receives information concerning balance from the vestibular nerve and possibly concerning sight through the tectocerebellar tract. All this information is fed into the cerebellar cortical circuitry by the mossy fibers and the climbing fibers (Fig. 9-3). After several synaptic relays in the cerebellar cortex, the afferent impulses converge on the Purkinje cells. The axons of the Purkinje cells project with few exceptions on the deep cerebellar nuclei. The output of the lateral cerebellar hemisphere projects to the dentate nucleus, the vermis projects to the fastigial nucleus, and the intermediate regions of the cortex project to the globose and emboliform nuclei. A few Purkinje cell axons pass directly out of the cerebellum and end on the lateral vestibular nucleus in the brainstem. Now it is generally believed that the Purkinje axons exert an inhibitory influence on the neurons of the cerebellar nuclei and the lateral vestibular nuclei.

The cerebellar output is conducted to the sites of origin of the descending pathways that influence motor activity at the segmental spinal level. In this respect, it is interesting to note that the cerebellum has no direct neuronal connections with the lower motor neurons but exerts its influence indirectly through the cerebral cortex and brainstem.

The cerebellum functions unconsciously as a coordinator of precise movements by continually comparing the output of the motor area of the cerebral cortex with the proprioceptive information received from the site of muscle action; it is then able to bring about the necessary adjustments by influencing the activity of the lower motor neurons. This is accomplished by controlling the sequence of firing of the alpha and gamma motor neurons. It is also believed that the cerebellum can send back information to the motor cerebral cortex, to inhibit the agonist muscles and stimulate the antagonist muscles, thus limiting the extent of voluntary movement.

FUNCTIONS OF THE CEREBELLUM IN RELATION TO ITS PHYLOGENETIC DEVELOPMENT

The **archicerebellum,** formed by the flocculonodular lobe, is phylogenetically the oldest part of the cerebellum and receives input from the vestibular nerve and the vestibular nuclei. The output to the lower motor neurons is transmitted through the vestibulospinal tract, the medial longitudinal fasciculus, and the reticulospinal fibers. This part of the cerebellum responds to vestibular stimuli from the inner ear and assists in maintaining equilibrium by bringing about modification in muscle tone.

The **paleocerebellum** is formed by the anterior lobe, uvula, and pyramid of the vermis. It receives input from the proprioceptive endings in muscles and tendons, and from touch and pressure receptors (spinocerebellar tracts, cuneocerebellar fibers, and spinoreticular and reticulocerebellar tracts). The output to the lower motor neurons, especially the gamma efferents, is transmitted through vestibulospinal, rubrospinal, and reticulospinal tracts. This part of the cerebellum is sensitive to changes in muscle and tendon tension and information on touch and deep pressure and responds by modifying muscle tone and aiding the synergistic action of groups of muscles. It thus plays an active role in the maintenance of posture and the performance of voluntary movements.

The **neocerebellum** is formed by the middle lobe (except for the uvula and pyramid). It receives a very large input through the corticopontocerebellar tracts from the cerebral cortex of the opposite side; it also receives information through the olivocerebellar fibers. The output to the lower motor neurons travels through the thalamus to the motor area of the cerebral cortex, then through the corticospinal and corticonuclear fibers to the lower motor neurons. The neocerebellum thus facilitates a smooth, coordinated voluntary movement and ensures that the force, direction, and extent of the movement are accurate.

CEREBELLAR DYSFUNCTION

There are two neuroanatomical features concerning the cerebellum that are of great clinical significance. First, the cortex of the cerebellum, unlike that of the cerebrum, has a uniform microscopic structure and physiological investigations show that the activities occurring are identical in all regions; functional localization, therefore, does not exist in the cerebellar cortex. Second, each cerebellar hemisphere is connected by nervous pathways principally with the same side of the body, so that a lesion in one cerebellar hemisphere gives rise to signs and symptoms that are limited to the same side of the body.

The classical signs and symptoms of cerebellar disease include **hypotonia, alteration of gait** with tendency to stagger toward the affected side, **intention tremor, decomposition of movement, pendular knee jerk, nystagmus,** and **dysarthria.**

NATIONAL BOARD TYPE QUESTIONS

In each of the following questions, answer:
A. If only (1) is correct
B. If only (2) is correct

C. If both (1) and (2) are correct
D. If neither (1) nor (2) is correct

1. Which of the following statements is (are) correct concerning the cerebellum?
   (1) The cerebellum lies in the posterior cranial fossa.
   (2) The cerebellum lies posterior to the fourth ventricle.
2. Which of the following statements is (are) correct concerning the fissures of the cerebellum?
   (1) The horizontal fissure separates the anterior lobe from the middle lobe.
   (2) The uvulonodular fissure separates the flocculonodular lobe from the middle lobe.
3. Which of the following general statements concerning the cerebellum is (are) correct?
   (1) The cortex of different parts of the cerebellum has a different microscopic structure.
   (2) The part of the cerebellum that lies in the midline is called the vermis.
4. Which of the following statements concerning the cerebellar peduncles is (are) correct?
   (1) The middle cerebellar peduncle contains the cuneocerebellar tract.
   (2) The superior cerebellar peduncle contains the posterior spinocerebellar tract.

Select the **best** response:

5. The following statements concerning the cerebellum are correct **except:**
   A. Each cerebellar hemisphere principally influences movement on the same side of the body.
   B. The middle cerebellar peduncle contains axons that arise from the pontine nuclei.
   C. The Purkinje cells are found in the most superficial layer of the cortex.
   D. The inferior cerebellar peduncles join the cerebellum to the medulla oblongata.
   E. The Golgi cells are found in the deepest layer of the cerebellar cortex.
6. The following statements concerning the intracerebellar nuclei are correct **except:**
   A. The nuclei are named from lateral to medial, fastigial, globose, emboliform, and dentate.
   B. Their axons form the main efferent outflow of the cerebellum.
   C. They are embedded in the white matter.
   D. They are located above the cavity of the fourth ventricle.
   E. The nuclei are made up of nerve cells supported by neuroglia.

In each of the following questions, answer:
A. If only (1), (2) and (3) are correct
B. If only (1) and (3) are correct
C. If only (2) and (4) are correct
D. If only (4) is correct
E. If all are correct

7. Which of the following statements concerning the functions of the cerebellum is (are) correct?
   (1) It influences the tone of smooth muscle.
   (2) It influences the tone of skeletal muscle.

(3) It influences the tone of cardiac muscle.

(4) It coordinates the force and extent of contraction of voluntary movements.

8. Which of the following signs or symptoms are indicative of a cerebellar lesion?

(1) Dysdiadochokinesis.

(2) Intention tremor.

(3) Ataxia.

(4) Resting tremor.

9. Efferent fibers leaving the deep cerebellar nuclei may synapse with the following:

(1) Cells of the red nucleus.

(2) Cells of the ventral lateral nucleus of the thalamus.

(3) Vestibular nucleus.

(4) Anterior gray column cells in the spinal cord.

10. Direct input to the cerebellar nuclei occurs from the following:

(1) Granule cells.

(2) Golgi cells.

(3) Vestibular nuclei.

(4) Purkinje cells.

11. Which of the following statements concerning the superior cerebellar peduncle is (are) correct?

(1) Contains fibers that synapse in the ventral lateral nucleus of the thalamus.

(2) Contains fibers that originate in the dentate nucleus.

(3) Conveys nervous impulses regulating skilled motor movements.

(4) Contributes fibers to the medial longitudinal fasciculus.

12. Which of the following statements concerning the structure and function of the cerebellum is (are) correct?

(1) The mossy fibers end by synapsing mainly with the stellate cells in the molecular layer of the cortex.

(2) The structure of the cortex of the anterior lobe of the cerebellum differs from that of the posterior lobe.

(3) Stimulation of the cerebellar cortex produces a sensory response.

(4) A tumor of the right cerebellar hemisphere causes the patient to lurch to the right on walking.

13. Which of the following statements concerning the structure and function of the cerebellum is (are) correct?

(1) The axons of the granular cells bifurcate at a T junction in the molecular layer of the cortex and run parallel to the long axis of the cerebellar folium.

(2) A lesion of the cerebellum causes muscular paralysis.

(3) Afferent fibers from muscles originate in the muscle spindles.

(4) The tendon spindles play no part in providing the cerebellum with information.

14. Inhibitory effects are produced in the cerebellum by

(1) Climbing fibers.

(2) Mossy fibers.

(3) Granule cell efferent fibers.

(4) Purkinje cell axons.

Match the pathways listed below on the left with the appropriate cerebellar peduncle through which they enter or leave the cerebellum listed below on the right.

15. Posterior spinocerebellar.   A. Superior cerebellar peduncle.
16. Pontocerebellar.   B. Middle cerebellar peduncle.
17. Dentorubral.   C. Inferior cerebellar peduncle.
18. Dentothalamic.
19. Anterior spinocerebellar.
20. Vestibulocerebellar.

ANSWERS AND EXPLANATIONS

1. C
2. B: (1) The horizontal fissure separates the superior surface from the inferior surface of the cerebellar hemisphere.
3. B: (1) The cortex of different parts of the cerebellum has an identical microscopic structure.
4. D: (1) The cuneocerebellar tract is situated in the inferior cerebellar peduncle. (2) The posterior spinocerebellar tract is situated in the inferior cerebellar peduncle.
5. C: The Purkinje cells lie in the middle layer of the cerebellar cortex.
6. A: The intracerebellar nuclei are named from medial to lateral, fastigial, globose, emboliform, and dentate.
7. C
8. A: (4) Resting tremor does not occur with cerebellar disease; it is characteristic of Parkinson's disease.
9. A: (4) The cerebellum, unlike the cerebrum, has no direct pathway to the lower motor neurons in the spinal cord.
10. D
11. A
12. D: (1) The mossy fibers end in the granular layer of the cerebellar cortex by synapsing with the granular cells. (2) All parts of the cerebellar cortex have the same microscopic structure. (3) The function of the cerebellum is to control motor, not sensory, activities.
13. B: (2) Although the cerebellum plays a very important role in muscle activity, it does not directly innervate a muscle. (4) The cerebellum receives afferent information from muscles that originates in both the muscle spindles and neurotendinous spindles.
14. D
15. C
16. B
17. A
18. A
19. A
20. C

10 Reticular Formation

SUGGESTED PLAN FOR REVIEW OF CHAPTER 10

1. Understand that the reticular formation consists of a network of nerve cells and fibers that extend from the spinal cord up through the brain to the cerebrum.
2. Appreciate that throughout its length the reticular formation has connections to all parts of the central nervous system including the cerebral cortex and the cerebellum.
3. Learn the main afferent and efferent connections.
4. Learn the six main functions of the reticular formation outlined in this chapter.

INTRODUCTION

The reticular formation, as its name would suggest, resembles a net (reticular) that is made up of nerve cells and nerve fibers. The net extends up through the axis of the central nervous system from the spinal cord to the cerebrum. It receives input from most of the sensory systems and has efferent fibers that descend and influence nerve cells at all levels of the central nervous system. The exceptionally long dendrites of the neurons of the reticular formation permit input from widely placed ascending and descending pathways. Through its many connections it can influence skeletal muscle activity, somatic and visceral sensations, the autonomic and endocrine systems, and even the level of consciousness.

The purpose of this chapter is to provide a brief overview of the structure and function of the reticular formation.

GENERAL ARRANGEMENT

The reticular formation consists of a deeply placed continuous network of nerve cells and fibers that extend from the spinal cord, through the medulla, the pons, the midbrain, the subthalamus, the hypothalamus, and the thalamus. The diffuse network may be divided into three longitudinal columns, the first occupying the median plane, called the **median column,** and consisting of intermediate-sized neurons, the second called the **medial column** containing large neurons, and the third or **lateral column** containing mainly small neurons (Fig. 10-1).

The groups of neurons are poorly defined and it is difficult to trace an anatomical pathway through the network. Nevertheless, experiments have shown that polysynaptic pathways exist and that both crossed and uncrossed ascending and descending pathways are present, involving many neurons that serve both somatic and visceral functions.

Fig. 10-1

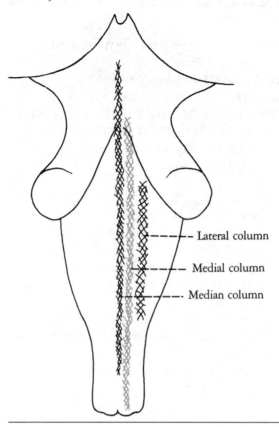

Lateral column

Medial column

Median column

Inferiorly, the reticular formation is continuous with the interneurons of the gray matter of the spinal cord, while superiorly impulses are relayed to the whole cerebral cortex; a substantial projection of fibers also leaves the reticular formation to enter the cerebellum.

AFFERENT PROJECTIONS

Many different afferent pathways project onto the reticular formation from most parts of the central nervous system. From the spinal cord there are the spinoreticular tracts, the spinothalamic tracts, and the medial lemniscus. From the cranial nerve nuclei there are ascending afferent tracts that will include the vestibular, acoustic, and visual pathways. From the cerebellum, there is the cerebelloreticular pathway. From the subthalamic, hypothalamic, and thalamic nuclei, and from the corpus striatum and the limbic system, there are further afferent tracts. Other important afferent fibers arise in the primary motor cortex of the frontal lobe and from the somesthetic cortex of the parietal lobe.

EFFERENT PROJECTIONS

Multiple efferent pathways extend down to the brainstem and spinal cord through the reticulobulbar and reticulospinal tracts to neurons in the motor nuclei of the cranial nerves and the anterior horn cells of the spinal cord. Other descending pathways extend to the sympathetic outflow and the craniosacral parasympathetic outflow of the autonomic nervous system. Additional pathways extend to the corpus striatum, the cerebellum, the red nucleus, the substantia nigra, the tectum, and the nuclei of the thalamus, subthalamus and hypothalamus. Most regions of the cerebral cortex also receive efferent fibers.

FUNCTIONS OF THE RETICULAR FORMATION

From the previous description of the vast number of connections of the reticular formation to all parts of the nervous system, it is not surprising to find that the functions are many. A few of the more important functions will be considered here.

1. **Control of skeletal muscle.** Through the reticulospinal and reticulobulbar tracts, the reticular formation can influence the activity of the alpha and gamma motor neurons. Thus the reticular formation can modulate muscle tone and reflex activity. It can also bring about reciprocal inhibition, so that, for example, when the flexor muscles contract the antagonistic extensors relax. The reticular formation, assisted by the vestibular apparatus of the inner ear and the vestibular spinal tract, plays an important role in maintaining the tone of the antigravity muscles when standing. The so-called respiratory centers of the brainstem, described by neurophysiologists in the control of the respiratory muscles, are now considered to be part of the reticular formation.
2. **Control of somatic and visceral sensations.** The reticular formation by virtue of its central location in the cerebrospinal axis can influence all ascending pathways passing to supraspinal levels. The influence may be facilitory or inhibitory. In particular, the reticular formation may play a leading role in the "gating mechanism" for the control of the perception of pain (see p. 71).
3. **Control of the autonomic nervous system.** Higher control of the autonomic nervous system, from the cerebral cortex, hypothalamus, and other subcortical nuclei, can be exerted by the reticulobulbar and reticulospinal tracts, which descend to the sympathetic outflow and the parasympathetic craniosacral outflow.
4. **Control of the endocrine nervous system.** The reticular formation either directly or indirectly through the hypothalamic nuclei can influence the synthesis or release of releasing or release-inhibiting factors and thus control the activity of the hypophysis cerebri.
5. **Influence on the biological clocks.** The reticular formation by means of its multiple afferent and efferent pathways to the hypothalamus probably influences the biological rhythms.
6. **The reticular activating system.** Multiple ascending pathways carrying sensory information to higher centers are channeled through the reticular formation, which in turn projects the information to different parts of the cerebral cortex, causing a sleeping person to awaken. In fact it has been suggested that the state of consciousness is dependent on the continuous projection to the cortex of sensory information. Different degrees of wakefulness seem to depend on the degree of activity of the reticular formation.

From the above description it must be apparent that the network of neurons in the cerebrospinal axis, almost totally ignored in the past, is now being shown to influence practically all activities of the body. Pathological lesions of the reticular formation may cause loss of consciousness and even coma. It has been suggested that loss of consciousness that occurs in epilepsy may be due to inhibition of the activity of the reticular formation in the upper part of the diencephalon.

In each of the following questions, answer:

A. If only (1) is correct
B. If only (2) is correct
C. If both (1) and (2) are correct
D. If neither (1) nor (2) is correct

1. Which of the following statements concerning the reticular formation is (are) correct?
   (1) It can influence the alpha motor neurons in the spinal cord.
   (2) It is an interrupted network that extends from the midbrain down to the spinal cord.

2. Which of the following statements concerning the structure of the reticular formation is (are) correct?
   (1) It consists of neurons with short dendritic processes.
   (2) It receives afferent fibers from most sensory pathways entering the central nervous system.

3. Which of the following statements concerning the function of the reticular formation is (are) correct?
   (1) It may influence the reception of pain.
   (2) It can affect the level of consciousness.

4. Which of the following statements concerning the arrangement of the reticular formation is (are) correct?
   (1) Its descending fibers extend into the peripheral spinal nerves.
   (2) The network can be divided into three longitudinal columns.

5. Which of the following statements concerning the function of the reticular formation is (are) correct?
   (1) It can influence the hypothalamic nuclei and thus indirectly control the activity of the hypophysis cerebri.
   (2) It influences the biological clock.

6. Which of the following statements concerning the nervous connections of the reticular formation is (are) correct?
   (1) The reticulobulbar fibers are connected to the sensory nuclei of the cranial nerves.
   (2) The highest levels of the reticular formation are connected to the cerebral cortex.

**ANSWERS AND
EXPLANATIONS**

1. A: (2) The reticular formation is a continuous network that extends downward from the cerebrum to the different levels of the entire length of the spinal cord.

2. B: (1) The reticular formation consists of neurons with long dendritic processes.

3. C

4. B: (1) The descending fibers of the reticular formation synapse on neurons at lower levels of the central nervous system but do not extend out into the peripheral nervous system.

5. C

6. B: (1) The reticulobulbar fibers are connected to the motor nuclei of the cranial nerves.

11 Diencephalon: The Hypothalamus

SUGGESTED PLAN FOR REVIEW OF CHAPTER 11

1. The hypothalamus, although small in size, is a very important part of the central nervous system. It controls the autonomic nervous system and the endocrine system and thus indirectly controls body homeostasis.
2. Understand the location and precise boundaries of the hypothalamus.
3. In general terms learn the names and position of the various nuclei of the hypothalamus.
4. Have an understanding of the main afferent and efferent connections of the hypothalamus.
5. Learn in detail the hypothalamohypophyseal tract and the hypophyseal portal system. These are very important.
6. Learn the functions of the hypothalamus and be able to list some of the common clinical problems that may arise should dysfunction occur.

INTRODUCTION

The diencephalon forms the central core of the cerebrum, while the remainder of the cerebrum forms the laterally placed cerebral hemispheres. The diencephalon consists of the third ventricle and the structures that form its boundaries. It extends posteriorly to the point where the third ventricle becomes continuous with the cerebral aqueduct and anteriorly as far as the interventricular foramina (Fig. 11-1). The diencephalon may be divided up, for purposes of description, into four major parts: (1) the thalamus, (2) the subthalamus, (3) the epithalamus, and (4) the hypothalamus.

   The purpose of this chapter is to describe the hypothalamus, its connections, and its functions; the remaining parts of the diencephalon will be described elsewhere.

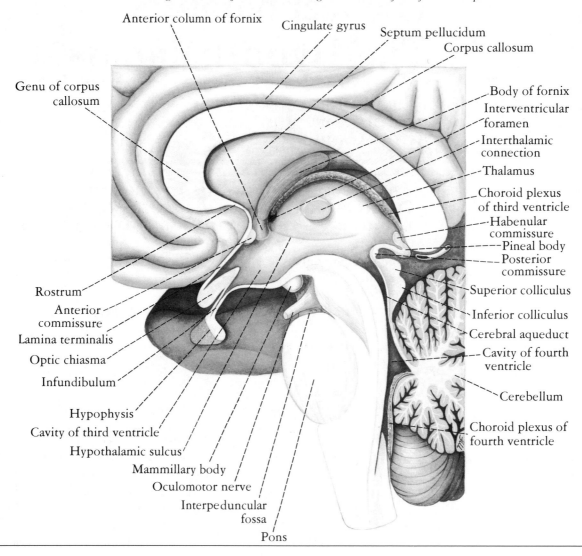

Anterior column of fornix — Cingulate gyrus — Septum pellucidum — Corpus callosum

Genu of corpus callosum — Body of fornix — Interventricular foramen — Interthalamic connection — Thalamus — Choroid plexus of third ventricle — Habenular commissure — Pineal body — Posterior commissure — Superior colliculus — Inferior colliculus — Cerebral aqueduct — Cavity of fourth ventricle — Cerebellum — Choroid plexus of fourth ventricle

Rostrum — Anterior commissure — Lamina terminalis — Optic chiasma — Infundibulum — Hypophysis — Cavity of third ventricle — Hypothalamic sulcus — Mammillary body — Oculomotor nerve — Interpeduncular fossa — Pons

HYPOTHALAMUS

The hypothalamus is that part of the diencephalon that extends from the region of the optic chiasma to the caudal border of the mammillary bodies. It lies below the thalamus and forms the floor and the inferior part of the lateral walls of the third ventricle (Fig. 11-1). Anterior to the hypothalamus is an area that for functional reasons is often included in the hypothalamus. Because it extends forward from the optic chiasma to the lamina terminalis and the anterior commissure, it is referred to as the **preoptic area.** Caudally, the hypothalamus merges into the tegmentum of the midbrain. The lateral boundary of the hypothalamus is formed by the internal capsule.

When observed from below, the hypothalamus is seen to be related to the following structures, from anterior to posterior: (1) the optic chiasma, (2) the tuber cinereum and the infundibulum, and (3) the mammillary bodies.

It is thus seen that anatomically the hypothalamus is a relatively small area of the brain that is strategically well placed close to the limbic system, the thalamus, the ascending and descending tracts, and the hypophysis. Physiologically there is hardly any activity in the body that is not influenced by the hypothalamus.

Microscopically, the hypothalamus is composed of small nerve cells that are arranged in groups or nuclei, many of which are not clearly segregated from one another. For purposes of description, the nuclei are divided by an imaginary parasagittal plane into medial and lateral zones. Lying within the plane are the columns of the fornix and the mammillothalamic tract, which serve as markers (Fig. 11-2).

Fig. 11-2

Sagittal section of the brain, showing the hypothalamic nuclei. (A) Medial zone nuclei lying medial to the plane of the fornix and the mammillothalamic tract. (B) Lateral zone nuclei lying lateral to the plane of the fornix and the mammillothalamic tract.

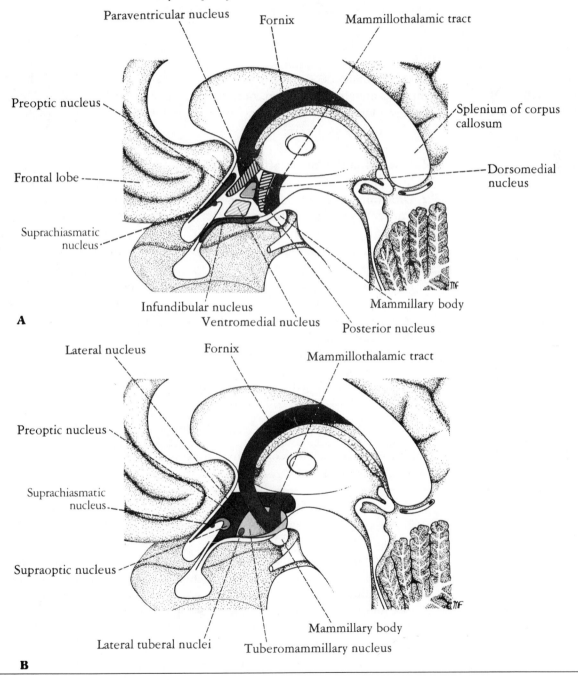

Medial Zone. In the medial zone, the following hypothalamic nuclei may be recognized, from anterior to posterior: (1) the **preoptic nucleus,** (2) the **paraventricular nucleus,** (3) the **dorsomedial nucleus,** (4) the **ventromedial nucleus,** (5) the **infundibular nucleus,** and (6) the **posterior nucleus** (Fig. 11-2).

Lateral Zone. In the lateral zone, the following hypothalamic nuclei may be recognized, from anterior to posterior: (1) the **supraoptic nucleus,** (2) the large **lateral nucleus,** (3) the **tuberomammillary nucleus,** and (4) the **lateral tuberal nuclei** (Fig. 11-2).

Some of the nuclei, for example, the preoptic nucleus, extend into both the medial and lateral zones. The mammillary body with its medial and lateral mammillary nuclei overlaps both zones. The **suprachiasmatic nucleus** also overlaps both zones and consists of a small group of neurons lying just above the optic chiasma; it receives nerve fibers from the retina.

AFFERENT CONNECTIONS OF THE HYPOTHALAMUS

The hypothalamus receives many afferent fibers from the viscera, the olfactory mucous membrane, the cerebral cortex, and the limbic system. The afferent connections are numerous and complex, and only the main pathways (Fig. 11-3) are described here:

1. **Visceral and somatic afferents** reach the hypothalamus through collateral branches of the lemniscal afferent fibers and through the reticular formation.
2. **Olfaction** travels through the medial forebrain bundle.
3. **Corticohypothalamic fibers** arise from the frontal lobe of the cerebral cortex and pass directly to the hypothalamus.
4. **Hippocampohypothalamic fibers** pass from the hippocampus through the fornix to the mammillary body. Many neurophysiologists regard the hypothalamus as the main output pathway of the limbic system.
5. **Amygdalohypothalamic fibers** pass from the amygdaloid complex to the hypothalamus through the stria terminalis and by a route that passes inferior to the lentiform nucleus.
6. **Thalamohypothalamic fibers** arise from the dorsomedial and midline thalamic nuclei.
7. **Tegmental fibers** arise from the midbrain.

EFFERENT CONNECTIONS OF THE HYPOTHALAMUS

The efferent connections of the hypothalamus are also numerous and complex, and only the main pathways (Fig. 11-3) are described here:

1. The **mammillothalamic tract** arises in the mammillary body and terminates in the anterior nucleus of the thalamus. Here the pathway is relayed to the cingulate gyrus.
2. The **mammillotegmental tract** arises from the mammillary body and terminates in the cells of the reticular formation in the tegmentum of the midbrain.
3. **Descending fibers to the brainstem and spinal cord** influence the peripheral neurons of the autonomic nervous system. Through the reticular formation, the hypothalamus is connected to the parasympathetic nuclei of the oculomotor, facial, glossopharyngeal, and vagus nerves in the brainstem. In a similar manner, the reticulospinal fibers connect the hypothalamus with sympathetic cells of origin in the lateral gray horns of the first thoracic segment to

Fig. 11-3

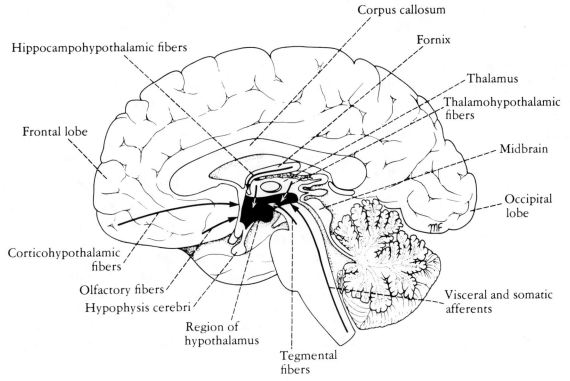

Corpus callosum

Fornix

Hippocampohypothalamic fibers

Thalamus

Thalamohypothalamic fibers

Frontal lobe

Midbrain

Occipital lobe

Corticohypothalamic fibers

Olfactory fibers

Hypophysis cerebri

Region of hypothalamus

Tegmental fibers

Visceral and somatic afferents

A

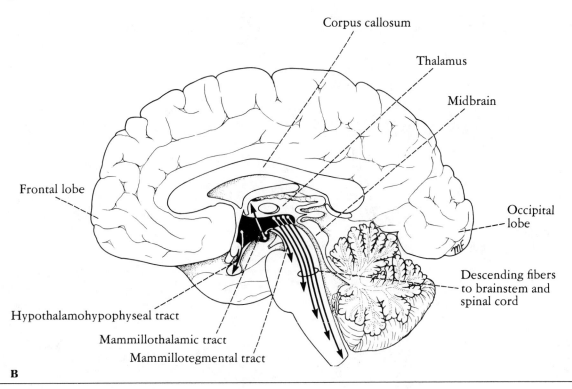

Corpus callosum

Thalamus

Midbrain

Frontal lobe

Occipital lobe

Descending fibers to brainstem and spinal cord

Hypothalamohypophyseal tract

Mammillothalamic tract

Mammillotegmental tract

B

the second lumbar segment of the spinal cord and the sacral parasympathetic outflow at the level of the second, third, and fourth sacral segments of the spinal cord.

CONNECTIONS OF THE HYPOTHALAMUS WITH THE HYPOPHYSIS CEREBRI

The hypothalamus is connected to the hypophysis cerebri (pituitary gland) by two pathways: (1) nerve fibers that travel from the supraoptic and paraventricular nuclei to the posterior lobe of the hypophysis, and (2) long and short portal blood vessels that connect sinusoids in the median eminence and infundibulum with capillary plexuses in the anterior lobe of the hypophysis (Fig. 11-4). These pathways enable the hypothalamus to influence the activities of the endocrine glands.

Hypothalamohypophyseal Tract. The hormones **vasopressin** and **oxytocin** are synthesized in the nerve cells of the supraoptic and paraventricular nuclei. The hormones are passed along the axons together with carrier proteins called **neurophysins** and released at the axon terminals (Fig. 11-4). Here the hormones are absorbed into the bloodstream in the capillaries of the posterior lobe of the hypophysis. The hormone vasopressin is produced mainly in the nerve cells of the supraoptic nucleus. Its function is to cause vasoconstriction. It also has an important antidiuretic function, causing an increased absorption of water in the distal convoluted tubules and collecting tubules of the kidney. The other hor-

Fig. 11-4   *A. Hypothalamohypophyseal tract. B. Hypophyseal portal system.*

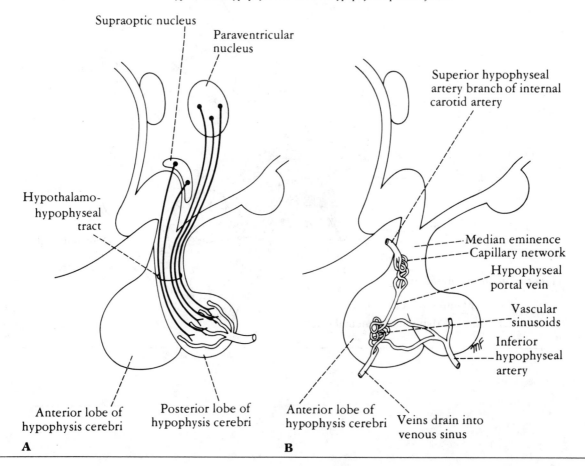

Supraoptic nucleus

Paraventricular nucleus

Superior hypophyseal artery branch of internal carotid artery

Hypothalamo-hypophyseal tract

Median eminence
Capillary network
Hypophyseal portal vein
Vascular sinusoids
Inferior hypophyseal artery

Anterior lobe of hypophysis cerebri

Posterior lobe of hypophysis cerebri

Anterior lobe of hypophysis cerebri

Veins drain into venous sinus

A   **B**

mone is oxytocin, which is mainly produced in the paraventricular nucleus. Oxytocin stimulates the contraction of the smooth muscle of the uterus and causes contraction of the myoepithelial cells that surround the alveoli of the mammary gland.

The supraoptic nucleus, which produces vasopressin, acts as an **osmoreceptor.** Should the osmotic pressure of the blood circulating through the nucleus be too high, the nerve cells increase their production of vasopressin and the antidiuretic effect of this hormone will increase the reabsorption of water from the kidney. By this means, the osmotic pressure of the blood will return to normal limits.

Hypophyseal Portal System. The hypophyseal portal system is formed on each side from the superior hypophyseal artery, which is a branch of the internal carotid artery (Fig. 11–4). The artery enters the median eminence and divides into tufts of capillaries. These capillaries drain into long and short descending vessels that end in the anterior lobe of the hypophysis by dividing into vascular sinusoids that pass between the secretory cells of the anterior lobe.

The portal system carries **releasing hormones** and **release-inhibiting hormones,** which are produced in the neurons of the hypothalamus, to the secretory cells of the anterior lobe of the hypophysis. The releasing hormones stimulate the production and release of **adrenocorticotropic hormone** (ACTH), **follicle-stimulating hormone** (FSH), **luteinizing hormone** (LH), **thyrotropic hormone** or **thyroid-stimulating hormone** (TSH), and **growth hormone** (GH). The release of inhibiting hormones inhibits the release of the **melanocyte-stimulating hormone** (MSH) and **luteotropic hormone** (LTH). LTH (also known as the **lactogenic hormone** or **prolactin**) stimulates the corpus luteum to secrete progesterone and the mammary gland to produce milk. The growth hormone inhibitory hormone (somatostatin) inhibits the release of growth hormone (GH).

The neurons of the hypothalamus that are responsible for the production of the releasing hormones and the release-inhibiting hormones are influenced by the afferent fibers passing to the hypothalamus. They also are influenced by the level of the hormone produced by the target organ controlled by the hypophysis. Should the level of thyroxin in the blood, for example, fall, then the releasing factor for the thyrotropic hormone would be produced in increased quantities.

FUNCTIONS OF THE HYPOTHALAMUS	**Autonomic Control.** The hypothalamus has a controlling influence on the autonomic nervous system and integrates the autonomic and neuroendocrine systems, thus preserving body homeostasis. The hypothalamus should be regarded as a higher nervous center for the control of lower autonomic centers in the brainstem and spinal cord.

Electrical stimulation of the hypothalamus in animal experiments shows that the anterior hypothalamic area and the preoptic area influence parasympathetic responses; these include lowering of the blood pressure, slowing of the heart rate, contraction of the bladder, increased motility of the gastrointestinal tract, increased acidity of the gastric juice, salivation, and pupillary constriction.

Stimulation of the posterior and lateral nuclei causes sympathetic responses, which include elevation of blood pressure, acceleration of the heart rate, cessation of peristalsis in the gastrointestinal tract, pupillary dilation, and hyperglycemia.

Endocrine Control. The nerve cells of the hypothalamus, by producing the **releasing factors** or **release-inhibiting factors,** control the production of ACTH, FSH, LH, TSH, GH, MSH, and LTH. Some of these hormones act directly on body tissues, while others, such as ACTH, act through an endocrine organ, which in turn produces further hormones that influence the activities of general body tissues. It should be pointed out that each stage is controlled by negative or positive feedback mechanisms.

Temperature Regulation. The anterior portion of the hypothalamus controls those mechanisms that dissipate heat loss. Experimental stimulation of this area causes dilation of skin blood vessels and sweating, which lower the body temperature. Stimulation of the posterior portion of the hypothalamus results in vasoconstriction of the skin blood vessels and inhibition of sweating; there also may be shivering, in which the skeletal muscles produce heat.

Regulation of Food and Water Intake. Stimulation of the lateral region of the hypothalamus initiates eating and increases food intake. This lateral region sometimes is referred to as the **hunger center.** Stimulation of the medial region of the hypothalamus inhibits eating and reduces food intake. This area is referred to as the **satiety center.**

Experimental stimulation of other areas in the lateral region of the hypothalamus causes an immediate increase in water intake; this area is referred to as the **thirst center.** The hypothalamus also exerts control on the osmolarity of the blood through the secretion of vasopressin by the posterior lobe of the hypophysis and its influence on the distal convoluted tubules and collecting tubules of the kidneys.

Emotion and Behavior. Emotion and behavior are a function of the hypothalamus, the limbic system, and the prefrontal cortex. The hypothalamus is the integrator of afferent information received from the other areas of the nervous system and brings about the physical expression of emotion; it can produce an increase in the heart rate, elevate the blood pressure, cause dryness of the mouth, flushing or pallor of the skin, and sweating, and can often produce a massive peristaltic activity of the gastrointestinal tract.

Control of Circadian Rhythms. The hypothalamus controls many circadian rhythms, including body temperature, adrenocortical activity, eosinophil count, and renal secretion. Sleeping and wakefulness, although dependent on the activities of the thalamus, the limbic system, and the reticular activating system, are also controlled by the hypothalamus. Lesions of the anterior part of the hypothalamus seriously interfere with the rhythm of sleeping and waking. The suprachiasmatic nucleus, which receives afferent fibers from the retina, appears to play an important role in controlling the biological rhythms. Nerve impulses generated in response to variations in the intensity of light are transmitted via this nucleus to influence the activities of many of the hypothalamic nuclei.

CLINICAL DISORDERS ASSOCIATED WITH HYPOTHALAMIC LESIONS	The most common abnormalities include severe obesity and wasting, genital hypoplasia, hyperthermia and hypothermia, diabetes insipidus, disturbances of sleep, and emotional disorders.
NATIONAL BOARD TYPE QUESTIONS	In each of the following questions, answer: A. If only (1), (2), and (3) are correct B. If only (1) and (3) are correct

C. If only (2) and (4) are correct
D. If only (4) is correct
E. If all are correct

1. Which of the following statements concerning the position of the hypothalamus is (are) correct?
   (1) The hypothalamus lies below the thalamus in the tectum of the midbrain.
   (2) The hypothalamus lies in the center of the limbic system.
   (3) The lateral boundary of the hypothalamus is formed by the external capsule.
   (4) The hypothalamus extends forward as far as the optic chiasma.

2. Which of the following statements concerning the nuclei of the hypothalamus is (are) correct?
   (1) The margins of the different nuclei cannot be seen with the naked eye.
   (2) The suprachiasmatic nucleus overlaps both the medial and lateral groups of nuclei.
   (3) The columns of the fornix and the mammillothalamic tract divide the nuclei of the hypothalamus into medial and lateral groups.
   (4) The medial nuclei of the hypothalamus are related medially to the cavity of the fourth ventricle.

3. Which of the following statements concerning the afferent fibers of the hypothalamus is (are) correct?
   (1) The limbic system sends fibers to the hypothalamus.
   (2) The pineal gland sends afferent fibers to the hypothalamus.
   (3) The olfactory mucous membrane sends fibers to the hypothalamus.
   (4) The majority of the afferent fibers reach the hypothalamus via the habenular commissure.

4. Which of the following statements concerning the functions of the hypothalamus is (are) correct?
   (1) The anterior hypothalamic area and the preoptic area can influence the parasympathetic part of the autonomic system.
   (2) The posterior and lateral nuclei of the hypothalamus can influence the activity of the sympathetic part of the autonomic system.
   (3) Stimulation of the anterior nuclei of the hypothalamus can lower the body temperature.
   (4) The medial nuclei of the hypothalamus can influence the intake of food.

5. Which of the following statements concerning the hypothalamus is (are) correct?
   (1) The hypothalamus integrates the functions of the autonomic and endocrine systems.
   (2) The visceral afferents to the hypothalamus reach their destination via the medial longitudinal fasciculus.
   (3) The nerve cells of the hypothalamus produce releasing factors that control the production of various pituitary hormones.
   (4) The mammillary bodies lie anterior to the tuber cinereum on the inferior aspect of the hypothalamus.

6. Which of the following statements concerning the hypophyseal portal system is (are) correct?
   (1) The portal system carries releasing hormones and release-inhibiting hormones to the secretory cells of the anterior lobe of the pituitary gland.
   (2) The blood vessels begin superiorly in the median eminence and end below in the posterior lobe of the hypophysis.
   (3) The afferent nerve fibers entering the hypothalamus can influence the production of releasing hormones by the nerve cells.

(4) The portal system is fed by arteries that are branches of the ophthalmic artery.

7. Which of the following statements concerning the hypothalamohypophyseal tract is (are) correct?
   (1) Vasopressin stimulates the distal convoluted tubules and collecting tubules of the kidney, causing a decreased absorption of water from the urine.
   (2) The hormones travel in the axoplasm of the neurons in the tract with neurophysins.
   (3) The nerve cells of the lateral hypothalamic nuclei produce the hormone vasopressin.
   (4) Oxytocin stimulates the contraction of the smooth muscle of the uterus.

8. Which of the following efferent connections of the hypothalamus is (are) correct?
   (1) The mammillotegmental tract connects the mammillary body to the reticular formation in the midbrain.
   (2) The parasympathetic nucleus of the oculomotor nerve receives descending fibers from the hypothalamus.
   (3) The anterior nucleus of the thalamus receives fibers from the mammillary body.
   (4) The supraoptic nucleus sends fibers to the cerebellar cortex.

9. The following nuclei of the hypothalamus lie only in the lateral zone:
   (1) The preoptic nucleus.
   (2) The infundibular nucleus.
   (3) The posterior nucleus.
   (4) The tuberomammillary nucleus.

10. Which of the following statements concerning the hypothalamus is (are) correct?
   (1) The portal system carries releasing hormones that stimulate the production and release of ACTH and FSH.
   (2) The portal system carries inhibiting hormones that inhibit the release of MSH.
   (3) The growth inhibitory hormone inhibits the release of growth hormone.
   (4) The neurons of the hypothalamus are sensitive to the blood level of the hormone produced by the target endocrine organ controlled by the hypophysis.

ANSWERS AND EXPLANATIONS

1. C: (1) The hypothalamus is situated in the diencephalon and does not lie in the midbrain. (3) The lateral boundary of the hypothalamus is the internal capsule.
2. A: (4) The medial nuclei of the hypothalamus are related medially to the lower part of the lateral wall of the third ventricle.
3. B: (2) The pineal gland sends no afferent fibers to the hypothalamus. (4) The habenular commissure does not serve as the main pathway for afferent fibers to the hypothalamus.
4. A: (4) Stimulation of the lateral nuclei of the hypothalamus can initiate eating and increase food intake.
5. B: (2) The visceral afferents to the hypothalamus reach their destination through collateral branches of the lemnisci and through the reticular formation. (4) The mammillary bodies lie posterior to the tuber cinereum on the inferior surface of the hypothalamus.

6. B: (2) The blood vessels begin above in the median eminence and end below in the anterior lobe of the hypophysis. (4) The portal system is fed by the superior hypophyseal artery, a branch of the internal carotid artery.

7. C: (1) Vasopressin stimulates the distal convoluted tubules and collecting tubules of the kidney, causing an increased absorption of water from the urine. (3) The hormone vasopressin is produced by the nerve cells of the supraoptic and paraventricular nuclei of the hypothalamus.

8. A: (4) The supraoptic nucleus does not send fibers to the cerebellar cortex.

9. D: (1) The preoptic nucleus lies in the medial zone. (2) The infundibular nucleus lies in the medial zone. (3) The posterior nucleus lies in the medial zone.

10. E

12 Diencephalon: The Thalamus

SUGGESTED PLAN FOR REVIEW OF CHAPTER 12

1. Realize that the thalamus is a very important relay station for the ascending sensory pathways to the cerebral cortex.
2. Using sagittal, coronal, and horizontal diagrams of the brain, accurately localize the thalamus. If possible, look at specimens of the brain in the laboratory.
3. Understand the subdivisions of the thalamus and the different nuclei.
4. Recognize the position of the ventral posterolateral nucleus of the thalamus and realize that it is the relay station for the important ascending sensory tracts.
5. Note the positions of the medial and lateral geniculate bodies and learn their functions.
6. Review the main connections of the thalamic nuclei. Note that, in contrast to all other sensory pathways, the olfactory afferent pathway reaches the cerebral cortex without synapsing in one of the thalamic nuclei.
7. Learn the functions of the thalamus.

INTRODUCTION

The thalamus is a large, ovoid mass of gray matter that forms the major part of the diencephalon. It is situated on each side of the third ventricle (Fig. 12-1). The anterior end of the thalamus is narrow and rounded and forms the posterior boundary of the interventricular foramen. The posterior end is expanded to form the **pulvinar.** The inferior surface is continuous with the tegmentum of the midbrain. The medial surface of the thalamus forms part of the lateral wall of the third ventricle and is usually connected to the opposite thalamus by a band of gray matter (Fig. 12-1), the **interthalamic connection** (interthalamic adhesion).

The purpose of this chapter is to describe briefly the structure of the thalamus, its connections, and its function.

SUBDIVISIONS OF THE THALAMUS

The thalamus is covered on its superior surface by a thin layer of white matter, called the **stratum zonale,** and on its lateral surface by another layer, the **exter-**

Fig. 12-1

(A) Coronal section of the cerebral hemispheres, showing the position and relations of the thalamus.
(B) The nuclei of the thalamus.

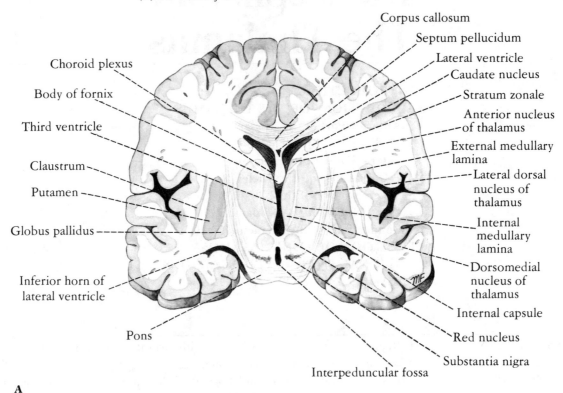

Corpus callosum
Septum pellucidum
Lateral ventricle
Caudate nucleus
Stratum zonale
Anterior nucleus of thalamus
External medullary lamina
Lateral dorsal nucleus of thalamus
Internal medullary lamina
Dorsomedial nucleus of thalamus
Internal capsule
Red nucleus
Substantia nigra

Choroid plexus
Body of fornix
Third ventricle
Claustrum
Putamen
Globus pallidus
Inferior horn of lateral ventricle
Pons
Interpeduncular fossa

A

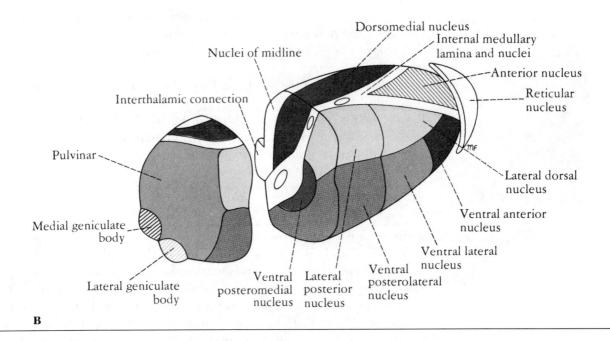

Dorsomedial nucleus
Nuclei of midline
Internal medullary lamina and nuclei
Anterior nucleus
Reticular nucleus
Interthalamic connection
Pulvinar
Lateral dorsal nucleus
Ventral anterior nucleus
Medial geniculate body
Ventral lateral nucleus
Lateral geniculate body
Ventral posteromedial nucleus
Lateral posterior nucleus
Ventral posterolateral nucleus

B

nal medullary lamina (Fig. 12-1). The gray matter of the thalamus is divided by a vertical sheet of white matter, the **internal medullary lamina,** into medial and lateral halves (Fig. 12-1). The internal medullary lamina consists of nerve fibers that pass from one thalamic nucleus to another. Anterosuperiorly, the internal medullary lamina splits so that it is Y-shaped. The thalamus thus is subdivided into three main parts; the **anterior part** lies between the limbs of the Y, and the **medial and lateral parts** lie on the sides of the stem of the Y.

Each of the three parts of the thalamus contains a group of thalamic nuclei (Fig. 12-1). Moreover, smaller nuclear groups are situated within the internal medullary lamina, and some are located on the medial and lateral surfaces of the thalamus.

Anterior Part of the Thalamus. This part of the thalamus contains the **anterior thalamic nuclei.** They receive the mammillothalamic tract from the mammillary nuclei. These anterior thalamic nuclei also receive reciprocal connections with the cingulate gyrus and hypothalamus. The function of the anterior thalamic nuclei is closely associated with that of the limbic system and is concerned with emotional tone and the mechanisms of recent memory.

Medial Part of the Thalamus. This part of the thalamus contains the large **dorsomedial nucleus** and several smaller nuclei. The dorsomedial nucleus has two-way connections with the whole prefrontal cortex of the frontal lobe of the cerebral hemisphere. It also has similar connections with the hypothalamic nuclei. It is interconnected with all other groups of thalamic nuclei. The medial part of the thalamus is responsible for the integration of a large variety of sensory information, including somatic, visceral, and olfactory information, and the relation of this information to one's emotional feelings and subjective states.

Lateral Part of the Thalamus. The nuclei are subdivided into a dorsal tier and a ventral tier (Fig. 12-1).

DORSAL TIER OF THE NUCLEI. This tier includes the **lateral dorsal nucleus,** the **lateral posterior nucleus,** and the **pulvinar.** The details of the connections of these nuclei are not clear. However, they are known to have interconnections with other thalamic nuclei and with the parietal lobe, cingulate gyrus, and occipital and temporal lobes.

VENTRAL TIER OF THE NUCLEI. This tier consists of the following in a craniocaudal sequence:

1. **Ventral anterior nucleus** (Fig. 12-1). This nucleus is connected to the reticular formation, the substantia nigra, the corpus striatum, and the premotor cortex as well as to many of the other thalamic nuclei. Since this nucleus lies on the pathway between the corpus striatum and the motor areas of the frontal cortex, it probably influences the activities of the motor cortex.
2. **Ventral lateral nucleus** (Fig. 12-1). This nucleus has connections similar to those of the ventral anterior nucleus but, in addition, has a major input from the cerebellum and a minor input from the red nucleus. Its main projections pass to the motor and premotor regions of the cerebral cortex. Here again this thalamic nucleus probably influences motor activity.
3. **Ventral posterior nucleus.** This nucleus is subdivided into the **ventral posteromedial nucleus** and the **ventral posterolateral nucleus** (Fig. 12-1). The ventral posteromedial nucleus receives the ascending trigeminal and gustatory pathways, while the ventral posterolateral nucleus receives the important ascending sensory tracts, the medial and spinal lemnisci.

The thalamocortical projections from these important nuclei pass through the posterior limb of the internal capsule and corona radiata to the primary somatic sensory areas of the cerebral cortex in the postcentral gyrus (areas 3, 1, and 2).

Other Nuclei of the Thalamus. These nuclei include the intralaminar nuclei, the midline nuclei, the reticular nucleus, and the medial and lateral geniculate bodies.

The **intralaminar nuclei** are small collections of nerve cells within the internal medullary lamina (Fig. 12-1). They receive afferent fibers from the reticular formation and also fibers from the spinothalamic and trigeminothalamic tracts; they send efferent fibers to other thalamic nuclei, which in turn project to the cerebral cortex, and fibers to the corpus striatum.

The **midline nuclei** consist of groups of nerve cells adjacent to the third ventricle and in the interthalamic connection (Fig. 12-1). They receive afferent fibers from the reticular formation. Their precise functions are unknown.

The **reticular nucleus** is a thin layer of nerve cells sandwiched between the external medullary lamina and the posterior limb of the internal capsule (Fig. 12-1). Afferent fibers converge on this nucleus from the cerebral cortex and the reticular formation, and its output is mainly to other thalamic nuclei. The function of this nucleus is not fully understood, but it may be concerned with a mechanism by which the cerebral cortex regulates thalamic activity.

The **medial geniculate body** forms part of the auditory pathway and is a swelling on the posterior surface of the thalamus beneath the pulvinar (Fig. 12-1). Afferent fibers to the medial geniculate body form the **inferior brachium** and come from the inferior colliculus. It will be remembered that the inferior colliculus receives the termination of the fibers of the lateral lemniscus. The medial geniculate body receives auditory information from both ears but predominantly from the opposite ear.

The efferent fibers leave the medial geniculate body to form the auditory radiation, which passes to the auditory cortex of the superior temporal gyrus.

The **lateral geniculate body** forms part of the visual pathway and is a swelling on the undersurface of the pulvinar of the thalamus (Fig. 12-1). The nucleus consists of six layers of nerve cells and is the terminus of all but a few fibers of the optic tract (except the fibers passing to the pretectal nucleus). The fibers are the axons of the ganglion cell layer of the retina and come from the temporal half of the ipsilateral eye and from the nasal half of the contralateral eye, the latter fibers crossing the midline in the optic chiasma. Each lateral geniculate body, therefore, receives visual information from the opposite field of vision.

The efferent fibers leave the lateral geniculate body to form the visual radiation, which passes to the visual cortex of the occipital lobe.

Connections of the Thalamic Nuclei. The main connections of the various thalamic nuclei are summarized in Figure 12-2.

FUNCTION OF THE THALAMUS

1. The thalamus is made up of collections of nerve cells that are centrally placed in the brain and are interconnected.
2. A vast amount of sensory information (except smell) converges on the thalamus and is integrated through the interconnections between the nuclei. The resulting information pattern is distributed to other parts of the central nervous system. It is probable that olfactory information is first integrated at a lower level with taste and other sensations and is relayed to the thalamus from the amygdaloid complex and hippocampus through the mammillothalamic tract.
3. The thalamus and the cerebral cortex are closely linked. The fiber connections have been established, and it is known that following removal of the cortex the thalamus can appreciate crude sensations. However, the cerebral

cortex is required for the interpretation of sensations based on past experiences.

4. The thalamus possesses certain very important nuclei that include the ventral posteromedial nucleus, the ventral posterolateral nucleus, the medial geniculate body, and the lateral geniculate body.

5. The large dorsomedial nucleus has extensive connections with the frontal lobe cortex and hypothalamus. There is considerable evidence that this nucleus lies on the pathway that is concerned with subjective feeling states and the personality of the individual.

6. The intralaminar nuclei are closely connected with the activities of the retic-

Fig. 12-2   *The main connections of the thalamus. The afferent fibers are shown on the left and the efferent fibers on the right.*

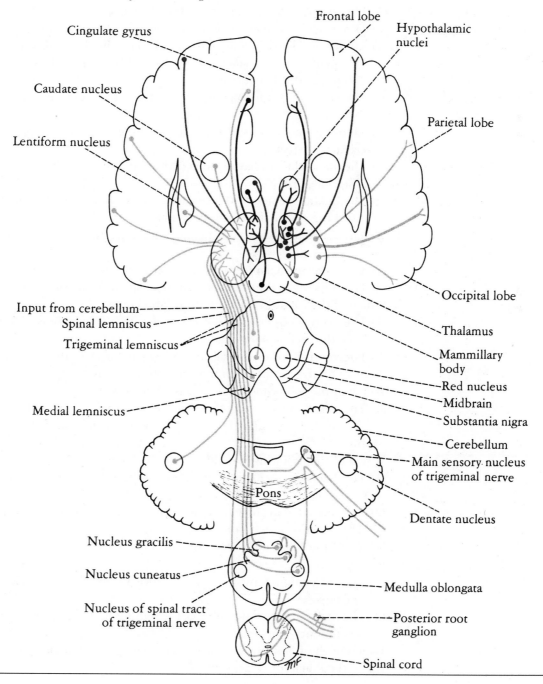

ular formation and they receive much of their information from this source. Their strategic position enables them to control the level of overall activity of the cerebral cortex. They are thus able to influence the levels of consciousness and alertness in an individual.

NATIONAL BOARD TYPE QUESTIONS

In each of the following questions, answer:

A. If only (1) is correct
B. If only (2) is correct
C. If both (1) and (2) are correct
D. If neither (1) nor (2) is correct

1. Which of the following statements concerning the position of the thalamus within the brain is (are) correct?
   (1) The thalamus lies in the floor of the third ventricle.
   (2) The thalamus is related laterally to the internal capsule.

2. Which of the following statements concerning the thalamus is (are) correct?
   (1) The right and left thalami are connected by a band of white matter that crosses the third ventricle.
   (2) The pulvinar of the thalamus is the name given to its expanded anterior end.

3. Which of the following statements concerning the subdivisions of the thalamus is (are) correct?
   (1) The internal medullary lamina divides up the thalamus into anterior and posterior parts.
   (2) The lateral surface of the thalamus is covered by a layer of gray mater called the external medullary lamina.

4. Which of the following statements concerning the thalamic nuclei is (are) correct?
   (1) The anterior thalamic nuclei are concerned with emotional tone.
   (2) The dorsomedial nucleus has connections with the prefrontal cortex.

5. Which of the following statements is (are) correct?
   (1) The ventral posterolateral nucleus receives afferent sensory information from the medial lemniscus.
   (2) The ventral posterolateral nucleus sends fibers to the postcentral gyrus through the posterior limb of the internal capsule.

6. Which of the following statements is (are) correct?
   (1) The intralaminar nuclei lie within the internal medullary lamina.
   (2) The medial geniculate body projects from the medial surface of the thalamus.

7. Which of the following statements is (are) correct?
   (1) The lateral geniculate body receives fibers from the optic tract of the same side.
   (2) The medial geniculate body is connected to the auditory area of the cerebral cortex on the same side.

8. Which of the following statements concerning the function of the thalamus is (are) correct?
   (1) The intralaminar nuclei can influence the levels of consciousness and alertness.
   (2) The thalamus can appreciate crude sensations if the cerebral cortex is not functioning.

9. Which of the following statements concerning the disability following damage to the thalamus is (are) correct?

(1) Destruction of the ventral posteromedial and the ventral posterolateral nuclei results in loss of all forms of sensation from the opposite side of the body.

(2) Destruction of the thalamus, caused by an arterial thrombosis, can produce spontaneous pain on the opposite side of the body.

10. Which of the following statements concerning the thalamus is (are) correct?

(1) The nuclei of the thalamus serve to integrate all sensations received via the afferent fibers.

(2) The thalamus receives a large amount of sensory information from the nasal mucous membrane.

ANSWERS AND EXPLANATIONS

1. B: (1) The medial surface of the thalamus forms part of the lateral wall of the third ventricle.

2. D: (1) The right and left thalami are usually connected across the third ventricle by a band of gray matter called the interthalamic connection. (2) The pulvinar of the thalamus is the name given to its expanded posterior end.

3. D: (1) The internal medullary velum divides up the thalamus into medial and lateral halves. (2) The lateral surface of the thalamus is covered by a layer of white matter called the external medullary lamina.

4. C

5. C

6. A: (2) The medial geniculate body is a swelling on the posterior surface of the thalamus beneath the pulvinar.

7. C

8. C

9. C

10. A: (2) The thalamus does not receive the sensation of smell.

13 Basal Ganglia (Basal Nuclei)

SUGGESTED PLAN FOR REVIEW OF CHAPTER 13

1. Be able to define the term *basal ganglia* and know the names of its parts.
2. Understand what is meant by the term *corpus striatum*.
3. Be able to locate on a specimen the caudate nucleus, the lentiform nucleus, the amygdaloid nucleus, and the claustrum.
4. Understand the main connections of the basal ganglia.
5. Learn the functions of the basal ganglia relative to muscular movements.
6. Read through the common clinical syndromes associated with disease of the basal ganglia. Learn about Parkinson's disease.

INTRODUCTION

The term *basal ganglia* is applied to a collection of masses of gray matter or nuclei situated within each cerebral hemisphere. They are the corpus striatum, the amygdaloid nucleus, and the claustrum. The basal ganglia play an important role in the control of posture and voluntary movement.

The purpose of this chapter is to describe briefly the basal ganglia, their connections, and their functions.

CORPUS STRIATUM

The corpus striatum is situated lateral to the thalamus. It is almost completely divided by a band of nerve fibers, the **internal capsule,** into the caudate nucleus and the lentiform nucleus (Fig. 13-1).

Fig. 13-1

Lateral view of the right cerebral hemisphere showing the lentiform nucleus, the caudate nucleus, the thalamus, and the hippocampus.

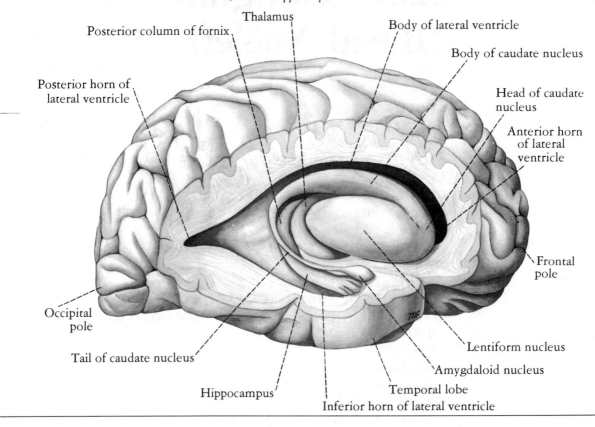

Caudate Nucleus. The caudate nucleus is a large **C**-shaped mass of gray matter that is closely related to the lateral ventricle and lies lateral to the thalamus (Fig. 13-1). The lateral surface of the nucleus is related to the internal capsule, which separates it from the lentiform nucleus. For purposes of description, it may be divided up into a head, a body, and a tail.

The **head** of the caudate nucleus is large and rounded and forms the lateral wall of the anterior horn of the lateral ventricle (Figs. 13-1 and 13-2). The head is continuous inferiorly with the putamen of the lentiform nucleus.* Just superiorly to this point of union, strands of gray matter pass through the internal capsule, giving the region a striated appearance; hence the term **corpus striatum.**

The **body** of the caudate nucleus is long and narrow and is continuous with the head in the region of the interventricular foramen. The body of the caudate nucleus forms part of the floor of the body of the lateral ventricle (Fig. 13-1).

The **tail** of the caudate nucleus is long and slender and is continuous with the body in the region of the posterior end of the thalamus (Fig. 13-2). It follows the contour of the lateral ventricle and continues forward in the roof of the inferior horn of the lateral ventricle. It terminates anteriorly in the **amygdaloid nucleus** (Fig. 13-1).

*The caudate nucleus and the putamen are sometimes referred to as the **neostriatum.**

Fig. 13-2

Horizontal section of the cerebrum as seen from above, showing the relationship between the lentiform nucleus, the caudate nucleus, the thalamus, and the internal capsule.

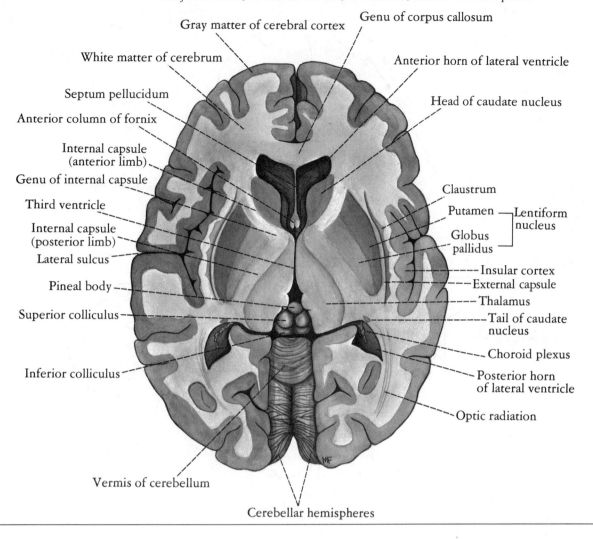

Lentiform Nucleus. The lentiform nucleus is a wedge-shaped mass of gray matter, whose broad convex base is directed laterally and its blade medially (Fig. 13-2). It is buried deep in the white matter of the cerebral hemisphere and is related medially to the internal capsule, which separates it from the caudate nucleus and the thalamus. The lentiform nucleus is related laterally to a thin sheet of white matter, the **external capsule,** that separates it from a thin sheet of gray matter, called the **claustrum.** The claustrum, in turn, separates the external capsule from the subcortical white matter of the insula. A vertical plate of white matter divides the nucleus into a larger, darker lateral portion, the **putamen,** and an inner lighter portion, the **globus pallidus** (Fig. 13-2). Inferiorly at its anterior end, the putamen is continuous with the head of the caudate nucleus.

AMYGDALOID NUCLEUS

The amygdaloid nucleus is situated in the temporal lobe close to the uncus (Fig. 13-1). The amygdaloid nucleus is considered to be part of the limbic system and is described in Chapter 15.

Fig. 13-3

Some of the main connections between the cerebral cortex, the basal nuclei, and the thalamic nuclei.

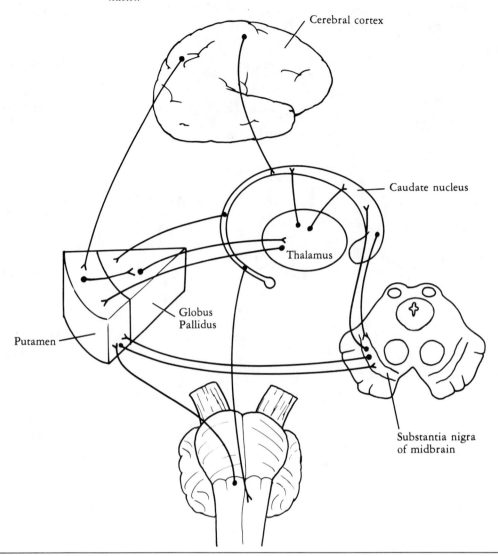

CLAUSTRUM

The claustrum is a thin sheet of gray matter that is separated from the lateral surface of the lentiform nucleus by the external capsule (Fig. 13-2). Lateral to the claustrum is the subcortical white matter of the insula. The function of the claustrum is unknown.

CONNECTIONS OF THE CORPUS STRIATUM

Afferent Fibers

CORTICOSTRIATE FIBERS. All parts of the cerebral cortex send axons to the caudate nucleus and the putamen (Fig. 13-3). Each part of the cerebral cortex projects to a specific part of the caudate-putamen complex. Most of the projections are from the cortex of the same side. The largest input is from the sensory-motor cortex. Glutamate is the neurotransmitter of the corticostriate fibers.

THALAMOSTRIATE FIBERS. Intralaminar nuclei of the thalamus send large numbers of axons to the caudate nucleus and the putamen (Fig. 13-3).

NIGROSTRIATE FIBERS. Cells in the substantia nigra send axons to the caudate nucleus and the putamen and liberate dopamine at their terminals as the neurotransmitter. It is believed that these fibers are inhibitory in function (Fig. 13-3).

BRAINSTEM STRIATAL FIBERS. Ascending fibers from the brainstem end in the caudate nucleus and putamen and liberate serotonin at their terminals at the neurotransmitter. It is thought that these fibers are inhibitory in function.

Efferent Fibers

STRIATOPALLIDAL FIBERS. These fibers pass from the caudate nucleus and putamen to the globus pallidus (Fig. 13-3). They have gamma-aminobutyric acid (GABA) as their neurotransmitter.

STRIATONIGRAL FIBERS. Fibers pass from the caudate nucleus and putamen to the substantia nigra (Fig. 13-3). Some of the fibers use GABA as the neurotransmitter, while others use substance P.

CONNECTIONS OF THE GLOBUS PALLIDUS

Afferent Fibers

STRIATOPALLIDAL FIBERS. These fibers pass from the caudate nucleus and putamen to the globus pallidus. As noted previously, these fibers have GABA as their neurotransmitter.

Efferent Fibers

PALLIDOFUGAL FIBERS. These fibers may be divided into four groups: (1) the ansa lenticularis, (2) the fasciculus lenticularis, (3) the pallidotegmental fibers, and (4) the pallidosubthalamic fibers.

FUNCTIONS OF THE BASAL GANGLIA

The basal ganglia are joined together and connected with many different regions of the nervous system by a very complex number of neurons.

Basically, the corpus striatum receives afferent information from most of the cerebral cortex, the thalamus, the subthalamus, and the brainstem, including the substantia nigra. The information is integrated within the corpus striatum and the outflow passes back to the areas listed above. This circular pathway is believed to function as follows.

The activity of the basal ganglia is initiated by information received from the sensory cortex, the thalamus, and the brainstem. The outflow from the basal ganglia is channeled through the globus pallidus, which then influences the activities of the motor areas of the cerebral cortex or other motor centers in the brainstem. Thus the basal ganglia can control muscular movements by influencing the cerebral cortex rather than through direct descending pathways to the brainstem and spinal cord.

Destruction of the motor cerebral cortex prevents the individual from performing fine discrete movements of the hands and feet on the opposite side of the body. However, the individual is still capable of performing gross crude movements. If destruction of the corpus striatum then occurs, paralysis of the remaining movements of the opposite side of the body takes place.

It has been shown that the globus pallidus plays a role in controlling the axial and girdle movements of the body and the positioning of the proximal parts of the limbs. The activity in the neurons of the globus pallidus changes before active movements take place in the limb muscles. This important function enables the motor part of the cerebral cortex to perform discrete movements of the hands and feet after the trunk and limbs have been placed in an appropriate position.

COMMON CLINICAL SYNDROMES ASSOCIATED WITH DISEASE OF THE BASAL GANGLIA

Chorea. In this syndrome the patient exhibits quick, jerky, irregular movements that are nonrepetitive. Swift grimaces and sudden movements of the head or limbs are good examples. In **Huntington's chorea** there is a degeneration of the GABA-secreting and acetylcholine-secreting neurons of the striatonigral inhibiting pathway. This results in the dopamine-secreting neurons of the substantia nigra becoming overactive so that the nigrostriatal pathway inhibits the caudate nucleus and the putamen. This inhibition produces the abnormal movements seen in this disease.

Athetosis. This consists of slow, sinuous, writhing movements that most commonly involve the distal segments of the limbs. Degeneration of the globus pallidus occurs with a breakdown of the circuitry involving the basal ganglia and the cerebral cortex.

Hemiballismus. This is a form of involuntary movement confined to one side of the body. It usually involves the proximal extremity musculature and the limb suddenly flies about in all directions out of control. The lesion occurs in the opposite subthalamic nucleus where normal smooth movements of different parts of the body are integrated.

Parkinson's Disease. This disease is associated with neuronal degeneration in the substantia nigra and to a lesser extent in the globus pallidus, putamen, and caudate nucleus. The degeneration of the inhibitory nigrostriate fibers results in a reduction in the release of the neurotransmitter dopamine within the corpus striatum. This leads to hypersensitivity of the dopamine receptors in the postsynaptic neurons in the corpus striatum, which become overactive. The signs and symptoms of the disease include tremor, cogwheel rigidity, and bradykinesis.

NATIONAL BOARD TYPE QUESTIONS

In each of the following questions, answer:
A. If only (1), (2), and (3) are correct
B. If only (1) and (3) are correct
C. If only (2) and (4) are correct
D. If only (4) is correct
E. If all are correct

1. Which of the following statements concerning the position of the basal ganglia is (are) true?

(1) The putamen lies medial to the globus pallidus.

(2) The lentiform nucleus is related medially to the external capsule.

(3) The head of the caudate nucleus lies lateral to the internal capsule.

(4) The head of the caudate nucleus is connected to the putamen.

2. Which of the following statements concerning the basal ganglia is (are) correct?

(1) The insula forms part of the basal ganglia.

(2) The corpus striatum is made up of the caudate nucleus and the lentiform nucleus.

(3) The pulvinar of the thalamus is considered to be part of the basal ganglia.

(4) The neostriatum is formed by the caudate nucleus and the putamen.

3. Which of the following statements concerning the caudate nucleus is (are) correct?

(1) It is a C-shaped mass of gray matter.

(2) It lies lateral to the thalamus.

(3) It has a head, a body, and a tail.

(4) The body lies in the roof of the lateral ventricle.

4. Which of the following statements concerning the afferent corticostriate fibers to the corpus striatum is (are) correct?

(1) All parts of the cerebral cortex send fibers to the corpus striatum.

(2) Glutamate is the neurotransmitter of the corticostriate fibers.

(3) Most of the corticostriate fibers come from the cortex of the same side.

(4) The largest input is from the sensory-motor cortex.

5. Which of the following statements concerning the nigrostriate fibers is (are) correct?

(1) The fibers exert a stimulatory effect on the putamen.

(2) The fibers liberate dopamine at their terminals.

(3) The caudate nucleus receives no fibers from the substantia nigra.

(4) Parkinson's disease is caused by degeneration of the nigrostriate fibers.

6. Which of the following statements concerning the efferent fibers of the corpus striatum is (are) correct?

(1) None of the efferent fibers descend directly to the motor nuclei of the cranial nerves or the anterior horn cells of the spinal cord.

(2) The striatopallidal fibers have GABA as their neurotransmitter.

(3) The striatonigral fibers pass from the caudate nucleus and putamen to the neurons in the substantia nigra.

(4) The efferent fibers have no effect on posture.

7. Which of the following statements concerning the functions of the basal ganglia is (are) correct?

(1) The corpus striatum integrates all information received from different parts of the nervous system.

(2) The outflow from the basal ganglia is channeled through the globus pallidus, which then influences the activities of the motor areas of the cerebral cortex.

(3) The basal ganglia are capable of producing gross crude movements in the absence of the motor areas of the cerebral cortex.

(4) The basal ganglia influence muscle movements on the opposite side of the body.

Match the numbered structures shown in Figure 13-4 with the appropriate lettered structure listed on the right.

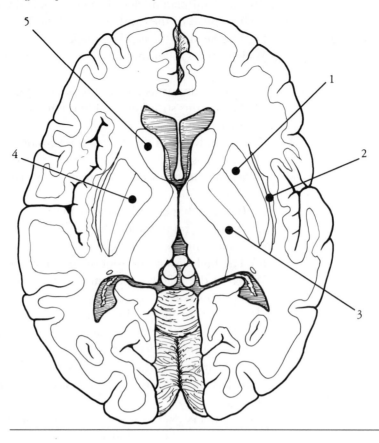

8. Structure 1.   A. Head of caudate nucleus.
9. Structure 2.   B. Internal capsule.
10. Structure 3.   C. Globus pallidus.
11. Structure 4.   D. Putamen.
12. Structure 5.   E. Claustrum.

ANSWERS AND EXPLANATIONS

1. D: (1) The putamen lies lateral to the globus pallidus. (2) The lentiform nucleus is related medially to the internal capsule. (3) The head of the caudate nucleus lies medial to the internal capsule.
2. C
3. A: (4) The body of the caudate nucleus lies in the floor of the lateral ventricle.
4. E
5. C: (1) The nigrostriate fibers exert an inhibitory effect on the putamen and the caudate nucleus. (3) The caudate nucleus receives nigrostriate fibers.
6. A: (3) The basal ganglia exert control on posture and voluntary movements. It will be remembered that posture depends on muscle tone, and the activity of the anterior horn cells of the spinal cord are indirectly influenced by the activities of the basal ganglia.
7. E
8. D
9. E
10. B
11. C
12. A

Cerebral Cortex

1. Learn the structure of the cerebral cortex including the names and character-istic features of the different layers. Know the differences between the gran-ular and agranular types of cortex. Note that the cerebral cortex varies in structure in different areas, whereas the cortex of the cerebellum is identical in structure in all areas.

2. Understand that the cerebral cortex is organized into vertical units of func-tional activity.

3. The section on the functional localization of the cerebral cortex must be care-fully read and learned. Each area of the cortex discussed in this chapter must be understood and committed to memory.

4. It is essential that the reader understands how the primary motor area and the premotor area control the movements of the contralateral side of the body. It is also important to understand how these areas on one side of the cerebral cortex control bilateral movements of the muscles of the upper part of the face, the tongue and the mandible, and the larynx and the pharynx.

5. The results of lesions of each of the cortical areas must be understood and learned. This material provides the examiners with a great many examples from which to construct suitable questions.

6. Understand what is meant by cerebral dominance.

INTRODUCTION

The cerebral cortex is the highest level of the central nervous system and always functions in association with the lower centers. It receives vast amounts of infor-mation and responds in a precise manner by bringing about appropriate changes. Many of the responses are influenced by inherited programs, while others are colored by programs learned during the individual's life and stored in the cerebral cortex.

The cerebral cortex is composed of gray matter and forms a complete cover-ing of the cerebral hemisphere. The surface area of the cortex has been in-creased by throwing it into **convolutions,** or **gyri,** separated by **fissures** or **sulci.**

STRUCTURE OF THE CEREBRAL CORTEX

Nerve Cells of the Cerebral Cortex. The following types of nerve cells are pres-ent in the cerebral cortex: (1) pyramidal cells, (2) stellate cells, (3) fusiform cells, (4) horizontal cells of Cajal, and (5) cells of Martinotti (Fig. 14-1).

The **pyramidal cells** measure 10 to 50 μm long. However, there are giant pyramidal cells, also known as **Betz cells,** whose cell bodies measure as much as 120 μm; these are found in the motor precentral gyrus of the frontal lobe.

From the apex of each cell a dendrite extends upward toward the pia, giving off collateral branches. From the basal angles, several basal dendrites pass lat-erally into the surrounding neuropil. The axon arises from the base of the cell body and either terminates in the deeper cortical layers or, more commonly, enters the white matter of the cerebral hemisphere.

The **stellate cells** are polygonal in shape and their cell bodies measure about 8 μm in diameter (Fig. 14-1). These cells have multiple branching dendrites and a short axon, which terminates on a nearby neuron.

The **fusiform cells** have their long axis vertical to the surface and are concen-trated mainly in the deepest cortical layers (Fig. 14-1). Dendrites arise from each pole of the cell body. The inferior dendrite branches within the same cellular layer, while the superficial dendrite ascends toward the surface of the cortex and branches in the superficial layers. The axon arises from the inferior part of the cell body and enters the white matter.

Fig. 14-1   *The neurons present in the cerebral cortex.*

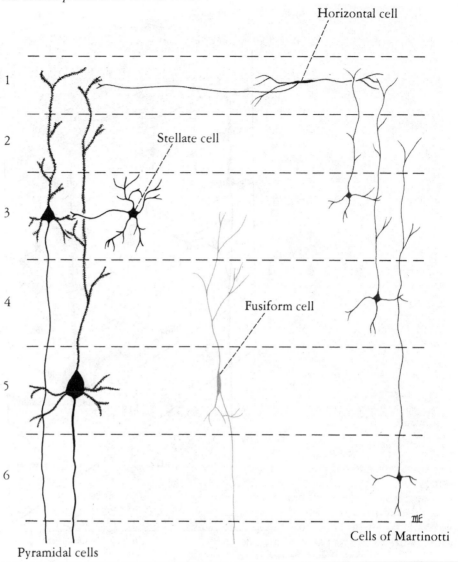

Pyramidal cells

The **horizontal cells of Cajal** are fusiform, horizontally oriented cells found in the most superficial layers of the cortex (Fig. 14-1). A dendrite emerges from each end of the cell and an axon runs parallel to the surface of the cortex, making contact with the dendrites of pyramidal cells.

The **cells of Martinotti** are small, multipolar cells that are present throughout the layers of the cortex (Fig. 14-1). The cell has short dendrites, but the axon is directed toward the pial surface of the cortex, where it ends in a more superficial layer. The axon gives origin to a few short collateral branches en route.

Nerve Fibers of the Cerebral Cortex. The nerve fibers of the cerebral cortex are arranged both radially and tangentially (Fig. 14-2). The **radial fibers** run at right angles to the cortical surface (Fig. 14-3). They include the afferent entering projection, association, and commissural fibers that terminate within the cortex, and the axons of pyramidal, stellate, and fusiform cells, which leave the cortex to become projection, association, and commissural fibers of the white matter of the cerebral hemisphere.

The **tangential fibers** run parallel to the cortical surface and are collateral and

Fig. 14-2 *Neuronal connections of the cerebral cortex.*

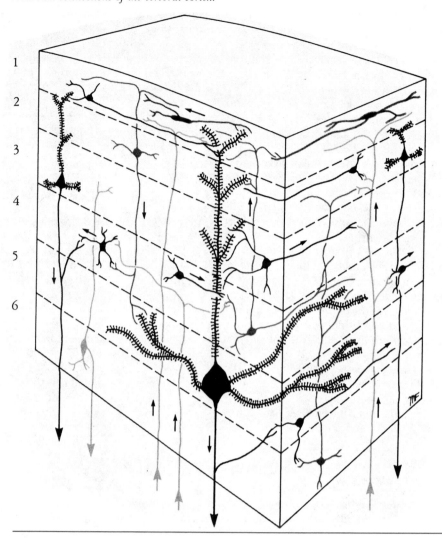

terminal branches of afferent fibers. They include also the axons of horizontal and stellate cells and collateral branches of pyramidal and fusiform cells. The tangential fibers are most concentrated in layer 4 and layer 5, where they are referred to as the outer and inner **bands of Baillarger,** respectively (Fig. 14-3). The bands of Baillarger are particularly well-developed in the sensory areas due to the high concentration of the terminal parts of the thalamocortical fibers. In the visual cortex the outer **band of Baillarger** is so thick it can be seen with the naked eye. Because of this the visual cortex is sometimes called the **striate cortex.**

Layers of the Cerebral Cortex. The names and characteristic features of the layers (Figs. 14-1 and 14-3) are as follows:

1. **Molecular layer (plexiform layer).** This is the most superficial layer; it consists of a dense network of tangentially oriented nerve fibers derived from the apical dendrites of the pyramidal cells and fusiform cells, the axons of the stellate cells, and the cells of Martinotti. Afferent fibers originating from the thalamus and from association and commissural fibers also are present. Scattered among these nerve fibers are the horizontal cells of Cajal.
2. **External granular layer.** This layer contains numerous small pyramidal cells

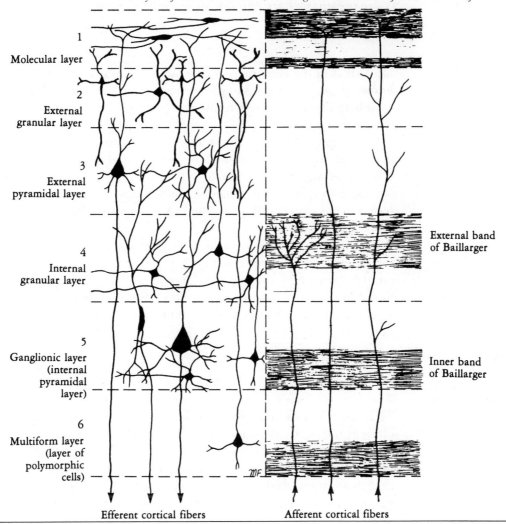

1
Molecular layer

2
External granular layer

3
External pyramidal layer

4
Internal granular layer

5
Ganglionic layer (internal pyramidal layer)

6
Multiform layer (layer of polymorphic cells)

External band of Baillarger

Inner band of Baillarger

Efferent cortical fibers   Afferent cortical fibers

and stellate cells (Figs. 14-1 and 14-3). The dendrites of these cells terminate in the molecular layer, and the axons enter deeper layers, where they terminate or pass on to enter the white matter of the cerebral hemisphere.

3. **External pyramidal layer.** This layer is composed of pyramidal cells, whose cell body size increases from the superficial to the deeper borders of the layer (Figs. 14-1 and 14-3). The apical dendrites pass into the molecular layer and the axons enter the white matter.

4. **Internal granular layer.** This layer is composed of closely packed stellate cells (Figs. 14-1 and 14-3). There is a high concentration of horizontally arranged fibers known collectively as the **external band of Baillarger.**

5. **Ganglionic layer (internal pyramidal layer).** This layer contains very large and medium-sized pyramidal cells (Figs. 14-1 and 14-3). Scattered among the pyramidal cells are stellate cells and cells of Martinotti. In addition, there are a large number of horizontally arranged fibers that form the **inner band of Baillarger.** In the motor cortex of the precentral gyrus, the pyramidal cells of this layer are very large and are known as Betz cells. These cells account for about 3 percent of the projection fibers of the **corticospinal** or **pyramidal tract.**

6. **Multiform layer (layer of polymorphic cells).** The majority of the cells are fusiform but many of the cells are triangular or ovoid (Figs. 14-1 and 14-3).

The cells of Martinotti also are conspicuous in this layer. Many nerve fibers are present that are entering or leaving the underlying white matter.

VARIATIONS IN CORTICAL STRUCTURE

Most areas of the cerebral cortex possess six layers and these are referred to as **homotypical.** Those areas of the cortex that have less than six layers are referred to as **heterotypical.** Two heterotypical areas will be described, the granular and the agranular type.

In the **granular type,** the granular layers are well-developed and contain densely packed stellate cells. Thus, layers 2 and 4 are well developed, so that layers 2 through 5 merge into a single layer of predominantly granular cells. It is these cells that receive thalamocortical fibers. The granular type of cortex is found in the postcentral gyrus, the superior temporal gyrus, and in parts of the hippocampal gyrus.

In the **agranular type** of cortex, the granular layers are poorly developed, so that layers 2 and 4 are practically absent. The pyramidal cells in layers 3 and 5 are densely packed and are very large in size. The agranular type of cortex is found in the precentral gyrus and other areas in the frontal lobe. These areas give rise to large numbers of efferent fibers that are associated with motor function.

MECHANISMS OF THE CEREBRAL CORTEX

The cerebral cortex is organized into vertical units of functional activity (Fig. 14-2). Such a functional unit possesses afferent fibers, internuncial neurons, and efferent fibers. An afferent fiber may synapse directly with an efferent neuron or may involve vertical chains of internuncial neurons. A single vertical chain of neurons may be involved or the wave of excitation may spread to adjacent vertical chains through short axon granular cells. The horizontal cells of Cajal permit activation of vertical units that lie some distance away from the incoming afferent fibers.

FUNCTIONAL LOCALIZATION OF THE CEREBRAL CORTEX

The simple division of cortical areas into motor and sensory is erroneous. The pre- and postcentral areas, for example, are both sensory and motor, the former predominantly motor and the latter predominantly sensory. Much of our understanding of the functional localization of the cerebral cortex is derived from clinicopathological studies in man and electrophysiological and ablation studies in animals.

Frontal Lobe. The **precentral area** is situated in the precentral gyrus and includes the anterior wall of the central sulcus and the posterior parts of the superior, middle, and inferior frontal gyri; it extends over the superomedial border of the hemisphere into the paracentral lobule (Fig. 14-4). Histologically, the characteristic feature of this area is the almost complete absence of the granular layers and the prominence of the pyramidal nerve cells. The giant pyramidal cells of Betz are concentrated in the superior part of the precentral gyrus and the paracentral lobule; their numbers diminish as one passes anteriorly in the precentral gyrus or inferiorly toward the lateral fissure. The great majority of the corticospinal and corticobulbar fibers originate from the small pyramidal cells in this area. It has been estimated that the number of Betz cells present is between 25,000 and 30,000 and accounts for only about 3 percent of the corti-

Fig. 14-4

Functional localization of the cerebral cortex. (A) Lateral view of left cerebral hemisphere. (B) Medial view of left cerebral hemisphere.

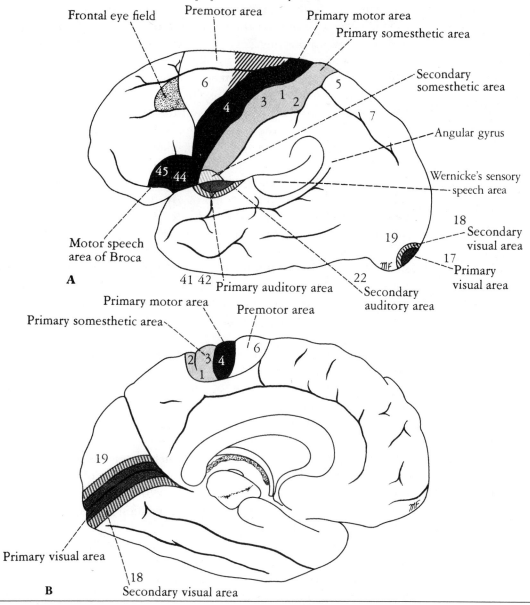

cospinal fibers. The postcentral gyrus and the second somatosensory areas, as well as the occipital and temporal lobes, give origin to descending tracts also; they control the sensory input to the nervous system and are not involved in muscular movement.

The precentral area may be divided into posterior and anterior regions. The posterior region—referred to as the **motor area, primary motor area,** or Brodmann's area 4—occupies the precentral gyrus extending over the superior border into the paracentral lobule (Fig. 14-4). The anterior area is known as the **premotor area, secondary motor area,** or Brodmann's area 6 and parts of areas 8, 44, and 45. It occupies the anterior part of the precentral gyrus and the posterior parts of the superior, middle, and inferior frontal gyri.

PRIMARY MOTOR AREA. The primary motor area if electrically stimulated produces isolated movements on the opposite side of the body and contraction of muscle groups concerned with the performance of a specific movement. Although isolated ipsilateral movements do not occur, bilateral movements of the extraocular muscles, the muscles of the upper part of the face, the tongue and the mandible, and the larynx and the pharynx do occur.

The movement areas of the body are represented in an inverted form in the precentral gyrus. Starting from below and passing superiorly are structures involved in swallowing, tongue, jaw, lips, larynx, eyelid, and brow. The next area is an extensive region for movements of the fingers, especially the thumb, hand, wrist, elbow, shoulder, and trunk. The movements of the hip, knee, and ankle are represented in the highest areas of the precentral gyrus and of the toes on the medial surface of the cerebral hemisphere in the paracentral lobule. The anal and vesical sphincters are also controlled in the paracentral lobule. The area of cortex controlling a particular movement is proportional to the skill involved in performing the movement.

The function of the primary motor area is to carry out the individual movements of different parts of the body. To assist in this function, it receives numerous afferent fibers from the premotor area, the sensory cortex, the thalamus, the cerebellum, and the basal ganglia. The primary motor cortex is not responsible for the design of the pattern of movement but is the final station for the conversion of the design into the execution of the movement.

Lesions of the primary motor cortex in one hemisphere result in paralysis of the contralateral extremities, the finer and more skilled movements suffering most.

The **Jacksonian epileptic seizure** is due to an irritative lesion of the primary motor area (area 4). The convulsion begins in the part of the body represented in the primary motor area that is being irritated. The convulsive movement may be restricted to one part of the body, such as the face or the foot, or it may spread to involve many regions.

PREMOTOR AREA. The premotor area, which is wider superiorly than below, has no giant pyramidal cells of Betz. Electrical stimulation of the premotor area produces muscular movements similar to those obtained by stimulation of the primary motor area; however, stronger stimulation is necessary to produce the same degree of movement.

The premotor area receives numerous inputs from the sensory cortex, the thalamus, and the basal ganglia. The function of the premotor area is to store programs of motor activity assembled as the result of past experience. The premotor area thus programs the activity of the primary motor area. It is particularly involved in the control of coarse postural movements through its connections with the basal ganglia.

Lesions of the secondary motor area produce difficulty in the performance of skilled movements, with little loss of strength.

MUSCLE SPASTICITY CAUSED BY LESIONS OF THE MOTOR CORTEX. A discrete lesion of the primary motor cortex (area 4) results in little change in the muscle tone. However, larger lesions involving the primary and secondary motor areas (areas 4 and 6), which are the most common, result in muscle spasm. The explanation for this is that the primary motor cortex gives origin to corticospinal and corticonuclear tracts and the secondary motor cortex gives origin to extrapyramidal tracts that pass to the basal ganglia and the reticular formation. The corticospinal and corticonuclear tracts tend to increase muscle tone, but the extrapyramidal fibers transmit inhibitory impulses that lower muscle tone. Destruction of the secondary motor area removes the inhibitory influence and, consequently, the muscles are spastic.

SUPPLEMENTARY MOTOR AREA. The supplementary motor area is situated in the medial frontal gyrus on the medial surface of the hemisphere and anterior to the paracentral lobule. Stimulation of this area results in movements of the contralateral limbs, but a stronger stimulus is necessary than when the primary motor area is stimulated. Removal of the supplementary motor area produces no permanent loss of movement.

FRONTAL EYE FIELD. The frontal eye field (Fig. 14-4) extends forward from the facial area of the precentral gyrus into the middle frontal gyrus (parts of Brodmann's areas 6, 8, and 9). Electrical stimulation of this region causes conjugate movements of the eyes, especially toward the opposite side. The nerve fibers from this area are thought to pass to the superior colliculus of the midbrain. The superior colliculus is connected to the nuclei of the extraocular muscles by the reticular formation. The frontal eye field controls voluntary scanning movements of the eye and is independent of visual stimuli. The involuntary following of moving objects by the eyes involves the visual area of the occipital cortex to which the frontal eye field is connected by association fibers.

Lesions of the Frontal Eye Field. Destructive lesions of the frontal eye field of one hemisphere cause the two eyes to deviate to the side of the lesion and an inability to turn the eyes to the opposite side. The involuntary tracking movement of the eyes when following moving objects is unaffected, since the lesion does not involve the visual cortex in the occipital lobe.

Irritative lesions of the frontal eye field of one hemisphere cause the two eyes to deviate periodically to the opposite side of the lesion.

MOTOR SPEECH AREA OF BROCA. The motor speech area of Broca (Fig. 14-4) is located in the inferior frontal gyrus between the anterior and ascending rami and the ascending and posterior rami of the lateral fissure (Brodmann's areas 44 and 45). In the majority of individuals, this area is important on the left or dominant hemisphere and ablation will result in paralysis of speech. In those individuals where the right hemisphere is dominant, the area on the right side is of importance. The ablation of this region in the nondominant hemisphere has no effect on speech.

Broca's speech area brings about the formation of words by its connections with the adjacent primary motor area, and the muscles of the larynx, mouth, tongue, soft palate, and the respiratory muscles are appropriately stimulated.

Lesions of the Motor Speech Area of Broca. Destructive lesions in the left inferior frontal gyrus result in the loss of ability to produce speech, i.e., **expressive aphasia.** The patients, however, retain the ability to think the words they wish to say, they can write the words, and they can understand their meaning when they see or hear them.

Lesions of the Sensory Speech Area of Wernicke. Destructive lesions restricted to Wernicke's speech area in the dominant hemisphere produce a loss of ability to understand the spoken and written word, i.e., **receptive aphasia.** Since Broca's area is unaffected, speech is unimpaired and the patient can produce fluent speech. However, he is unaware of the meaning of the words he uses and he uses incorrect words or even nonexistent words. The patient is also unaware of his mistakes.

Lesions of the Motor and Sensory Speech Areas. Destructive lesions involving both Broca's and Wernicke's speech areas result in the loss of the production of speech and the understanding of the spoken and written word, i.e., **global aphasia.**

Lesions of the Dominant Angular Gyrus. Destructive lesions in the angular gyrus in the posterior parietal lobe (often considered a part of Wernicke's area) divide the pathway between the visual association area and the anterior part of Wernicke's area. This results in the patient being unable to read (**alexia**) or write (**agraphia**).

PREFRONTAL CORTEX. The prefrontal cortex is an extensive area that lies anterior to the precentral area. It includes the greater parts of the superior, middle, and inferior frontal gyri, the orbital gyri, most of the medial frontal gyrus, and the anterior half of the cingulate gyrus (Brodmann's areas 9, 10, 11, and 12). Large numbers of afferent and efferent pathways connect the prefrontal area with other areas of the cerebral cortex, the thalamus, the hypothalamus, and the corpus striatum. The frontopontine fibers also connect this area to the cerebellum through the pontine nuclei. The commissural fibers of the forceps minor and genu of the corpus callosum unite these areas in both cerebral hemispheres.

The prefrontal area is concerned with the individual's personality. It also exerts its influence in determining the initiative and judgment of an individual. *Lesions of the Prefrontal Cortex.* Destruction of the prefrontal region does not produce any marked loss of intelligence. It is an area of the cortex that is capable of associating experiences that are necessary for the production of abstract ideas, judgment, emotional feeling, and personality. Tumors or traumatic destruction of the prefrontal cortex results in the person's losing initiative and judgment. Emotional changes that occur include a tendency to euphoria. The patient no longer conforms to the accepted mode of social behavior and becomes careless of dress and appearance.

Parietal Lobe

PRIMARY SOMESTHETIC AREA. The primary somesthetic area (Fig. 14-4) occupies the postcentral gyrus on the lateral surface of the hemisphere and the posterior part of the paracentral lobule on the medial surface (Brodmann's areas 3, 1, and 2). Histologically, the anterior part of the postcentral gyrus is the area that borders the central sulcus (area 3), is granular in type, and contains only scattered pyramidal cells. The **outer layer of Baillarger** is broad and very obvious. The posterior part of the postcentral gyrus (areas 1 and 2) possesses fewer granular cells. The primary somesthetic areas of the cerebral cortex receive projection fibers from the ventral posterior lateral and ventral posterior medial nuclei of the thalamus. The opposite half of the body is represented as inverted. The pharyngeal region, tongue, and jaws are represented in the most inferior part of the postcentral gyrus; this is followed by the face, fingers, hand, arm, trunk, and thigh. The leg and the foot areas are found on the medial surface of the hemisphere in the posterior part of the paracentral lobule. The anal and genital regions are also found in this latter area. The apportioning of the cortex for a particular part of the body is related to its functional importance. The face, lips, thumb, and index finger have particularly large areas assigned to them.

Although the majority of the sensations reach the cortex from the contralateral side of the body, some from the oral region go to the same side, and those from the pharynx, larynx, and perineum go to both sides.

SECONDARY SOMESTHETIC AREA. The secondary somesthetic area (Fig. 14-4) is in the superior lip of the posterior limb of the lateral fissure. The face area lies most anterior and the leg area is posterior. The body is bilaterally represented with the contralateral side dominant. The detailed connections of this area are unknown, but the spinothalamic tracts are believed to be associated with it. The functional significance of this area is not known.

Lesions of the Sensory Cortex. The sensory cortex is necessary for the appreciation of spatial recognition, recognition of relative intensity, and recognition of similarity and difference.

Lesions of the **primary somesthetic area** of the cortex result in contralateral sensory disturbances, which are most severe in the distal parts of the limbs. Crude painful, tactile, and thermal stimuli often return, but this is believed to be due to the function of the thalamus. The patient remains unable to judge degrees of warmth, unable to localize tactile stimuli accurately, and unable to judge weights of objects. Loss of muscle tone may also be a symptom of lesions of the sensory cortex.

Lesions of the **secondary somesthetic area** of the cortex do not cause recognizable sensory defects.

SOMESTHETIC ASSOCIATION AREA. The somesthetic association area (Fig. 14-4) occupies the superior parietal lobule extending onto the medial surface of the hemisphere (Brodmann's areas 5 and 7). This area has many connections with other sensory areas of the cortex. Its main function is to receive and integrate different sensory modalities. For example, it enables one to recognize objects placed in the hand without the help of vision. In other words, it not only receives information concerning the size and shape of an object but relates this to past sensory experiences, so that the information may be interpreted and recognition occurs.

Occipital Lobe

PRIMARY VISUAL AREA. The primary visual area (Brodmann's area 17) is situated in the walls of the posterior part of the calcarine sulcus and occasionally extends around the occipital pole onto the lateral surface of the hemisphere (Fig. 14-4). Macroscopically, this area can be recognized by the thinness of the cortex and the visual stria, and microscopically, it is seen to be a granular type of cortex with only a few pyramidal cells present.

The visual cortex receives afferent fibers from the lateral geniculate body. The fibers first pass forward in the white matter of the temporal lobe and then turn back to the primary visual cortex in the occipital lobe. The visual cortex receives fibers from the temporal half of the ipsilateral retina and the nasal half of the contralateral retina. The right half of the field of vision, therefore, is represented in the visual cortex of the left cerebral hemisphere and vice versa. It is also important to note that the superior retinal quadrants (inferior field of vision) pass to the superior wall of the calcarine sulcus, while the inferior retinal quadrants (superior field of vision) pass to the inferior wall of the calcarine sulcus.

The macula lutea, which is the central area of the retina and the area for most perfect vision, is represented on the cortex in the posterior part of area 17 and accounts for one-third of the visual cortex. The peripheral parts of the retina in the region of the orra serrata are represented in the anterior part of area 17.

Lesions of the Primary Visual Area. Lesions involving the walls of the posterior part of one calcarine sulcus result in a loss of sight in the opposite visual field **(crossed homonymous hemianopia).** It is interesting to note that the central part of the visual field, when tested, apparently is normal. This so-called macular sparing is probably due to the patient's shifting his eyes very slightly while the visual fields are being examined. The following clinical defects should be understood. Lesions of the upper half of one primary visual area, i.e., the area above the calcarine sulcus, result in **inferior quadrantic hemianopia,** whereas lesions involving one visual area below the calcarine sulcus result in **superior quadrantic hemianopia.** Lesions of the occipital pole produce central scotomas. The most

169

common causes of these lesions are vascular disorders, tumors, and injuries from gunshot wounds.

SECONDARY VISUAL AREA. The secondary visual area (Brodmann's areas 18 and 19) surrounds the primary visual area on the medial and lateral surfaces of the hemisphere (Fig. 14-4). This area receives afferent fibers from area 17 and other cortical areas, as well as from the thalamus. The function of the secondary visual area is to relate the visual information received by the primary visual area to past visual experiences, thus enabling the individual to recognize and appreciate what he is seeing.

The **occipital eye field** is thought to exist in the secondary visual area in man. Stimulation produces conjugate deviation of the eyes, especially to the opposite side. The function of this eye field is believed to be reflex and associated with movements of the eye when it is following an object. The occipital eye fields of both hemispheres are connected by nervous pathways and also are thought to be connected to the superior colliculus. The frontal eye field, on the other hand, controls voluntary scanning movements of the eye and is independent of visual stimuli.

Lesions of the Secondary Visual Area. Lesions of the secondary visual area result in a loss of ability to recognize objects seen in the opposite field of vision. The reason for this is that the area of cortex that stores past visual experiences has been lost.

Temporal Lobe

PRIMARY AUDITORY AREA. The primary auditory area (Brodmann's areas 41 and 42) includes the gyrus of Heschl and is situated in the inferior wall of the lateral sulcus (Fig. 14-4). Area 41 is a granular type of cortex; area 42 is homotypical and is mainly an auditory association area.

Projection fibers to the auditory area arise principally in the medial geniculate body and form the **auditory radiation of the internal capsule.** A unilateral lesion of the auditory area produces partial deafness in both ears, the greater loss being on the contralateral ear. This can be explained on the basis that the medial geniculate body receives fibers mainly from the organ of Corti of the opposite side as well as some fibers from the same side.

Lesions of the Primary Auditory Area. Because the primary auditory area in the inferior wall of the lateral sulcus receives nerve fibers from both cochleae, a lesion of one cortical area will produce slight bilateral loss of hearing, but the loss will be greatest in the opposite ear. The main defect noted is a loss of ability to locate the source of the sound. Bilateral destruction of the primary auditory areas causes complete deafness.

SECONDARY AUDITORY AREA. The secondary auditory area (auditory association cortex) is situated posterior to the primary auditory area (Fig. 14-4) in the lateral sulcus and in the superior temporal gyrus (Brodmann's area 22). This area is thought to be necessary for the interpretation of sounds.

Lesions of the Secondary Auditory Area. Lesions of the cortex posterior to the primary auditory area in the lateral sulcus and in the superior temporal gyrus result in an inability to interpret sounds, and the patient may experience **word deafness (acoustic verbal agnosia).**

SENSORY SPEECH AREA OF WERNICKE. The sensory speech area of Wernicke (Fig. 14-4) is localized in the left dominant hemisphere, mainly in the superior temporal gyrus, with extensions round the posterior end of the lateral sulcus into the parietal region. Wernicke's area is connected to Broca's area by a bundle of nerve fibers called the **arcuate fasciculus.** It receives fibers from the visual cortex in the occipital lobe and the auditory cortex in the superior temporal gyrus. Wernicke's area permits the understanding of the written and spoken language and allows a person to read a sentence, understand it, and say it out loud.

Other Cortical Areas

TASTE AREA. The taste area is probably situated at the lower end of the postcentral gyrus in the superior wall of the lateral sulcus or in the adjoining area of the insula (Brodmann's area 43). Ascending fibers from the nucleus solitarius ascend to the ventral posterior nucleus of the thalamus, where they synapse on neurons that send fibers to the cortex.

VESTIBULAR AREA. The vestibular area is thought to be situated near the part of the postcentral gyrus concerned with sensations of the face. Its exact location is unknown.

INSULA. The insula is an area of the cortex that is buried within the lateral sulcus and forms its floor. It can be examined only when the lips of the lateral sulcus are separated widely. Histologically, the posterior part is granular and the anterior part is agranular, thus resembling the adjoining cortical areas. It is believed to be associated with visceral functions.

Association Cortex. The primary sensory areas with their granular cortex and the primary motor areas with their agranular cortex form only a small part of the total cortical surface area. The remaining areas are referred to as association cortex. They have multiple inputs and outputs and are very much concerned with our behavior, discrimination, and interpretation of sensory experiences. Three main association areas are recognized: prefrontal, anterior temporal, and posterior parietal.

The prefrontal cortex is discussed on page 168. The anterior temporal cortex is thought to play a role in the storage of previous sensory experiences. Stimulation may cause the individual to recall objects seen or music heard in the past. In the posterior parietal cortex the sensory input of touch, pressure, and proprioception is integrated into concepts of size, form, and texture. This ability is known as **stereognosis.** An appreciation of the body image is also assembled in the posterior parietal cortex. An individual is able to develop a body scheme that he is able to appreciate consciously. The right side of the body is represented in the left hemisphere and the left side of the body in the right hemisphere.

LESIONS OF THE SOMESTHETIC ASSOCIATION AREA. Lesions of the superior parietal lobule interfere with the patient's ability to combine touch, pressure, and proprioceptive impulses, so he is unable to appreciate texture, size, and form. This loss of integration of sensory impulses is called **astereognosis.** For example, with the eyes closed, the individual would be unable to recognize a key placed in his hand.

Destruction of the posterior part of the parietal lobe, which integrates somatic and visual sensations, will interfere with the appreciation of the body image on the opposite side of the body. The individual may fail to recognize the opposite side of the body as his own. He may fail to wash it or dress it or shave that side of his face.

CEREBRAL DOMINANCE

An anatomical examination of the two cerebral hemispheres shows that the cortical gyri and fissures are almost identical. Moreover, nervous pathways projecting to the cortex do so largely contralaterally and equally to identical cortical areas. In addition, the cerebral commissures, especially the corpus callosum and the anterior commissure, provide a pathway for information that is received in one hemisphere to be transferred to the other. Nevertheless, we know that certain nervous activity is predominantly performed by one of the two cerebral hemispheres. Handedness, perception of language, and speech are functional areas of behavior that are in most individuals controlled by the dominant hemisphere. On the other hand, spatial perception and recognition of faces and music are interpreted by the nondominant hemisphere.

Over 90 percent of the adult population are right-handed and are therefore left hemisphere dominant. About 96 percent of the adult population are left hemisphere dominant for speech. During childhood, one hemisphere slowly comes to dominate the other, and it is only after the first decade that the dominance becomes fixed. This would explain why a 5-year-old child with damage to the dominant hemisphere can easily learn to become left-handed and speak well, whereas in the case of the adult this is almost impossible.

NATIONAL BOARD TYPE QUESTIONS

In each of the following questions, answer:
A. If only (1) is correct
B. If only (2) is correct
C. If both (1) and (2) are correct
D. If neither (1) nor (2) is correct

1. Which of the following statements concerning the cerebral cortex is (are) correct?
   (1) The cerebral cortex covers the entire cerebral hemisphere except for a small area at the bottom of each fissure.
   (2) The cerebral cortex is composed of a mixture of gray and white matter.
2. Which of the following statements concerning the structure of the cerebral cortex is (are) correct?
   (1) The cerebral cortex in all areas is made up of four layers of cells.
   (2) The Betz cells are found in the motor precentral gyrus.
3. Which of the following statements concerning the nerve cells of the cerebral cortex is (are) correct?
   (1) The horizontal cells of Cajal are found in the superficial layers of the cortex.
   (2) The cells of Martinotti are found in all the layers of the cerebral cortex.
4. Which of the following statements concerning the nerve fibers of the cerebral cortex is (are) correct?
   (1) The entering projection, association, and commissural fibers run at right angles to the cortical surface and are known as radial fibers.
   (2) The bands of Baillarger are tangential fibers that are most concentrated in layers 4 and 5.
5. Which of the following statements concerning the layers of the cerebral cortex is (are) correct?
   (1) In the cortex of the precentral gyrus, the pyramidal cells of the ganglionic layer are very large.
   (2) The granular layers are very well developed in the postcentral gyrus.

6. Which of the following statements concerning the mechanisms of the cerebral cortex is (are) correct?
   (1) The cerebral cortex is organized into vertical functional units.
   (2) The horizontal cells of Cajal permit activation of functional units some distance away from the incoming afferent fibers.

7. Which of the following statements concerning the cerebral cortex is (are) correct?
   (1) It sends no axons to the caudate nucleus.
   (2) It sends axons directly to the putamen.

Select the **best** response.

8. Concerning the cerebral cortex:
   A. The precentral gyrus is entirely motor in function.
   B. A homotypical cortex possesses four layers of cortex.
   C. In the agranular type of cortex, the pyramidal cells in layers three and five are densely packed.
   D. Clinicopathological studies are of little value in determining the functional localization of the cerebral cortex.
   E. Ablation studies of the cerebral cortex in animals have contributed very little to our understanding of the function of the different parts of the cerebral cortex.

9. Concerning the precentral area:
   A. It is located in the precentral gyrus and the anterior wall of the central sulcus and the posterior parts of the superior, middle, and inferior frontal gyri.
   B. The granular layers are conspicuous.
   C. The giant Betz cells are concentrated in the inferior part of the precentral gyrus.
   D. The majority of the corticospinal fibers arise from the large pyramidal cells in this area.
   E. Brodmann's area 4 occupies the anterior part of this area.

10. Concerning the primary motor area:
    A. It controls the contraction of groups of muscles.
    B. It is concerned with the performance of specific movements on the opposite side of the body.
    C. The movement areas of the body are represented in an inverted form in the precentral gyrus.
    D. There is an extensive area representing the movements of the thumb and fingers.
    E. All the above are correct.

11. The following information concerning the primary motor area is correct **except:**
    A. Movements of the toes are represented on the medial surface of the cerebral hemisphere.
    B. The anal and urethral sphincters are represented on the paracentral lobule.
    C. The primary motor area receives afferent fibers from the thalamus.
    D. The primary motor area is responsible for the design of the pattern of the muscular movement.
    E. The area of cortex controlling a particular movement is proportional to the skill involved in performing the movement.

12. The insula of the cerebrum is located in which area?
    A. Medial to the corpus striatum.
    B. In the longitudinal fissure.
    C. In the parietal lobe.
    D. Deep in the lateral fissure between the parietal and temporal lobes.
    E. Between the temporal and occipital lobes.
13. Which of the following is **not** true regarding the visual cortex?
    A. Areas 18 and 19 are visual association areas.
    B. Primary area 17 surrounds the calcarine sulcus.
    C. It is called the striate cortex because of the bands of Baillarger.
    D. Inferior retinal quadrants are projected onto the superior visual cortex.
    E. Because of the large number of stellate cells, the cortex is called granular.
14. Which of the following statements concerning the association fibers of the cerebrum is (are) correct?
    A. They cross from one hemisphere to the other.
    B. They remain in the same hemisphere but pass from place to place within the hemisphere.
    C. They project from motor areas of the cortex to the tegmentum of the midbrain.
    D. They conduct impulses from the spinal cord to the sensory areas of the cortex.
    E. They run from the deep layers of the cerebral cortex to the superficial layers.
15. During brain surgery under local anesthesia, a surgeon exposes the left postcentral gyrus 7 cm lateral to the midline, stimulates this area with an electrode, and asks the patient what he feels. The patient might reply:
    A. That he feels pain in his left leg.
    B. That he feels as if something is touching his right index finger.
    C. That he hears a ringing noise.
    D. That he sees flashes of light in both eyes.
    E. The patient would not reply because he would lose consciousness.
16. Lesions of the posterior part of the parietal lobe (area 7) of the right hemisphere may result in:
    A. Paralysis of the left side of the face.
    B. Anesthesia of the left arm.
    C. Receptive aphasia.
    D. Paralysis of the right leg.
    E. Inability to recognize objects in the left visual half-fields.
17. The olfactory association cortex includes the:
    A. Parahippocampal gyrus.
    B. Superior temporal gyrus.
    C. Hypothalamus.
    D. Paracentral gyrus.
    E. Cuneus.
18. The corticospinal tracts originate from:
    A. Cells of Martinotti.
    B. Pyramidal cells.
    C. Horizontal cells.
    D. Stellate cells.
    E. Golgi type II cells.
19. The cerebral cortex is an essential component of the pathway included in:
    A. Pupillary light reflex.
    B. Consensual light reflex.

C. Corneal reflex.

D. Gag reflex.

E. Accommodation reflex.

20. Stimulation of the middle frontal cortex (area 8) of the cerebral cortex would most likely produce:

    A. Contraction of the muscles of the contralateral leg.

    B. Visual agnosia.

    C. Auditory hallucinations.

    D. Conjugate eye movements.

    E. Fasciculations in the muscles of the ipsilateral hand.

21. The prefrontal cortex receives projection fibers from the following areas of the nervous system **except** the:

    A. Thalamus.

    B. Putamen.

    C. Caudate nucleus.

    D. Hypothalamus.

    E. Substantia nigra.

22. Motor seizures limited to the right arm with no loss of consciousness are often due to lesions of which cortical area?

    A. Wernicke's area on the left hemisphere.

    B. Striate cortex on the right hemisphere (area 17).

    C. Precentral gyrus on the left hemisphere (area 4).

    D. Broca's area on the left hemisphere.

    E. Posterior parietal cortex on the right hemisphere (area 7).

23. Which of the following connects Wernicke's area in the temporal lobe to Broca's area in the frontal lobe?

    A. Inferior longitudinal fasciculus.

    B. Corpus callosum.

    C. Arcuate fasciculus.

    D. Corona radiata.

    E. Cingulum.

Match the areas of the cerebral hemisphere listed below on the left with the appropriate gyri or lobes listed below on the right. An answer may be used more than once.

24. Area 17.   A. Occipital lobe.

25. Area 4.   B. Precentral gyrus.

26. Area 41.   C. Superior temporal gyrus.

27. Area 3, 1, 2.   D. Parahippocampal gyrus.

28. Area 19.   E. None of the above.

In each of the following questions, answer:

A. If only (1), (2), and (3) are correct

B. If only (1) and (3) are correct

C. If only (2) and (4) are correct

D. If only (4) is correct

E. If all are correct

29. Which of the following regions of the body has the largest representation in cortical area 4?

    (1) Trunk muscles.

    (2) Muscles of the forearm.

(3) Muscles of mastication.

(4) Muscles of the thumb.

30. Representation of the body parts (somatotopic representation) is found in the:

(1) Postcentral gyrus.

(2) Precentral gyrus.

(3) Paracentral lobule.

(4) Angular gyrus.

31. In the maintenance of normal posture, the alpha motor neurons may receive direct or indirect nervous input from:

(1) Labyrinth and neck muscles.

(2) Cerebellum.

(3) Muscles, joints, and skin receptors.

(4) Cerebral cortex.

32. The precentral gyrus receives inputs either directly or indirectly from the following areas of the nervous system when voluntary movements are performed:

(1) Limbic system.

(2) Ascending tracts in the medial lemniscus.

(3) Eyes.

(4) Cerebellum.

33. The hand area on the motor cortex:

(1) Is rarely involved in Jacksonian epilepsy.

(2) Is smaller than the thoracic area.

(3) Is on the medial surface of the cerebral hemisphere.

(4) Is one of the largest areas on the precentral gyrus.

Match the numbers listed below on the left in Figure 14-5 with the most likely functional areas listed below on the right.

34. Number 1.   A. Primary motor area.
35. Number 2.   B. Secondary motor area.
36. Number 3.   C. Secondary auditory area.
37. Number 4.   D. Secondary somesthetic area.
38. Number 5.   E. None of the above.
39. Number 6.
40. Number 7.

ANSWERS AND EXPLANATIONS

1. D: (1) The cerebral cortex covers the entire cerebral hemisphere and there are no exceptions. (2) The cerebral cortex is composed entirely of gray matter.

2. B: (1) Most areas of the cerebral cortex are made up of six layers; however, there are some important exceptions (see p. 164).

3. C

4. C

5. C

6. C

7. B

8. C: A. The precentral gyrus has both motor and sensory functions but the motor function predominates. B. A homotypical cortex possesses six layers. D. Clinicopathological studies have been of great value in determining the functional significance of different areas of the cerebral cortex. E. Experi-

Fig. 14-5

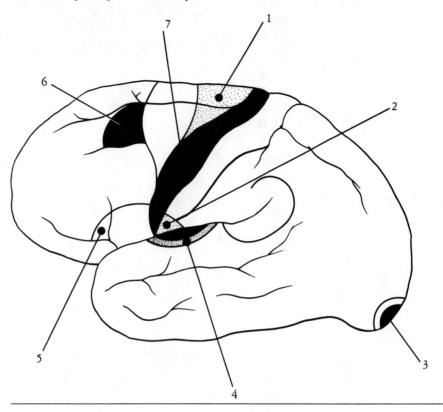

mental ablation studies in animals have provided a great deal of important information regarding cerebral cortical function.

9. A: B. The granular layers are inconspicuous. C. The giant cells of Betz are concentrated in the superior part of the precentral gyrus. D. The majority of the corticospinal fibers arise from the small pyramidal cells. E. Brodmann's area 4 is the primary motor area and occupies the posterior part of the precentral gyrus.

10. E

11. D: The primary motor area is not responsible for the design of the pattern of muscular movement but is the final station for the conversion of the design into the execution of the movement.

12. D

13. D: The inferior retinal quadrants are projected onto the inferior visual cortex.

14. B.

15. B: Stimulation of the left postcentral gyrus 7 cm lateral to the midline would excite the cortical area for the right index finger.

16. E

17. A

18. B

19. E. For further details see page 213.

20. D.

21. E

22. C

23. C

24. A

25. B

26. C
27. E
28. A
29. D
30. A
31. E
32. E
33. D
34. B
35. D
36. E
37. C
38. E
39. E
40. A

15 Limbic System

SUGGESTED PLAN FOR REVIEW OF CHAPTER 15

1. Understand that the limbic system consists of a group of structures clustered around the hypothalamus. Learn the names of these structures and know their position.
2. Understand what is meant by such terms as alveus, fimbria, dentate gyrus, and indusium griseum.
3. Learn the position of the parts of the fornix; they are commonly asked in spot examinations when brain specimens are used.
4. Understand how the different parts of the limbic system are connected to the remainder of the nervous system.
5. Learn the functions of the limbic system.

INTRODUCTION

The word *limbic* means border or margin and the term *limbic system* was loosely used to include a group of structures that lie in the border zone between the cerebral cortex and the hypothalamus. Now it is recognized, as the result of research, that the limbic system is involved with many other structures beyond the border zone in the control of emotion, behavior, and drive; it also appears to be important to memory.

Anatomically the limbic structures include the subcallosal, cingulate, and parahippocampal gyri, the hippocampal formation, amygdaloid nucleus, mammillary bodies, and the anterior thalamic nucleus (Fig. 15-1).

HIPPOCAMPAL FORMATION

The hippocampal formation consists of the hippocampus, the dentate gyrus, and the parahippocampal gyrus.

The **hippocampus** is a curved elevation of gray matter that extends throughout the entire length of the floor of the inferior horn of the lateral ventricle. It is named hippocampus because it resembles a "sea horse" in coronal section. Its anterior end is expanded to form the **pes hippocampus.** The convex ventricular surface is covered with ependyma, beneath which lies a thin layer of white matter called the **alveus.** The alveus consists of nerve fibers that have originated in the hippocampus and these converge medially to form a bundle called the **fimbria.** The fimbria in turn becomes continuous with the crus of the fornix. The hippocampus terminates posteriorly beneath the splenium of the corpus callosum.

Fig. 15-1

The medial surface of the right cerebral hemisphere showing the parts of the limbic system.

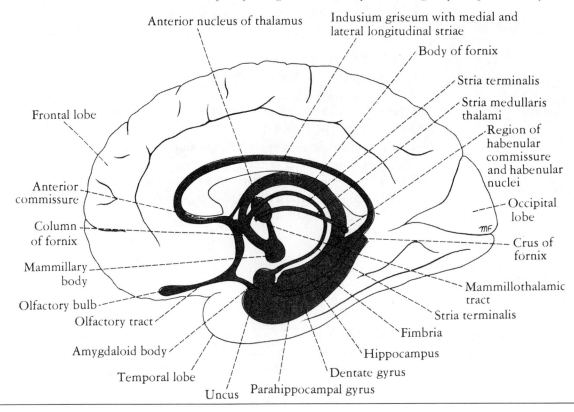

The **dentate gyrus** is a narrow, notched band of gray matter that lies between the fimbria of the hippocampus and the parahippocampal gyrus (Fig. 15-1). Posteriorly, the gyrus accompanies the fimbria almost to the splenium of the corpus callosum and becomes continuous with the **indusium griseum.** The indusium griseum is a thin, vestigial layer of gray matter that covers the superior surface of the corpus callosum. Anteriorly, the dentate gyrus is continued into the **uncus.**

The **parahippocampal gyrus** lies between the hippocampal fissure and the collateral sulcus and is continuous with the hippocampus along the medial edge of the temporal lobe.

AMYGDALOID NUCLEUS

The amygdaloid nucleus (body) resembles an almond. It is situated partly anterior and partly superior to the tip of the inferior horn of the lateral ventricle (Fig. 15-1). It is fused with the tip of the tail of the caudate nucleus, which has passed anteriorly in the roof of the inferior horn of the lateral ventricle. The stria terminalis emerges from its posterior aspect.

CONNECTING PATHWAYS OF THE LIMBIC SYSTEM

These pathways are the alveus, the fimbria, the fornix, the mammillothalamic tract, and the stria terminalis.

The **alveus** consists of nerve fibers that originate in the hippocampal cortex. The fibers converge on the medial border of the hippocampus to form a bundle called the **fimbria.**

The fimbria now leaves the posterior end of the hippocampus as the **crus of the fornix.** This curves posteriorly and superiorly beneath the splenium of the corpus callosum and around the posterior surface of the thalamus. The two crura now converge to form the **body of the fornix.** As the two crura come together they are connected by transverse fibers called the **commissure of the fornix.** These fibers decussate and join the hippocampi of the two sides.

The body of the fornix splits anteriorly into two anterior **columns of the fornix.** Each column then joins the mammillary body.

The **mammillothalamic tract** provides important connections between the mammillary body and the anterior nuclear group of the thalamus.

The **stria terminalis** emerges from the posterior aspect of the amygdaloid nucleus and runs as a bundle of nerve fibers posteriorly in the roof of the inferior horn of the lateral ventricle on the medial side of the tail of the caudate nucleus. It follows the curve of the caudate nucleus and comes to lie in the floor of the body of the lateral ventricle.

STRUCTURE OF THE HIPPOCAMPUS AND THE DENTATE GYRUS	The cortical structure of the parahippocampal gyrus is six-layered. As the cortex is traced into the hippocampus there is a gradual transition from a six- to a three-layered arrangement. These three layers are the superficial **molecular layer,** consisting of nerve fibers and scattered small neurons; the **pyramidal layer,** consisting of many large pyramidal shaped neurons; and the inner **polymorphic layer,** which is similar in structure to the polymorphic layer of the cortex seen elsewhere.

The dentate gyrus also has three layers but the pyramidal layer is replaced by the granular layer.

Afferent Connections of the Hippocampus. Afferent connections of the hippocampus may be divided into six groups (Fig. 15-2).

1. Fibers arising in the cingulate gyrus passing to the hippocampus.
2. Fibers arising from the septal nuclei (nuclei lying within the midline close to the anterior commissure) pass posterior in the fornix to the hippocampus.
3. Fibers arising from one hippocampus pass across the midline to the opposite hippocampus in the commissure of the fornix.
4. Fibers from the indusium griseum pass posteriorly in the longitudinal striae to the hippocampus.
5. Fibers from the entorhinal area or olfactory association cortex pass to the hippocampus.
6. Fibers arising from the dentate and parahippocampal gyri travel to the hippocampus.

Efferent Connections of the Hippocampus. Axons of the large pyramidal cells of the hippocampus form the alveus and the fimbria and continue as the crus of the fornix. The fibers within the fornix are distributed to the following regions (Fig. 15-2):

1. Fibers pass posterior to the anterior commissure to enter the mammillary body, where they end in the medial nucleus.
2. Fibers pass posterior to the anterior commissure to end in the anterior nuclei of the thalamus.
3. Fibers pass posterior to the anterior commissure to enter the tegmentum of the midbrain.

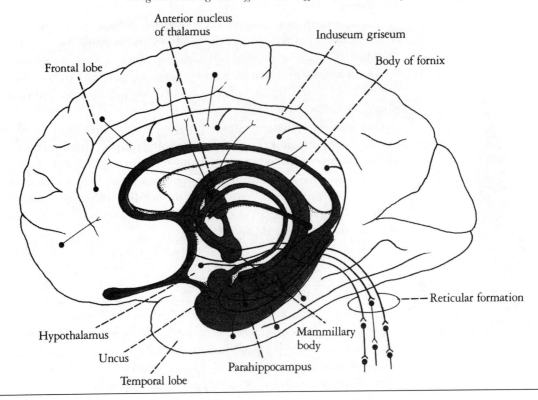

4. Fibers pass anterior to the anterior commissure to end in the septal nuclei, the lateral preoptic area, and the anterior part of the hypothalamus.
5. Fibers join the stria medullaris thalami to reach the habenular nuclei.

Consideration of the above complex anatomical pathways indicates that the structures comprising the limbic system are not only interconnected, but send projection fibers to many different parts of the nervous system. Physiologists now recognize the importance of the hypothalamus as being the major output pathway of the limbic system. The hypothalamus, by means of its connections through the reticular formation with the outflow of the autonomic nervous system, and its control of the endocrine system, is able to influence many aspects of emotional behavior.

FUNCTIONS OF THE LIMBIC SYSTEM

There is considerable evidence to indicate that the limbic system is concerned with emotional behavior, particularly the reactions of fear and anger and the emotions associated with sexual behavior. There also is evidence that the hippocampus is concerned with recent memory. Memory for remote past events usually is unaffected by lesions of this structure. There is no evidence that the limbic system has an olfactory function.

NATIONAL BOARD TYPE QUESTIONS

In each of the following questions, answer:
A. If only (1) is correct
B. If only (2) is correct

C. If both (1) and (2) are correct
D. If neither (1) nor (2) is correct

1. Which of the following statements concerning the limbic system is (are) correct?
    (1) The limbic structures are phylogenetically among the oldest parts of the brain.
    (2) The gyri of the limbic system form a ring that surrounds the upper end of the brainstem.
2. Which of the following statements concerning the limbic system is (are) correct?
    (1) In the past the limbic system was considered to be an important part of the olfactory system.
    (2) The hypothalamus is considered to be part of the outflow of the limbic system.
3. Which of the following statements concerning the afferent connections of the hippocampus is (are) correct?
    (1) Fibers arise from the cingulate gyrus and pass to the hippocampus.
    (2) Fibers arise in the nucleus gracilis and cuneatus and ascend to the cortex of the hippocampus.
4. Which of the following statements concerning the efferent connections of the hippocampus is (are) correct?
    (1) They travel through the fornix.
    (2) They originate in the large pyramidal cells of the cortex.
5. Which of the following statements concerning the functions of the limbic system is (are) correct?
    (1) The hippocampus is concerned with past memory.
    (2) It is concerned with emotions, such as the reactions of fear and anger.
6. Which of the following statements concerning the functions of the limbic system is (are) correct?
    (1) The limbic system is capable of producing changes in blood pressure and respiration.
    (2) Sexual behavior is unaffected by the activities of the limbic system.

ANSWERS AND EXPLANATIONS

1. C
2. C
3. A
4. C
5. B: (1) The hippocampus is concerned with recent memory.
6. A: (2) Sexual behavior is definitely affected by the limbic system.

16 Blood Supply of the Brain

SUGGESTED PLAN FOR REVIEW OF CHAPTER 16

1. The blood supply to the brain is important since many clinical problems arise as the result of arterial hemorrhage or thrombosis. It follows, therefore, that examination questions in this area are common.

2. Be able to make simple diagrams of (a) the circulus arteriosus and (b) the arterial supply to the cortex on the lateral and medial surfaces of the cerebral hemispheres.

3. Know the blood supply to the internal capsule. This important structure contains the major ascending and descending pathways to the cerebral cortex and it is commonly disrupted as the result of arterial hemorrhage or thrombosis (stroke).

4. Understand the venous drainage of the brain; the details need not be committed to memory.

INTRODUCTION

The normal cerebral blood flow averages 50 to 60 ml/100 g of brain per minute. The main arterial inflow is provided by four arteries: two internal carotids and two vertebrals. The two vertebral arteries unite to form the basilar artery, and the basilar artery and the carotids unite to form an important arterial circle. The hemispheres are supplied by branches from this circle. The blood is drained by thin-walled valveless cerebral veins into the cranial venous sinuses. The cerebral blood flow is related to the metabolic activity of the nerve tissue and is mainly regulated locally by the concentrations of carbon dioxide, oxygen, and hydrogen ions. Unconsciousness occurs within 10 seconds after the cessation of cerebral blood flow and irreversible brain damage rapidly follows.

ARTERIES OF THE BRAIN

The brain is supplied by the two internal carotid and the two vertebral arteries. The four arteries lie within the subarachnoid space and their branches anastomose on the inferior surface of the brain to form the **circulus arteriosus.**

Internal Carotid Artery. The internal carotid artery begins at the bifurcation of the common carotid artery. It ascends the neck and enters the skull by passing through the carotid canal of the temporal bone. After horizontally running forward through the cavernous sinus, it emerges on the medial side of the anterior clinoid process by perforating the dura mater. It now enters the subarachnoid space and divides into the **anterior** and **middle cerebral arteries** (Fig. 16-1).

BRANCHES OF THE CEREBRAL PORTION OF THE INTERNAL CAROTID ARTERY
1. The **ophthalmic artery** arises as the internal carotid artery emerges from the cavernous sinus.
2. The **posterior communicating artery** is a vessel that arises from the internal carotid artery close to its terminal bifurcation (Fig. 16-1). It runs posteriorly above the oculomotor nerve to join the posterior cerebral artery, thus forming part of the **circulus arteriosus.**
3. The **choroidal artery,** a small branch, originates from the internal carotid artery close to its terminal bifurcation. The choroidal artery enters the choroid

Fig. 16-1   *The arteries of the inferior surface of the brain. Note the formation of the circulus arteriosus.*

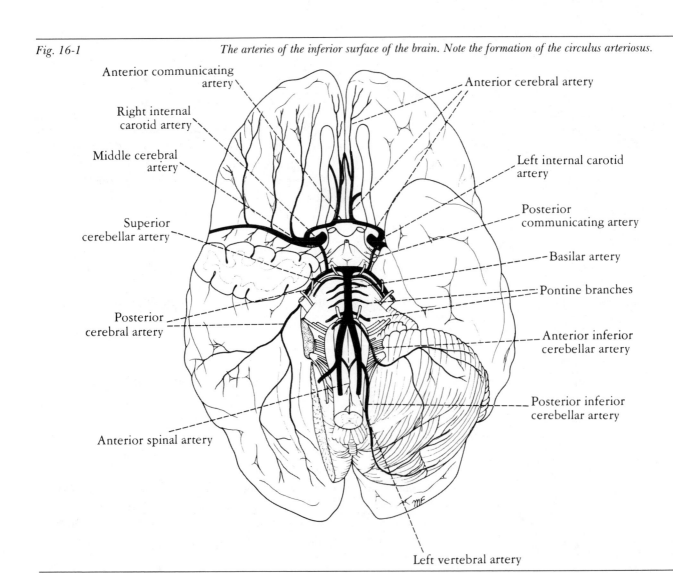

Anterior communicating artery

Right internal carotid artery

Middle cerebral artery

Superior cerebellar artery

Posterior cerebral artery

Anterior spinal artery

Anterior cerebral artery

Left internal carotid artery

Posterior communicating artery

Basilar artery

Pontine branches

Anterior inferior cerebellar artery

Posterior inferior cerebellar artery

Left vertebral artery

plexus of the inferior horn of the lateral ventricle. It gives off small branches to the crus cerebri, the lateral geniculate body, the optic tract, and the internal capsule.

4. The **anterior cerebral artery** is the smaller terminal branch of the internal carotid artery (Fig. 16-1). It runs forward and medially to enter the longitudinal fissure between the cerebral hemispheres. Here, it is joined to the anterior cerebral artery of the opposite side by the **anterior communicating artery.** It curves backward over the corpus callosum and, finally, anastomoses with the posterior cerebral artery (Fig. 16-1). The **cortical branches** supply all the medial surface of the cerebral cortex as far back as the parieto-occipital sulcus (Fig. 16-2). They also supply a strip of cortex about 1 inch (2.5 cm)

Fig. 16-2   *Areas of the cortex supplied by the cerebral arteries. A. The lateral surface of the right cerebral hemisphere. B. The medial surface of the right cerebral hemisphere.*

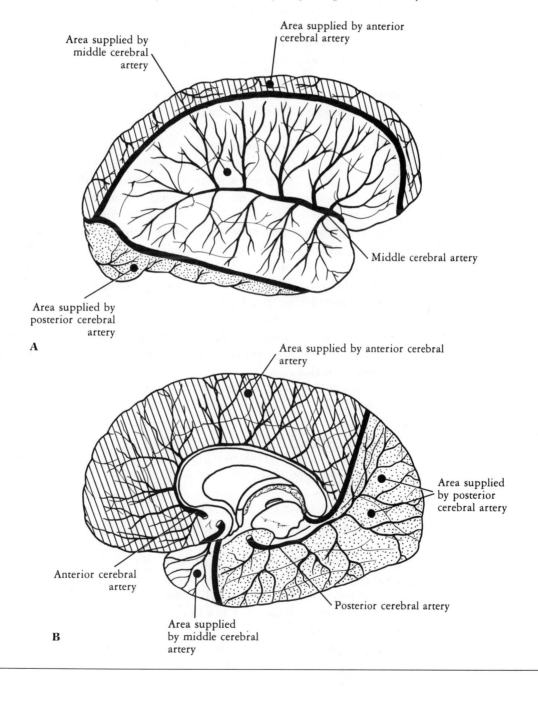

187

wide on the adjoining lateral surface. The anterior cerebral artery thus supplies the "leg area" of the precentral gyrus. A group of **central branches** pierces the anterior perforated substance and helps to supply parts of the lentiform and caudate nuclei and the internal capsule.

5. The **middle cerebral artery,** the largest branch of the internal carotid, runs laterally in the lateral cerebral sulcus (Fig. 16-1). **Cortical branches** supply the entire lateral surface of the hemisphere, except for the narrow strip supplied by the anterior cerebral artery, the occipital pole, and the inferolateral surface of the hemisphere, which are supplied by the posterior cerebral artery (Fig. 16-2). This artery thus supplies all the motor area except the "leg area." **Central branches** supply the lentiform and caudate nuclei and the internal capsule.

Vertebral Artery. The vertebral artery, a branch of the first part of the subclavian artery, ascends the neck through the foramina in the transverse processes of the upper six cervical vertebrae. It enters the skull through the foramen magnum and pierces the meninges to enter the subarachnoid space. It then passes upward, forward, and medially on the medulla oblongata. At the lower border of the pons, it joins the vessel of the opposite side to form the **basilar artery.**

BRANCHES OF THE CRANIAL PORTION OF THE VERTEBRAL ARTERY
1. The **meningeal branches** supply the bone and dura in the posterior cranial fossa.
2. The **posterior spinal artery** may arise from the vertebral artery or the posterior inferior cerebellar artery. It descends close to the posterior roots of the spinal nerves. The arteries are reinforced by radicular arteries that enter the vertebral canal through the intervertebral foramina.
3. The **anterior spinal artery** is formed from a contributory branch from each vertebral artery near its termination (Fig. 16-1). The single artery descends on the anterior surface of the medulla oblongata and spinal cord along the anterior median fissure. The artery is reinforced by radicular arteries that enter the vertebral canal through the intervertebral foramina. For the detailed distribution of the spinal arteries, see page 61.
4. The **posterior inferior cerebellar artery** supplies the inferior surface of the vermis, nuclei of the cerebellum, and the undersurface of the cerebellar hemisphere; it also supplies the medulla oblongata and the choroid plexus of the fourth ventricle.
5. The **medullary arteries** are small branches that are distributed to the medulla oblongata.

Basilar Artery. The basilar artery, formed by the union of the two vertebral arteries (Fig. 16-1), ascends in a groove on the anterior surface of the pons and ends by dividing into the two posterior cerebral arteries.

BRANCHES OF THE BASILAR ARTERY
1. The **pontine arteries** are several small vessels that enter the substance of the pons (Fig. 16-1).
2. The **labyrinthine artery** accompanies the facial and the vestibulocochlear nerves into the internal acoustic meatus and supplies the internal ear.
3. The **anterior inferior cerebellar artery** supplies the anterior and inferior parts of the cerebellum. A few branches pass to the pons and the upper part of the medulla oblongata.
4. The **superior cerebellar artery** arises close to the termination of the basilar

artery and supplies the superior surface of the cerebellum. It also supplies the pons and the pineal gland.

5. The **posterior cerebral artery** curves backward around the midbrain and is joined by the posterior communicating branch of the internal carotid artery (Fig. 16-1). **Cortical branches** supply the inferolateral and medial surfaces of the temporal lobe and the lateral medial surfaces of the occipital lobe (Fig. 16-2) including the visual cortex. **Central branches** pierce the brain substance and supply parts of the thalamus and the lentiform nucleus, and the midbrain, the pineal, and the medial geniculate bodies. A **choroidal branch** supplies the choroid plexuses of the lateral ventricle and third ventricle.

Circulus Arteriosus. The circulus arteriosus lies in the interpeduncular fossa at the base of the brain. It is formed by the anastomosis between the two internal carotid arteries and the two vertebral arteries (Figs. 16-1 and 16-3). The anterior communicating, anterior cerebral, internal carotid, posterior communicating, posterior cerebral, and basilar arteries all contribute to the circle. The circulus arteriosus allows blood that enters by either internal carotid or vertebral arteries to be distributed to any part of both cerebral hemispheres. Cortical and central branches arise from the circle and supply the brain substance.

Although the cerebral arteries anastomose with one another at the circulus arteriosus and by means of branches on the surface of the cerebral hemispheres, once they enter the brain substance no further anastomoses occur.

Arteries to Specific Brain Areas. The **corpus striatum** and the **internal capsule** are supplied mainly by the medial and lateral striate central branches of the middle cerebral artery; the central branches of the anterior cerebral artery supply the remainder of these structures.

The **thalamus** is supplied mainly by branches of the posterior communicating, basilar, and posterior cerebral arteries.

The **midbrain** is supplied by the posterior cerebral, superior cerebellar, and basilar arteries.

The **pons** is supplied by the basilar and the anterior, inferior, and superior cerebellar arteries.

Fig. 16-3   *The circulus arteriosus (circle of Willis) showing the distribution of blood from the four main arteries.*

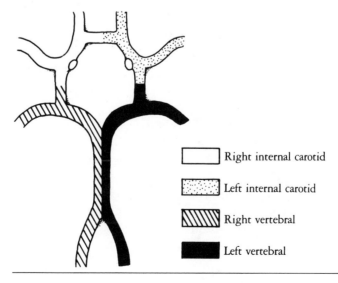

☐	Right internal carotid
▦	Left internal carotid
▨	Right vertebral
■	Left vertebral

The **medulla oblongata** is supplied by the vertebral, anterior and posterior spinal, posterior inferior cerebellar, and basilar arteries.

The **cerebellum** is supplied by the superior cerebellar, anterior inferior cerebellar, and posterior inferior cerebellar arteries.

Nerve Supply to the Cerebral Arteries. Although the cerebral arteries are innervated by sympathetic postganglionic nerve fibers, they apparently play no part in the control of cerebral vascular resistance in humans. They do, however, protect the brain from hypertension during severe exercise, by causing vasoconstriction.

The most powerful vasodilator substances for cerebral blood vessels are raised carbon dioxide and hydrogen ion concentrations and reduced oxygen concentrations. Products of metabolism, such as lactic and pyruvic acids, also cause cerebral vasodilation.

INTERRUPTION OF THE CEREBRAL CIRCULATION	Irreversible brain damage with death of nervous tissue rapidly follows complete arrest of cerebral blood flow. It has been estimated that neuronal function ceases after about 1 minute and that irreversible changes start to occur after about 4 minutes, although this time may be longer if the patient's body has been cooled. Cardiac arrest due to coronary thrombosis is the most common cause of this condition.
VEINS OF THE BRAIN	The veins of the brain have very thin walls and possess no valves. They emerge from the brain and lie in the subarachnoid space. They pierce the arachnoid mater and the meningeal layer of the dura and drain into the cranial venous sinuses.

External Cerebral Veins. The **superior cerebral veins** ascend over the lateral surface of the cerebral hemisphere and drain into the superior sagittal sinus.

The **superficial middle cerebral vein** drains the lateral surface of the cerebral hemisphere. It empties into the cavernous sinus.

The **deep middle cerebral vein** drains the insula and is joined by the **anterior cerebral and striate veins** to form the **basal vein.** The basal vein joins the great cerebral vein, which drains into the straight sinus.

Internal Cerebral Veins. The two internal cerebral veins are formed by the union of the **thalamostriate vein** and the **choroid vein** at the interventricular foramen. The two veins run posteriorly and unite to form the **great cerebral vein,** which empties into the straight sinus.

Veins of Specific Brain Areas. The **midbrain** is drained by veins that open into the basal or great cerebral veins.

The **pons** is drained by veins that open into the basal vein, cerebellar veins, or neighboring venous sinuses.

The **medulla oblongata** is drained by veins that open into the spinal veins and neighboring venous sinuses.

The **cerebellum** is drained by veins that empty into the great cerebral vein or adjacent venous sinuses.

In each of the following questions, answer:

A. If only (1), (2), and (3) are correct
B. If only (1) and (3) are correct
C. If only (2) and (4) are correct
D. If only (4) is correct
E. If all are correct

1. Which of the following statements concerning cerebral blood flow is (are) correct?
   (1) The blood flow is related to the local metabolic activity of the nervous tissue.
   (2) A high oxygen tension in the cerebral blood causes vasodilation of the cerebral blood vessels.
   (3) The sympathetic nerve fibers have very little control over the diameter of the cerebral arteries.
   (4) Numerous anastomoses take place between the cerebral arteries once they have gained entrance to the nervous tissue.

2. Which of the following statements concerning the interruption of cerebral blood flow is (are) correct?
   (1) Unconsciousness takes place within about 10 seconds.
   (2) Cooling of the patient's body speeds up neuronal degeneration.
   (3) Irreversible brain damage starts to occur after the blood flow has ceased for about 4 minutes.
   (4) Cardiac arrest is not a common cause of this condition.

3. Which of the following statements concerning the arterial supply to the brain is (are) correct?
   (1) The main arteries that supply the brain lie within the subarachnoid space.
   (2) The basilar artery is formed by the union of the two vertebral arteries.
   (3) The cerebral arteries anastomose on the surface of the brain.
   (4) The nuclei of the cerebral hemispheres receive their nourishment by diffusion of tissue fluid from the blood vessels situated on the surface of the brain.

4. Which of the following statements concerning the circus arteriosus is (are) correct?
   (1) It lies in the interpeduncular fossa at the base of the brain.
   (2) It lies within the subarachnoid space.
   (3) It permits the arterial blood to flow across the midline to the opposite side of the brain.
   (4) It permits the arterial blood to flow forward or backward should the internal carotid or vertebral artery be occluded.

5. Which of the following statements concerning the blood supply to the internal capsule is (are) correct?
   (1) It is supplied by the central branches of the middle cerebral artery.
   (2) It is supplied by central branches of the anterior cerebral artery.
   (3) It is a common site for cerebral hemorrhage.
   (4) It is supplied by perforating branches of the posterior cerebral artery.

Match the areas of the cerebral cortex numbered in Figure 16-4 and listed below on the left with the most likely cerebral arterial supply, listed below on the right. Answers may be used more than once.

Fig. 16-4

The lateral surface of the right cerebral hemisphere.

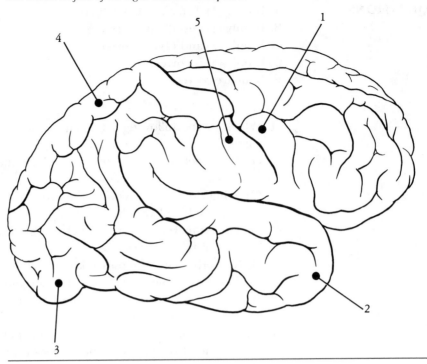

6. Number 1.   A. Anterior cerebral artery.
7. Number 2.   B. Middle cerebral artery.
8. Number 3.   C. Posterior cerebral artery.
9. Number 4.   D. None of the above.
10. Number 5.

Match the arteries listed below on the left with the most likely main stem arteries from which they arose, listed below on the right. Answers may be used more than once.

11. Pontine arteries.   A. Internal carotid artery.
12. Posterior inferior cerebellar artery.   B. External carotid artery.
13. Posterior communicating artery.   C. Basilar artery.
14. Anterior communicating artery.   D. Vertebral artery.
15. Superior cerebellar artery.   E. None of the above.

Match the veins listed below on the left with the most likely cranial venous sinuses into which they ultimately drain, listed below on the right. Answers may be used more than once.

16. Great cerebral vein.   A. Transverse sinus.
17. Internal cerebral vein.   B. Superior sagittal sinus.
18. Superior cerebral vein.   C. Straight sinus.
19. Superficial middle cerebral vein.   D. Inferior sagittal sinus.
20. Thalamostriate vein.   E. None of the above.

ANSWERS AND EXPLANATIONS

1. B: (2) A low oxygen tension in the cerebral blood causes vasodilation of the cerebral blood vessels. (4) Once a cerebral artery enters the substance of the brain it does not anastomose with another artery.

2. B: (2) Cooling of the patient's body slows down neuronal degeneration. (4) Cardiac arrest is one of the commonest causes of the interruption of cerebral blood flow.

3. A: (4) The nuclei that lie deep within the cerebral hemispheres receive their arterial supply from the central branches of the cerebral arteries.

4. E

5. A: (4) The posterior cerebral artery does not supply the internal capsule.

6. B

7. B

8. C

9. A

10. B

11. C

12. D

13. A

14. E

15. C

16. C

17. C

18. B

19. E

20. C

17 The Cerebrospinal Fluid, the Ventricles of the Brain, and the Brain Barriers

SUGGESTED PLAN FOR REVIEW OF CHAPTER 17

1. Know the composition and function of the cerebrospinal fluid (CSF).
2. Be able to describe the formation, circulation, and absorption of the CSF. Know the sites where the circulation is commonly obstructed.
3. Learn the boundaries and openings of the lateral, third, and fourth ventricles. Be able to identify the structures that lie beneath the floor of the fourth ventricle.
4. Understand the subarachnoid space and know the locations of the main cisterns.
5. Learn in detail the anatomy of lumbar puncture; this is a common clinical procedure.
6. Know the CSF pressure and remember that it is expressed in millimeters (mm) of water and **not** mercury. What is the Queckenstedt's sign?
7. Be able to define the following: (a) hydrocephalus, (b) blood-brain barrier, and (c) blood–cerebrospinal fluid barrier.
8. Learn the detailed structure of the blood-brain barrier.

INTRODUCTION

The cerebrospinal fluid is a clear, colorless fluid that fills the ventricles of the brain and bathes the external surface of the brain and spinal cord. It is formed from the choroid plexuses within the ventricles and circulates through the three openings in the roof of the fourth ventricle to reach the subarachnoid space. The fluid is produced continuously at a rate of about 0.5 ml per minute and with a total volume of about 130 ml; this corresponds to a turnover time of about 5 hours.

COMPOSITION AND PRESSURE OF CEREBROSPINAL FLUID

The cerebrospinal fluid has a specific gravity of about 1.007. It possesses, in solution, inorganic salts similar to those in the blood plasma. The glucose content is about half that of blood and there is only a trace of protein. A few cells are present and these are lymphocytes. The normal lymphocyte count is 0 to 3 cells/mm^3. In the lateral recumbent position the cerebrospinal fluid pressure, as measured by lumbar puncture, is about 60 to 150 mm water. This pressure may be easily raised by straining, coughing, or compressing the internal jugular veins in the neck.

FUNCTIONS OF THE CEREBROSPINAL FLUID

The cerebrospinal fluid serves as a protective cushion between the central nervous system and the surrounding bones. The close relationship of the fluid to the nervous tissue and the blood enables it to serve as a reservoir and assist in the regulation of the contents of the skull. The cerebrospinal fluid is an ideal physiological substrate and probably plays an active part in the nourishment of the nervous tissue; it almost certainly assists in the removal of products of neuronal metabolism. The secretions of the pineal gland possibly influence the activities of the pituitary gland by circulating through the cerebrospinal fluid in the third ventricle.

FORMATION OF CEREBROSPINAL FLUID

The cerebrospinal fluid is formed in the choroid plexuses of the lateral, third, and fourth ventricles; some may originate as tissue fluid in the brain substance.

The choroid plexuses have a folded surface and consist of a core of vascular connective tissue covered with cuboidal epithelium of the ependyma. The blood of the capillaries is separated from the ventricular lumen by fenestrated endothelium, a basement membrane, and the surface epithelium. The ependymal cells of the choroid plexuses actively secrete the cerebrospinal fluid.

CIRCULATION OF CEREBROSPINAL FLUID

The fluid passes from the lateral ventricles into the third ventricle through the interventricular foramina (Fig. 17-1). It then passes into the fourth ventricle through the cerebral aqueduct. The circulation is aided by the arterial pulsations of the choroid plexuses.

From the fourth ventricle, the fluid passes through the median aperture and the lateral foramina of the lateral recesses of the fourth ventricle and enters the subarachnoid space. The fluid then flows superiorly through the interval in the tentorium cerebelli to reach the inferior surface of the cerebrum (Fig. 17-1). It now moves superiorly over the lateral aspect of each cerebral hemisphere. Some of the cerebrospinal fluid moves inferiorly in the subarachnoid space around the

Fig. 17-1   *The circulation of the cerebrospinal fluid.*

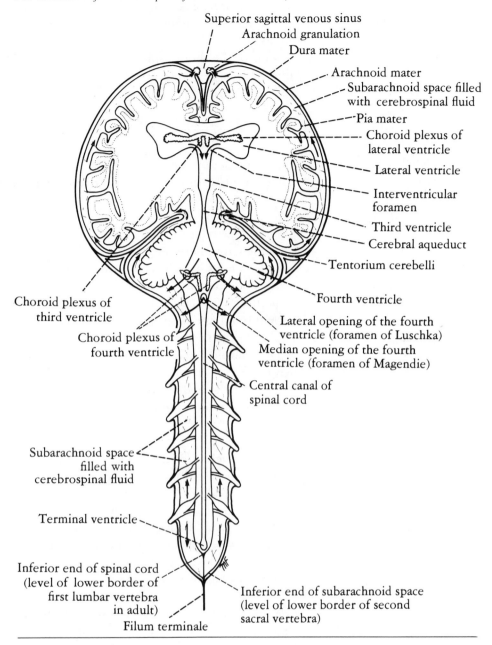

Superior sagittal venous sinus
Arachnoid granulation
Dura mater

Arachnoid mater
Subarachnoid space filled with cerebrospinal fluid
Pia mater
Choroid plexus of lateral ventricle
Lateral ventricle
Interventricular foramen
Third ventricle
Cerebral aqueduct
Tentorium cerebelli
Fourth ventricle
Lateral opening of the fourth ventricle (foramen of Luschka)
Median opening of the fourth ventricle (foramen of Magendie)
Central canal of spinal cord

Choroid plexus of third ventricle
Choroid plexus of fourth ventricle
Subarachnoid space filled with cerebrospinal fluid
Terminal ventricle
Inferior end of spinal cord (level of lower border of first lumbar vertebra in adult)
Filum terminale
Inferior end of subarachnoid space (level of lower border of second sacral vertebra)

spinal cord and cauda equina. The pulsations of the cerebral and spinal arteries and the movements of the vertebral column facilitate this flow of fluid.

ABSORPTION OF CEREBROSPINAL FLUID	The cerebrospinal fluid is absorbed into the **arachnoid villi** that project into the dural venous sinuses, especially the **superior sagittal sinus** (Fig. 17-1). The arachnoid villi are grouped together to form **arachnoid granulations.** Each arachnoid villus is a diverticulum of the subarachnoid space that pierces the dura mater.

Absorption of cerebrospinal fluid into the venous sinuses occurs when the cerebrospinal fluid pressure exceeds that in the sinus. Studies of the arachnoid villi indicate that fine tubules lined with endothelium permit a direct flow of fluid from the subarachnoid space into the lumen of the venous sinuses. Should the venous pressure rise and exceed the cerebrospinal fluid pressure, compression of the villi closes the tubules and prevents the reflux of blood into the subarachnoid space.

Some of the cerebrospinal fluid is absorbed directly into the veins in the subarachnoid space and escapes through the perineural lymph vessels of the cranial and spinal nerves.

VENTRICULAR SYSTEM	The ventricles are developmentally derived from the cavity of the neural tube. They are lined throughout with **ependyma** and are filled with **cerebrospinal fluid.**

Lateral Ventricles. There are two lateral ventricles and one is present in each cerebral hemisphere (Fig. 17-2). Each ventricle is a roughly C-shaped cavity and includes a **body,** which occupies the parietal lobe and from which **anterior, posterior,** and **inferior horns** extend into the frontal, occipital, and temporal lobes, respectively. The lateral ventricle communicates with the cavity of the third ventricle through the **interventricular foramen** (Fig. 17-1), which lies in the medial wall of the ventricle.

The **choroid plexus of the lateral ventricle** projects into the ventricle on its medial aspect between the fornix superiorly and the thalamus inferiorly. At the junction of the body of the lateral ventricle and the inferior horn, the choroid plexus is continued into the inferior horn and projects through the choroidal fissure.

Third Ventricle. The third ventricle is a slitlike cleft between the two thalami. It communicates anteriorly with the lateral ventricles through the interventricular foramina (of Monro) and posteriorly with the fourth ventricle through the cerebral aqueduct (of Sylvius) (Fig. 17-1). The **choroid plexuses of the third ventricle** hang from the roof.

The blood supply of the choroid plexuses of the third and lateral ventricles is derived from the choroidal branches of the internal carotid and basilar arteries. The venous blood drains into the internal cerebral veins.

Cerebral Aqueduct (Aqueduct of Sylvius). The cerebral aqueduct, a narrow channel about ¾ inch (1.8 cm) long, connects the third with the fourth ventricle (Fig. 17-1). It is lined with ependyma and is surrounded by a layer of gray matter called the **central gray.** The direction of flow of cerebrospinal fluid is from the third to the fourth ventricle. There is no choroid plexus in the cerebral aqueduct.

Fourth Ventricle. The fourth ventricle is a cavity situated anterior to the cerebellum and posterior to the pons and the superior half of the medulla oblongata (Fig. 17-2). It is continuous above with the cerebral aqueduct and below with the central canal of the spinal cord. The fourth ventricle possesses lateral boundaries, a roof, and a rhomboid-shaped floor. The lateral boundaries are formed by the **superior and inferior cerebellar peduncles.**

The tent-shaped roof projects into the cerebellum. It is formed by the **superior medullary velum** above and the **inferior medullary velum** below. The inferior medullary velum is pierced in the midline by a large opening, the **median aperture, the foramen of Magendie.**

Fig. 17-2

A cast of the ventricular cavities of the brain as seen from (A) lateral view, (B) anterior view, and (C) superior view.

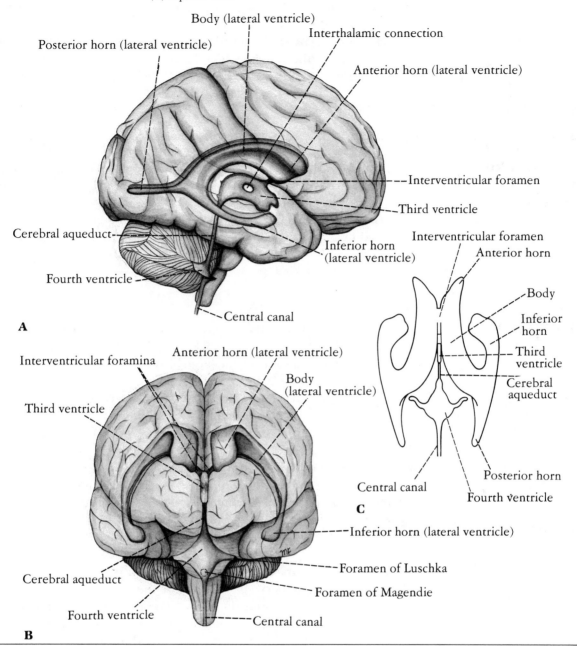

The floor is formed by the posterior surface of the pons and the cranial half of the medulla oblongata (see Fig. 8-6). In the midline is the **median sulcus.** On each side of this sulcus is the **median eminence,** which is bounded laterally by the **sulcus limitans.** Lateral to the sulcus limitans there is the **vestibular area,** beneath which lie the vestibular nuclei. The **facial colliculus,** produced by the fibers of the facial nerve looping over the abducens nucleus, lies at the inferior end of the medial eminence.

Strands of nerve fibers, the **stria medullaris,** emerge from the median sulcus and pass laterally to enter the inferior cerebellar peduncle. Inferior to the stria lies the **hypoglossal triangle** formed by the underlying hypoglossal nucleus and lateral to this lies the **vagal triangle** produced by the underlying dorsal motor nucleus of the vagus.

Lateral recesses extend around the sides of the medulla and open anteriorly as the **lateral openings of the fourth ventricle,** or the **foramina of Luschka** (Fig. 17-1). It is through these two openings and the foramen of Magendie that the cerebrospinal fluid enters the subarachnoid space.

The **choroid plexus of the fourth ventricle** is suspended from the interior half of the roof of the ventricle. The blood supply to the plexus is from the posterior inferior cerebellar arteries.

CENTRAL CANAL OF THE SPINAL CORD AND MEDULLA OBLONGATA	The central canal opens superiorly into the fourth ventricle. Inferiorly, it extends through the inferior half of the medulla oblongata and through the entire length of the spinal cord. In the conus medullaris of the spinal cord, it expands to form the **terminal ventricle.** The central canal is closed at its lower end, is filled with cerebrospinal fluid, and is lined with ependyma. The central canal is surrounded by gray matter, the **gray commissure.** There is no choroid plexus in the central canal.
SUBARACHNOID SPACE	The subarachnoid space is the interval between the arachnoid mater and pia mater and envelops the brain and spinal cord (Fig. 17-1). The space is filled with cerebrospinal fluid and contains the large blood vessels of the brain. Inferiorly, the subarachnoid space extends beyond the lower end of the spinal cord and invests the **cauda equina.** The subarachnoid space ends below at the level of the interval between the second and third sacral vertebrae.

Subarachnoid Cisterns. In certain locations around the base of the brain, the arachnoid does not closely follow the surface of the brain so that the subarachnoid space expands to form cisterns. The **cerebellomedullary cistern** lies between the cerebellum and the medulla oblongata, the **pontine cistern** lies on the anterior surface of the pons, and the **interpeduncular cistern** lies on the anterior surface of the midbrain between the crura cerebri.

Extensions of the Subarachnoid Space. A sleeve of the subarachnoid space extends around the optic nerve to the back of the eyeball. Here the arachnoid mater and pia mater fuse with the sclera. The central artery and vein of the retina cross this extension of the subarachnoid space to enter the optic nerve and they may be compressed in patients with raised cerebrospinal fluid pressure. Small extensions of the subarachnoid space also occur around the other cranial and spinal nerves.

The subarachnoid space also extends around the arteries and veins of the brain and spinal cord at points where they penetrate the nervous tissue. The pia mater, however, quickly fuses with the outer coat of the blood vessel below the surface of the brain and spinal cord, thus closing off the subarachnoid space.

LUMBAR PUNCTURE	Lumbar puncture may be performed to withdraw a sample of cerebrospinal fluid for microscopic or bacteriological examination or to inject drugs to combat infection or induce anesthesia. Fortunately, the spinal cord terminates inferiorly at the level of the lower border of the first lumbar vertebra in the adult. (In the

infant it may reach inferiorly to the third lumbar vertebra.) The subarachnoid space extends inferiorly as far as the lower border of the second sacral vertebra.

With the patient lying on his side with the vertebral column well flexed, the space between adjoining laminae in the lumbar region is opened to a maximum. An imaginary line joining the highest points on the iliac crests passes over the fourth lumbar spine. Using a careful aseptic technique and local anesthesia, the physician passes the lumbar puncture needle, fitted with a stylet, into the vertebral canal above or below the fourth lumbar spine. The needle will pass through the following anatomical structures before it enters the subarachnoid space: (1) skin, (2) superficial fascia, (3) supraspinous ligament, (4) interspinous ligament, (5) ligamentum flavum, (6) areolar tissue containing the internal vertebral venous plexus, (7) dura mater, and (8) arachnoid mater. The depth to which the needle will have to pass will vary from 1 inch (2.5 cm) or less in a child to as much as 4 inches (10 cm) in an obese adult.

The cerebrospinal fluid pressure may be measured by attaching a manometer to the needle. When the patient is in the recumbent position, the **normal pressure is about 60 to 150 mm water.** The pressure shows oscillations corresponding to the movements of respiration and the arterial pulse.

A block of the subarachnoid space in the vertebral canal, which may be caused by a tumor of the spinal cord or the meninges, may be detected by compressing the internal jugular veins in the neck. This raises the cerebral venous pressure and inhibits the absorption of cerebrospinal fluid in the arachnoid granulations, thus producing a rise in the manometer reading of the cerebrospinal fluid pressure. If this rise fails to occur, the subarachnoid space is blocked and the patient is said to exhibit a positive **Queckenstedt's sign.**

HYDROCEPHALUS

Hydrocephalus is an abnormal increase in the volume of the cerebrospinal fluid within the skull. If the hydrocephalus is accompanied by a raised cerebrospinal fluid pressure, then it is due to either (1) an abnormal increase in the formation of the fluid, (2) a blockage of the circulation of the fluid, or (3) a diminished absorption of the fluid. Rarely, hydrocephalus occurs with a normal cerebrospinal fluid pressure and in these patients there is a compensatory hypoplasia or atrophy of the brain substance.

BLOOD-BRAIN BARRIER

The blood-brain barrier protects the brain from toxic compounds. In the newborn child or premature infant, where these barriers are not fully developed, toxic substances such as bilirubin can readily enter the central nervous system and produce yellowing of the brain and **kernicterus.**

In certain situations, however, it is important that the nerve cells be exposed without a barrier to the circulating blood. This enables neuronal receptors to sample the plasma directly and to respond and maintain the normal internal environment of the body within very fine limits. There is no blood-brain barrier in the pineal gland, the hypothalamus, the posterior lobe of the pituitary, the tuber cinereum, the wall of the optic recess, and the area postrema at the lower end of the fourth ventricle.

The blood-brain barrier is formed by the tight junctions between the endothelial cells of the blood capillaries. In those areas where the blood-brain barrier is absent, the capillary endothelium contains fenestrations across which proteins and small organic molecules may pass from the blood to the nervous tissue.

BLOOD–CEREBROSPINAL FLUID BARRIER

There is free passage of water, gases, and lipid-soluble substances from the blood to the cerebrospinal fluid. Macromolecules such as proteins and most hexoses other than glucose are unable to enter the cerebrospinal fluid. It has been suggested that a barrier similar to the blood-brain barrier exists in the choroid plexuses and it is probable that the tight junctions between the choroidal epithelial cells serve as the barrier.

CEREBROSPINAL FLUID–BRAIN INTERFACE

There is no physiological barrier between the cerebrospinal fluid and the extracellular compartment of the central nervous system so that the extracellular spaces of the nervous tissue are in almost direct continuity with the subarachnoid space.

NATIONAL BOARD TYPE QUESTIONS

In each of the following questions, answer:
A. If only (1) is correct
B. If only (2) is correct
C. If both (1) and (2) are correct
D. If neither (1) nor (2) is correct

1. Which of the following statements is (are) correct?
   (1) The cerebrospinal fluid is a clear, greenish fluid.
   (2) The cerebrospinal fluid has a specific gravity of about 1.007.
2. Which of the following statements is (are) correct?
   (1) The total volume of cerebrospinal fluid is about 130 ml.
   (2) The cerebrospinal fluid is produced continuously by the choroid plexuses.
3. Which of the following statements is (are) correct?
   (1) The normal lymphocyte count in cerebrospinal fluid is 20 to 30 cells/mm^3.
   (2) The normal glucose concentration is about half that of blood.
4. Which of the following statements is (are) correct?
   (1) The normal cerebrospinal fluid pressure in the lateral recumbent position is about 60 to 150 mm water.
   (2) Compression of the internal jugular veins lowers the CSF pressure.
5. Which of the following statements is (are) correct?
   (1) The cerebrospinal fluid is found in the ventricles of the brain and in the subarachnoid space.
   (2) The choroid plexuses are located in the lateral, third, and fourth ventricles.
6. Which of the following statements concerning the ventricles of the brain is (are) correct?
   (1) The third ventricle is joined to the fourth ventricle by the interventricular foramen.
   (2) The lateral ventricles communicate directly with one another through the foramen of Monro.

Select the **best** response.

7. The following statements concerning the lateral ventricle are correct **except:**
   A. The ventricle is C-shaped and follows the curve of the caudate nucleus.
   B. It is present in the frontal, parietal, occipital, and temporal lobes of the cerebral hemisphere.

C. It communicates with the third ventricle through its medial wall.

D. The choroid plexus projects into the ventricle through the lateral wall.

E. The posterior horn arises at the junction of the body with the inferior horn.

8. Which of the following statements concerning the third ventricle is (are) correct?

A. The optic chiasma is placed in its floor.

B. The choroid plexus is situated in the floor.

C. The cavity is lined with pia mater.

D. The cavity is restricted to an area below the interthalamic connection.

E. The hypothalamus lies in its anterior wall.

9. The following statements concerning the fourth ventricle are correct **except:**

A. The cerebellum is located in its roof.

B. The foramen of Magendie is situated in the inferior medullary velum.

C. The facial colliculus lies in the floor of the upper part of the ventricle.

D. The foramina of Luschka allow the cerebrospinal fluid to escape into the subarachnoid space.

E. The nucleus of the fourth cranial nerve lies beneath the floor.

10. The following statements concerning the subarachnoid space are correct **except:**

A. The space is the interval between the arachnoid and the dura mater.

B. It is expanded to form cisterns.

C. The space receives cerebrospinal fluid through three holes in the fourth ventricle.

D. It terminates below in the adult at the level of the interval between the second and third sacral vertebrae.

E. It surrounds the cauda equina.

11. Which of the following statements concerning the formation of the cerebrospinal fluid is (are) correct?

A. The choroid plexuses actively secrete cerebrospinal fluid.

B. The cells responsible for the formation of the cerebrospinal fluid are the endothelial cells of the choroidal blood capillaries.

C. The tissue fluid of the brain does not contribute to the cerebrospinal fluid.

D. There is extensive diffusion of fluid from the cerebral veins situated in the subarachnoid space.

E. The arachnoid villi actively secrete cerebrospinal fluid.

12. The following statements concerning the circulation of the cerebrospinal fluid are correct **except:**

A. The arterial pulsations of the choroidal arteries and the cerebral arteries aid the circulation of the fluid.

B. The fluid reaches the cerebral hemispheres by passing through the notch in the tentorium cerebelli.

C. The fluid escapes from the central canal of the spinal cord through an aperture in the roof of the terminal ventricle.

D. Some of the fluid moves inferiorly around the spinal cord in the subarachnoid space.

E. The movements of the vertebral column assist in the mixing of the cerebrospinal fluid.

In each of the following questions, answer:

A. If only (1), (2), and (3) are correct

B. If only (1) and (3) are correct

C. If only (2) and (4) are correct

D. If only (4) is correct

E. If all are correct

13. Which of the following statements concerning the procedure of lumbar puncture is (are) correct?
    (1) With the patient lying on his side with the vertebral column well flexed, the space between adjoining laminae in the lumbar region is opened to a maximum.
    (2) The needle is inserted above or below the fourth lumbar spine.
    (3) The needle will pierce the supraspinous and interspinous ligaments and the ligamentum flavum before penetrating the meninges.
    (4) An imaginary line joining the highest points of the iliac crests is used to locate the level of the fourth lumbar spine.

14. Which of the following statements concerning the cerebrospinal fluid pressure is (are) correct?
    (1) The pressure shows oscillations corresponding to the respiratory movements and the arterial pulse.
    (2) Queckenstedt's sign may be positive if the spinal part of the subarachnoid space is blocked by a tumor.
    (3) The pressure will rise if the arachnoid villi are blocked by inflammatory exudate.
    (4) The pressure is lowered when one coughs.

15. Which of the following statements concerning hydrocephalus is (are) correct?
    (1) It is caused by an increase in the volume of cerebrospinal fluid in the subarachnoid space.
    (2) It can be caused by a blockage of the circulation of the cerebrospinal fluid.
    (3) It is never accompanied by a hypoplasia of the brain.
    (4) It may be caused by a diminished absorption of the cerebrospinal fluid.

16. Which of the following statements is (are) correct concerning the blood-brain barrier?
    (1) The blood-brain barrier protects the brain from toxic compounds.
    (2) The blood-brain barrier is absent from the hypothalamus.
    (3) The blood-brain barrier is incompletely formed in the newborn.
    (4) The blood-brain barrier is formed by the tight junctions between the endothelial cells of the blood capillaries.

17. Which of the following statements is (are) correct?
    (1) The cerebrospinal fluid can flow directly into the venous blood at the arachnoid granulations.
    (2) The cerebrospinal fluid flows directly into the neuropil of the central nervous system from the ventricles.
    (3) The cerebrospinal fluid flows directly into the neuropil through the pia mater.
    (4) The cerebrospinal fluid that extends along the spinal nerves is absorbed into the perineurial lymph vessels.

Match the numbers in Figure 17-3 and listed below on the left with the appropriate letters listed below on the right. The letters may be used more than once.

18. Number 1.	A. Sulcus limitans.
19. Number 2.	B. Vestibular area.
20. Number 3.	C. Hypoglossal triangle.
21. Number 4.	D. Facial colliculus.
22. Number 5.	E. None of the above.

Fig. 17-3   *The floor of the fourth ventricle.*

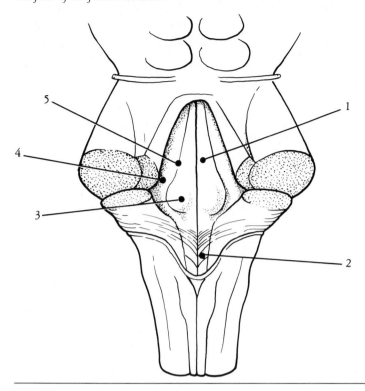

ANSWERS AND EXPLANATIONS

1. B: (1) The normal cerebrospinal fluid is colorless.
2. C
3. B: (1) The normal lymphocyte count of cerebrospinal fluid is 0 to 3 cells/mm³.
4. A: (2) Compression of the internal jugular vein in the neck raises the CSF pressure because it impedes the reabsorption of the fluid into the venous sinuses.
5. C
6. D: (1) The third ventricle is joined to the fourth ventricle by the cerebral aqueduct. (2) The lateral ventricles do not communicate directly with one another; they each communicate with the third ventricle via the foramen of Monro.
7. D: The choroid plexus projects into the lateral ventricle through the choroidal fissure on the medial wall.
8. A: B. The choroid plexus is situated in the roof of the third ventricle. C. The cavity of the ventricle is lined with ependyma. D. The interthalamic connection crosses the third ventricle so that part of the cavity lies above and part of the cavity lies below the connection. E. The hypothalamus lies in the floor of the third ventricle.
9. E: The nucleus of the fourth cranial nerve lies in the midbrain.
10. A: The subarachnoid space is the interval between the arachnoid mater and the pia mater.
11. A: B. The choroidal ependymal cells actively secrete CSF. C. The tissue fluid of the brain substance contributes slightly to the CSF. D. The cerebral veins do not contribute to the CSF. E. The arachnoid villi are sites where the CSF enters the venous blood.
12. C: The cerebrospinal fluid does not escape through the roof of the terminal ventricle in the spinal cord since there is no opening.

13. E
14. A: (4) The CSF pressure is raised when one coughs.
15. C: (1) Hydrocephalus is an increase in the volume of the CSF within the skull. (3) Hydrocephalus sometimes produces atrophy of the cerebral cortex.
16. E
17. E
18. E
19. C
20. D
21. B
22. A

18 Cranial Nerves I-IV

SUGGESTED PLAN FOR REVIEW OF CHAPTER 18

1. The cranial nerves are clinically important and testing for their integrity forms part of every physical examination. Moreover, each cranial nerve provides the examiner with many possible good questions.
2. Understand the basic information regarding the motor and sensory nuclei of the cranial nerves and note their location.
3. The optic nerve and lesions of the optic pathway must be learned. The possible lesions are tricky but with patience you will understand and master them.
4. Know the various visual reflexes.
5. Because the third and fourth nerves are of small diameter and are relatively long, they frequently are damaged in head injuries. Questions are commonly directed to the defects found after injury.

INTRODUCTION

There are 12 pairs of cranial nerves, which leave the brain and pass through foramina and fissures in the skull. All the nerves are distributed in the head and neck except the tenth, which also supplies structures in the thorax and abdomen. The cranial nerves are named as follows:

  1. Olfactory
  2. Optic
  3. Oculomotor
  4. Trochlear
  5. Trigeminal

6. Abducent
7. Facial
8. Vestibulocochlear
9. Glossopharyngeal
10. Vagus
11. Accessory
12. Hypoglossal

ORGANIZATION OF CRANIAL NERVES

The olfactory, optic, and vestibulocochlear nerves are entirely sensory. The oculomotor, trochlear, abducent, accessory, and hypoglossal nerves are entirely motor. The trigeminal, facial, glossopharyngeal, and vagus nerves are both sensory and motor nerves. The cranial nerves have central motor and/or sensory nuclei within the brain and peripheral nerve fibers that emerge from the brain and exit from the skull to reach their effector or sensory organs.

The different components of the cranial nerves, their functions, and the openings in the skull through which the nerves leave the cranial cavity are summarized in Table 18-1.

MOTOR NUCLEI OF THE CRANIAL NERVES

Somatic Motor and Branchomotor Nuclei. The somatic motor and branchomotor nerve fibers of a cranial nerve are the axons of nerve cells situated within the brain. These nerve cell groups form motor nuclei and they innervate striated muscle. Each nerve cell with its processes is referred to as a **lower motor neuron.** Such a nerve cell is, therefore, equivalent to the motor cells found in the anterior gray columns of the spinal cord.

The motor nuclei of the cranial nerves receive impulses from the cerebral cortex through the corticonuclear fibers. These fibers originate from the pyramidal cells in the inferior part of the precentral gyrus (area 4) and from the adjacent part of the postcentral gyrus. The corticonuclear fibers descend through the **corona radiata** and the **genu of the internal capsule.** They pass through the midbrain just medial to the corticospinal fibers in the **basis pedunculi** and end

Table 18-1		Cranial Nerves		
	Name	Components	Function	Opening in Skull
I.	Olfactory	Sensory	Smell	Openings in cribriform plate of ethmoid
II.	Optic	Sensory	Vision	Optic canal
III.	Oculomotor	Motor	Lifts upper eyelid, turns eyeball upward, downward, and medially; constricts pupil; accommodates eye	Superior orbital fissure
IV.	Trochlear	Motor	Assists in turning eyeball downward and laterally	Superior orbital fissure
V.	Trigeminal			
	Ophthalmic division	Sensory	Cornea, skin of forehead, scalp, eyelids, and nose; also mucous membrane of paranasal sinuses and nasal cavity	Superior orbital fissure

Table 18-1. (Continued)

	Name	Components	Function	Opening in Skull
	Maxillary division	Sensory	Skin of face over maxilla; teeth of upper jaw; mucous membrane of nose, the maxillary sinus, and palate	Foramen rotundum
	Mandibular division	Motor	Muscles of mastication, mylohyoid, anterior belly of digastric, tensor veli palatini, and tensor tympani	Foramen ovale
		Sensory	Skin of cheek, skin over mandible and side of head, teeth of lower jaw and temporomandibular joint; mucous membrane of mouth and anterior part of tongue	
VI.	Abducent	Motor	Lateral rectus muscle—turns eyeball laterally	Superior orbital fissure
VII.	Facial	Motor	Muscles of face and scalp, stapedius muscle, posterior belly of digastric and stylohyoid muscles	Internal acoustic meatus, facial canal, stylomastoid foramen
		Sensory	Taste from anterior two-thirds of tongue, floor of mouth and palate	
		Secretomotor parasympathetic	Submandibular and sublingual salivary glands, the lacrimal gland, and glands of nose and palate	
VIII.	Vestibulocochlear			
	Vestibular	Sensory	Position and movement of head	Internal acoustic meatus
	Cochlear	Sensory	Hearing	
IX.	Glossopharyngeal	Motor	Stylopharyngeus muscle—assists in swallowing	
		Secretomotor parasympathetic	Parotid salivary gland	Jugular foramen
		Sensory	Posterior one-third of tongue, pharynx, carotid sinus and carotid body	
X.	Vagus	Motor and sensory	Heart and great thoracic vessels; larynx, trachea, bronchi, and lungs; alimentary tract from pharynx to splenic flexure of colon; liver, kidneys, and pancreas	Jugular foramen
XI.	Accessory			
	Cranial root	Motor	Muscles of soft plate, pharynx, and larynx	Jugular foramen
	Spinal root	Motor	Sternocleidomastoid and trapezius muscles	
XII.	Hypoglossal	Motor	Muscles of tongue (except palatoglossus) controlling its shape and movement	Hypoglossal canal

by synapsing either directly with the lower motor neurons within the cranial nerve nuclei or indirectly through the **internuncial neurons.**

The majority of the corticonuclear fibers to the motor cranial nerve nuclei cross the median plane before reaching the nuclei. Bilateral connections are present for all the cranial motor nuclei except for part of the facial nucleus that supplies the muscles of the lower part of the face and a part of the hypoglossal nucleus that supplies the genioglossus muscle.

General Visceral Motor Nuclei. The general visceral motor nuclei form the cranial outflow of the parasympathetic portion of the autonomic nervous system. They are the Edinger-Westphal nucleus of the oculomotor nerve, the superior salivatory nucleus of the facial nerve, the inferior salivatory nucleus of the glossopharyngeal nerve, and the dorsal motor nucleus of the vagus. These nuclei receive numerous afferent fibers including descending pathways from the hypothalamus.

SENSORY NUCLEI OF THE CRANIAL NERVES	These include somatic and visceral afferent nuclei. The sensory or afferent parts of a cranial nerve are the axons of nerve cells outside the brain and are situated in ganglia on the nerve trunks (equivalent to posterior root ganglion of a spinal nerve) or may be situated in a sensory organ such as the nose, eye, or ear. The central processes of these cells enter the brain and terminate by synapsing with cells forming the sensory nuclei. Axons from the nuclear cells now cross the midline and ascend to other sensory nuclei (e.g., the thalamus), where they synapse. The nerve cells of these nuclei send their axons to terminate in the cerebral cortex.
OLFACTORY NERVES (CRANIAL NERVE I)	The olfactory nerves arise from olfactory receptor nerve cells in the olfactory mucous membrane located in the upper part of the nasal cavity above the level of the superior concha. Bundles of these nerve fibers pass through the openings of the cribriform plate of the ethmoid bone to enter the **olfactory bulb** inside the skull. **Olfactory Bulb.** The incoming olfactory nerve fibers synapse with the dendrites of the **mitral cells** and form rounded areas known as **synaptic glomeruli.** Smaller nerve cells called **tufted cells** and **granular cells** also synapse with the mitral cells. The olfactory bulb, in addition, receives axons from the contralateral olfactory bulb through the olfactory tract. **Olfactory Tract.** This is a narrow band of white matter that runs from the posterior end of the olfactory bulb and divides into **medial and lateral olfactory striae.** The lateral stria carries the axons to the **olfactory area of the cerebral cortex,** namely, the **periamygdaloid and prepiriform areas** (Fig. 18-1). The medial olfactory stria carries the fibers that cross the median plane in the anterior commissure to pass to the olfactory bulb of the opposite side. The periamygdaloid and prepiriform areas of the cerebral cortex are often known as the **primary olfactory cortex.** The **entorhinal area (area 28) of the** parahippocampal gyrus, which receives numerous connections from the primary olfactory cortex, is called the **secondary olfactory cortex.** These areas of the cortex are responsible for the appreciation of olfactory sensations. Note that, in contrast to all other sensory pathways, the olfactory afferent pathway has only

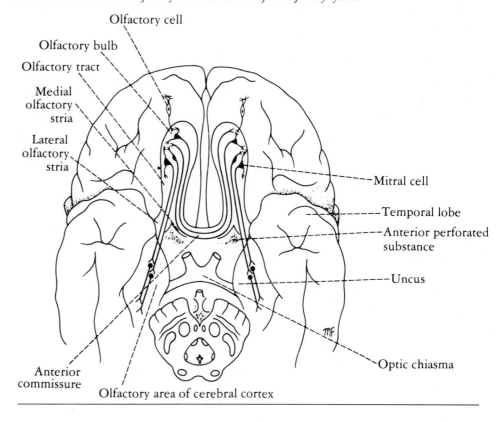

Olfactory cell

Olfactory bulb

Olfactory tract

Medial olfactory stria

Lateral olfactory stria

Mitral cell

Temporal lobe

Anterior perforated substance

Uncus

Optic chiasma

Anterior commissure

Olfactory area of cerebral cortex

two neurons and reaches the cerebral cortex without synapsing in one of the thalamic nuclei.

OPTIC NERVE (CRANIAL NERVE II)	The optic nerve is composed of axons from the ganglion cell layer of the retina. The nerve emerges from the back of the eyeball and leaves the orbital cavity of the skull through the optic canal. It unites with the optic nerve of the opposite side to form the **optic chiasma** (Fig. 18-2).

In the chiasma, the fibers from the medial (nasal) half of each retina cross the midline and enter the **optic tract** of the opposite side, while the fibers from the lateral (temporal) half of each retina pass posteriorly in the optic tract of the same side. Most of the fibers of the optic tract terminate by synapsing with nerve cells in the **lateral geniculate body,** which is a small projection from the posterior part of the thalamus. New fibers pass to the **pretectal nucleus** and **superior colliculus** of the midbrain and are concerned with the light reflexes (see below and p. 81).

The axons from the lateral geniculate body pass posteriorly as the **optic radiation** and terminate in the **visual cortex (area 17)** of the cerebral hemisphere (Fig. 18-2). This cortex occupies the upper and lower lips of the calcarine sulcus on the medial surface of the cerebral hemisphere. The visual association cortex (areas 18 and 19) is responsible for recognition of objects and perception of color. Note that the macula lutea is represented on the posterior part of area 17, and the periphery of the retina is represented anteriorly.

Visual Reflexes

DIRECT AND CONSENSUAL LIGHT REFLEXES. If a light is shone into one eye, the pupils of both eyes normally constrict. The constriction of the pupil upon which

Fig. 18-2   *The optic pathway.*

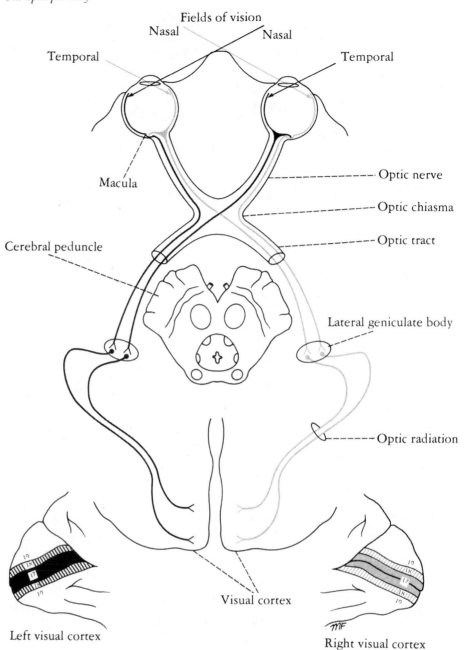

Fields of vision
Nasal   Nasal
Temporal   Temporal

Macula

Optic nerve

Optic chiasma

Optic tract

Cerebral peduncle

Lateral geniculate body

Optic radiation

Visual cortex

Left visual cortex

Right visual cortex

the light is shone is called the **direct light reflex;** the constriction of the opposite pupil even though no light fell upon that eye is called the **consensual light reflex** (Fig. 18-3).

The afferent impulses travel through the optic nerve, optic chiasma, and optic tract. Here a small number of fibers leave the optic tract and synapse on nerve cells in the **pretectal nucleus,** which lies close to the superior colliculus. The impulses are passed by axons of the pretectal nerve cells to the parasympathetic nuclei (**Edinger-Westphal nuclei**) of the third cranial nerve on both sides. Here the fibers synapse and the parasympathetic nerves travel through the third cranial nerve to the ciliary ganglion in the orbit (Fig. 18-3). Finally, postganglionic parasympathetic fibers pass through the **short ciliary nerves** to the eyeball and the **constrictor pupillae muscle** of the iris. Both pupils constrict in the consen-

Fig. 18-3   *The optic pathways and the visual reflexes.*

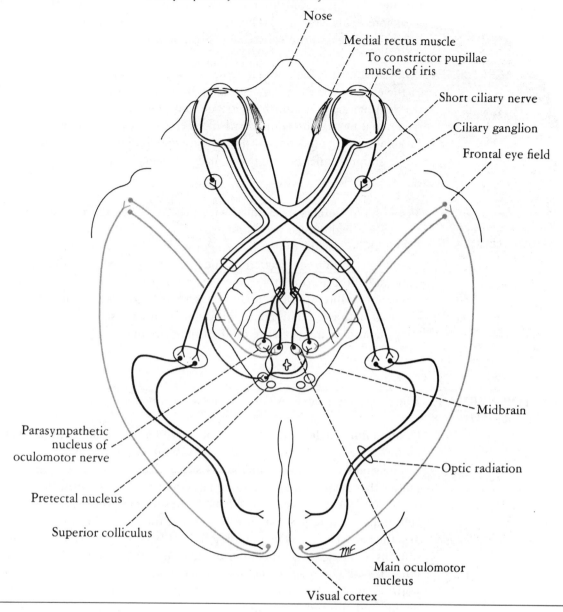

Nose

Medial rectus muscle

To constrictor pupillae
muscle of iris

Short ciliary nerve

Ciliary ganglion

Frontal eye field

Midbrain

Optic radiation

Parasympathetic
nucleus of
oculomotor nerve

Pretectal nucleus

Superior colliculus

Main oculomotor
nucleus

Visual cortex

sual light reflex because the pretectal nucleus sends fibers to the parasympathetic nuclei on both sides of the midbrain (Fig. 18-3). The fibers that cross the median plane do so close to the cerebral aqueduct in the posterior commissure.

ACCOMMODATION REFLEX. When the eyes are directed from a distant to a near object, contraction of the medial recti brings about convergence of the ocular axes, the lens thickens to increase its refractive power by contraction of the ciliary muscle, and the pupils constrict to restrict the light waves to the thickest central part of the lens. The afferent impulses travel through the optic nerve, the optic chiasma, the optic tract, the lateral geniculate body, and the optic radiation to the visual cortex. The visual cortex is connected to the eye field of the frontal cortex (Fig. 18-3). From here, cortical fibers descend through the internal capsule to the oculomotor nuclei in the midbrain. The oculomotor nerve travels to the medial recti muscles. Some of the descending cortical fibers synapse with the parasympathetic nuclei (Edinger-Westphal nuclei) of the third cranial nerve on both sides. Here the fibers synapse and the parasympathetic nerves travel through the third cranial nerve to the ciliary ganglion in the orbit. Finally, postganglionic parasympathetic fibers pass through the short ciliary nerves to the **ciliary muscle** and the **constrictor pupillae muscle** of the iris (Fig. 18-3).

CORNEAL REFLEX. Light touching of the cornea or conjunctiva results in blinking of the eyelids. Afferent impulses from the cornea or conjunctiva travel through the ophthalmic division of the trigeminal nerve to the sensory nucleus of the trigeminal nerve. Internuncial neurons connect with the motor nucleus of the facial nerve on both sides through the medial longitudinal fasciculus. The facial nerve and its branches supply the orbicularis oculi muscle, which causes closure of the eyelids.

Visual Field Defects Associated with Lesions of the Optic Pathways. The various visual field defects are summarized in Figure 18-4. Note that circumferential blindness may be due to hysteria or optic neuritis. Total blindness of one eye would follow complete section of one optic nerve. Lesions of the optic tract and optic radiation produce the same hemianopia for both eyes, i.e., homonymous hemianopia. Bitemporal hemianopia is a loss of the lateral halves of the fields of vision of both eyes. This condition is commonly caused by a tumor of the pituitary gland exerting pressure on the optic chiasma.

| OCULOMOTOR NERVE (CRANIAL NERVE III) | The oculomotor nerve is entirely motor in function. |

Oculomotor Nuclei. The oculomotor nerve has two motor nuclei: (1) the main motor nucleus and (2) the accessory parasympathetic nucleus.

The **main oculomotor nucleus** is situated in the anterior part of the gray matter that surrounds the **cerebral aqueduct of the midbrain** (Fig. 18-5). It lies at the level of the superior colliculus. The nucleus consists of groups of nerve cells that supply all the extrinsic muscles of the eye except the superior oblique and the lateral rectus. The outgoing nerve fibers pass anteriorly through the red nucleus and emerge on the anterior surface of the midbrain in the **interpeduncular fossa.** The main oculomotor nucleus receives corticonuclear fibers from both cerebral hemispheres. It receives tectobulbar fibers from the superior colliculus and through this route receives information from the visual cortex. It also receives fibers from the medial longitudinal fasciculus, by which it is connected to the nuclei of the fourth, sixth, and eighth cranial nerves.

The **accessory parasympathetic nucleus (Edinger-Westphal nucleus)** is situated posterior to the main oculomotor nucleus (Fig. 18-5). The axons of the nerve cells, which are preganglionic, accompany the other oculomotor fibers to the orbit. Here they synapse in the **ciliary ganglion** and postganglionic fibers pass through the **short ciliary nerves** to the constrictor pupillae of the iris and the ciliary muscles. The accessory parasympathetic nucleus receives corticonuclear fibers for the accommodation reflex and fibers from the pretectal nucleus for the direct and consensual light reflexes.

Oculomotor Nerve. The oculomotor nerve emerges on the anterior surface of the midbrain. It passes forward in the middle cranial fossa in the lateral wall of the cavernous sinus. Here, it divides into a superior and an inferior ramus, which enter the orbital cavity through the superior orbital fissure.

The oculomotor nerve supplies the following extrinsic muscles of the eye: levator palpebrae superioris, superior rectus, medial rectus, inferior rectus, and

Fig. 18-4

Visual field defects associated with lesions of the optic pathways. (1) Right-sided circumferential blindness due to retrobulbar neuritis. (2) Total blindness of right eye due to division of right optic nerve. (3) Right nasal hemianopia due to partial lesion of right side of optic chiasma. (4) Bitemporal hemianopia due to complete lesion of optic chiasma. (5) Left temporal hemianopia and right nasal hemianopia due to lesion of right optic tract. (6) Left temporal and right nasal hemianopia due to lesion of right optic radiation. (7) Left temporal and right nasal hemianopia due to lesion of right visual cortex.

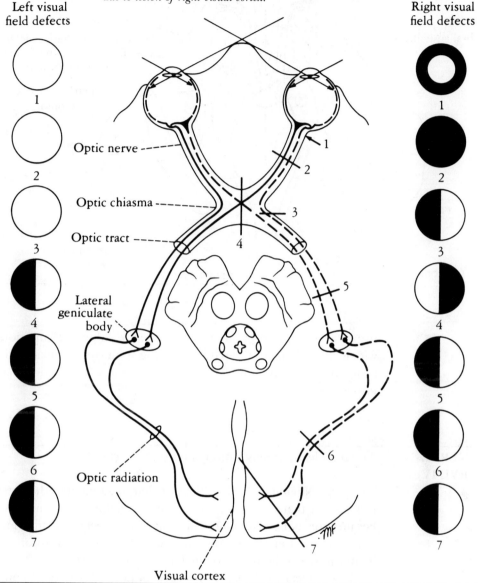

Left visual
field defects

Right visual
field defects

Optic nerve ---

Optic chiasma ---

Optic tract ---

Lateral
geniculate
body

Optic radiation

Visual cortex

inferior oblique. It also supplies through its branch to the ciliary ganglion and the short ciliary nerves parasympathetic nerve fibers to the following intrinsic muscles: the constrictor pupillae of the iris and the ciliary muscles.

The oculomotor nerve is therefore entirely motor and is responsible for lifting the upper eyelid, turning the eye upward, downward, and medially, constricting the pupil, and accommodating the eye.

Oculomotor Paralysis. In complete oculomotor paralysis the eye cannot be moved upward, downward, or inward. At rest the eye looks laterally (external strabismus) owing to the activity of the lateral rectus and downward due to the activity of the superior oblique. The patient has diplopia. There is ptosis of the

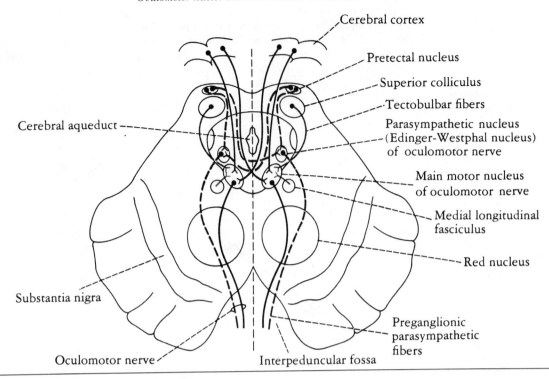

upper eyelid due to paralysis of the levator palpebrae superioris. The pupil is widely dilated due to the paralysis of the sphincter pupillae and the unopposed action of the dilator pupillae (supplied by the sympathetic). Accommodation is impossible.

TROCHLEAR NERVE (CRANIAL NERVE IV)

The trochlear nerve is entirely motor in function.

Trochlear Nucleus. The trochlear nucleus is situated in the anterior part of the gray matter that surrounds the cerebral aqueduct of the midbrain (Fig. 18-6). It lies inferior to the oculomotor nucleus at the level of the inferior colliculus. The nerve fibers, after leaving the nucleus, pass posteriorly around the central gray matter to reach the posterior surface of the midbrain.

The trochlear nucleus receives corticonuclear fibers from both cerebral hemispheres. It receives the tectobulbar fibers, which connect it to the visual cortex through the superior colliculus. It also receives fibers from the medial longitudinal fasciculus, by which it is connected to the nuclei of the third, sixth, and eighth cranial nerves.

Trochlear Nerve. The trochlear nerve, the most slender of the cranial nerves, and the only one to leave the posterior surface of the brainstem, emerges from the midbrain and **immediately decussates** with the nerve of the opposite side. The trochlear nerve passes forward through the middle cranial fossa in the lateral wall of the cavernous sinus and enters the orbit through the superior orbital fissure. The nerve supplies the superior oblique muscle of the eyeball. The trochlear nerve is entirely motor and assists in turning the eye downward and laterally.

Fig. 18-6   *Trochlear nerve nucleus and its central connections.*

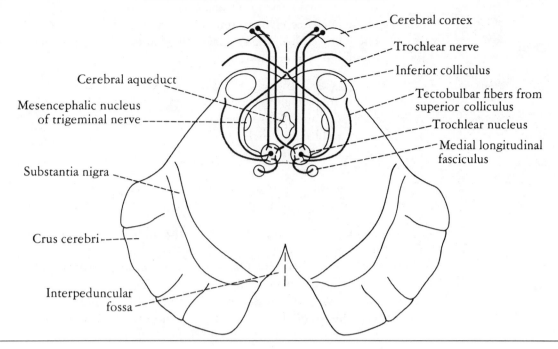

Cerebral cortex
Trochlear nerve
Inferior colliculus
Tectobulbar fibers from superior colliculus
Trochlear nucleus
Medial longitudinal fasciculus
Cerebral aqueduct
Mesencephalic nucleus of trigeminal nerve
Substantia nigra
Crus cerebri
Interpeduncular fossa

Trochlear Nerve Paralysis. In trochlear nerve paralysis, the patient complains of double vision on looking straight downward. This is because the superior oblique is paralyzed, and the eye turns medially as well as downward. The patient has great difficulty in turning the eye downward and laterally.

NATIONAL BOARD TYPE QUESTIONS

In each of the following questions, answer:
A. If only (1) is correct
B. If only (2) is correct
C. If both (1) and (2) are correct
D. If neither (1) nor (2) is correct

1. Which of the following statements concerning the cranial nerves is (are) correct?
   (1) All the cranial nerves are only distributed to structures in the head and neck.
   (2) All the cranial nerves leave the skull through foramina and fissures.
2. Which of the following statements concerning the cranial nerves is (are) correct?
   (1) The oculomotor, trochlear, and hypoglossal nerves are entirely motor in function.
   (2) The facial, glossopharyngeal, and vagus nerves are both sensory and motor in function.
3. Which of the following statements concerning the motor cranial nerve nuclei is (are) correct?
   (1) All motor neurons of the cranial nerve nuclei receive descending motor fibers from both cerebral hemispheres.
   (2) The corticonuclear fibers pass through the midbrain lateral to the corticospinal fibers to the lower limb.

4. Which of the following statements concerning the general visceral motor nuclei of the cranial nerves is (are) correct?
   (1) These nuclei receive afferent fibers from the hypothalamus.
   (2) These nuclei form the cranial outflow of the parasympathetic part of the autonomic nervous system.

In each of the following questions, answer:
A. If only (1), (2), and (3) are correct
B. If only (1) and (3) are correct
C. If only (2) and (4) are correct
D. If only (4) is correct
E. If all are correct

5. Which of the following statements concerning the sensory nuclei of cranial nerves is (are) correct?
   (1) Some of the afferent fibers to the nuclei are derived from nerve cells situated in ganglia outside the brain.
   (2) The axons of the nuclei cross the midline of the brain.
   (3) With the exception of the olfactory input, all ascending fibers from the nuclei synapse with nerve cells in the thalamus.
   (4) Most of the information from the cranial nerve nuclei ultimately terminates in the postcentral gyrus of the cerebral cortex.
6. Which of the following statements concerning the olfactory nerve is (are) correct?
   (1) The receptor cells lie in the mucous membrane in the upper part of the nasal cavity.
   (2) The axons of the olfactory nerves synapse with mitral cells in the olfactory bulbs.
   (3) The lateral olfactory stria carries the axons of the mitral cells to the olfactory area of the cortex.
   (4) The periamygdaloid and prepiriform areas form the primary olfactory cortex.
7. Which of the following statements concerning the optic nerve is (are) correct?
   (1) The axons arise from the ganglionic layer of the retina.
   (2) At the optic chiasma, the fibers from the medial half of each retina cross the midline and enter the optic tract of the opposite side.
   (3) The optic nerve leaves the orbital cavity through the optic canal.
   (4) The optic nerve is surrounded by the three meninges and an extension into the orbital cavity of the subarachnoid space.
8. Which of the following statements concerning the optic tract is (are) correct?
   (1) Most of the fibers in the optic tract terminate in the lateral geniculate body.
   (2) The optic tract contains fibers from the nasal and temporal halves of the retina on the same side.
   (3) A few fibers of the optic tract pass to the pretectal nucleus and are concerned with light reflexes.
   (4) The optic tract contains postganglionic sympathetic fibers derived from the superior cervical sympathetic ganglion.
9. Which of the following statements concerning the optic radiation is (are) correct?
   (1) It is located in the anterior part of the internal capsule.
   (2) It contains axons derived from nerve cells in the lateral geniculate body.

(3) The axons pass directly to the area of Wernicke.

(4) The axons terminate in area 17 of the cerebral cortex.

10. Which of the following statements concerning the direct light reflex is (are) correct?

(1) The nerve impulses travel through the optic nerve, the optic chiasma, and the optic tract.

(2) The pretectal nucleus is an important relay station.

(3) The Edinger-Westphal nuclei on both sides of the midbrain are stimulated.

(4) The ciliary ganglia of both eyes are stimulated.

11. Which of the following statements concerning the consensual light reflex is (are) correct?

(1) The parasympathetic nuclei of both oculomotor nerves are involved.

(2) The fibers from the pretectal nuclei cross the midline close to the cerebral aqueduct in the posterior commissure.

(3) With an Argyll Robertson pupil the pretectal fibers passing to the oculomotor nucleus are destroyed by syphilis.

(4) The optic radiation is involved with this reflex.

12. The cerebral cortex plays an essential role in the following reflexes:

(1) Pupillary light reflex.

(2) Corneal reflex.

(3) Consensual light reflex.

(4) Accommodation reflex.

13. The nasal field of vision of the left eye is projected to:

(1) Right lateral geniculate body.

(2) Left lateral geniculate body.

(3) Nasal retina of the left eye.

(4) Both banks of the left calcarine fissure.

Match the numbered lesions of the optic pathways shown in Figure 18-7 and listed below on the left with the appropriate lettered visual defects shown on the right. An answer may be used more than once.

14. Number 1.   A. Bitemporal hemianopia.
15. Number 2.   B. Left temporal hemianopia and right nasal hemianopia.
16. Number 3.   C. Right nasal hemianopia (only).
17. Number 4.   D. Left nasal hemianopia (only).
                    E. None of the above.

Select the **best** response:

18. Which of the following statements concerning the oculomotor nerve is correct?

A. The nerve has three nuclei.

B. It contains both motor and sensory fibers.

C. The nuclei lie in the midbrain at the level of the superior colliculus.

D. The nerve fibers pass posteriorly around the red nucleus.

E. The somatic motor nucleus receives corticobulbar fibers only from the contralateral cerebral cortex.

19. The following statements concerning the oculomotor nerve are correct **except:**

A. The motor nucleus receives tectobulbar fibers from the superior colliculus.

B. The nerve may be found in the interpeduncular fossa.

Fig. 18-7   *The optic pathway.*

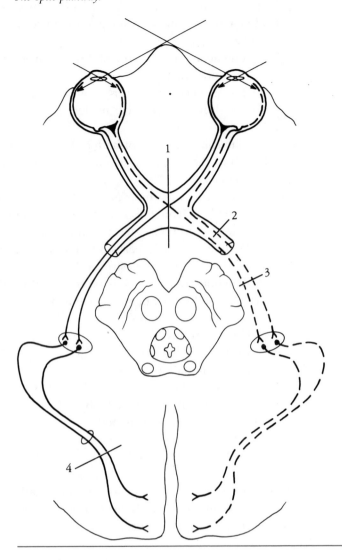

C. The motor nucleus is connected to the nuclei of the fourth, sixth, and eighth cranial nerves.

D. The nerve passes into the orbital cavity through the inferior orbital fissure.

E. The motor nucleus receives nerve fibers from the medial longitudinal fasciculus.

20. The following statements concerning the function of the oculomotor nerve are correct **except:**

    A. It accommodates the eye.

    B. It raises the upper eyelid.

    C. It innervates the lateral rectus muscle and thus turns the eye laterally.

    D. It turns the eye downward.

    E. It constricts the pupil.

21. The following statements concerning the trochlear nerve are correct **except:**

    A. It supplies the superior oblique muscle.

    B. It immediately decussates with the nerve of the opposite side on emerging from the brain.

    C. The nucleus is located in the midbrain at the level of the inferior colliculus.

D. The nucleus receives corticobulbar fibers from both cerebral hemispheres.

E. It is a large nerve that is rarely damaged in patients with head injuries.

22. The following statements concerning a lesion of the trochlear nerve are correct **except:**

A. The patient's eye tends to turn medially.

B. The nerve lesion is of the upper motor neuron type.

C. The nerve lesion is of the lower motor neuron type.

D. The patient has great difficulty in turning the eye downward and laterally.

E. The patient complains of double vision.

ANSWERS AND EXPLANATIONS

1. B: (1) All the cranial nerves are distributed in the head and neck except the tenth, which also supplies structures in the thorax and abdomen.

2. C

3. D: (1) All motor neurons of the cranial nerve nuclei receive descending motor fibers from both cerebral hemispheres, except those of the facial nerve nucleus that supply the muscles of the lower part of the face and those of the hypoglossal nucleus that supply the genioglossus muscle. These exceptional motor neurons only receive descending fibers from the cortex of the opposite cerebral hemisphere. (2) The descending corticonuclear (corticobulbar) fibers pass through the crus cerebri of the midbrain along with the corticospinal fibers; the corticonuclear fibers are situated medial to the corticospinal fibers.

4. C

5. E

6. E

7. E

8. B: (1) the optic tract contains fibers from the nasal half of the retina of the opposite side and the temporal half of the retina of the same side. (2) There are no sympathetic fibers in the optic tract.

9. C: (1) The optic radiation is located in the posterior part of the internal capsule. (3) No fibers of the optic radiation pass to the area of Wernicke.

10. E

11. A: (4) The optic radiation is not involved with this reflex.

12. D

13. C

14. A

15. C

16. B

17. E

18. C: A. The nerve has two nuclei, a somatic motor nucleus and a parasympathetic autonomic motor nucleus (Edinger-Westphal nucleus). B. It contains only motor fibers. D. The nerve fibers pass anteriorly through the red nucleus. E. The somatic motor nucleus receives corticobulbar fibers from the cerebral cortex of both cerebral hemispheres.

19. D: The oculomotor nerve enters the orbital cavity through the superior orbital fissure.

20. C: The lateral rectus muscle is innervated by the sixth cranial nerve.

21. E: The trochlear nerve is long and slender and is commonly damaged in head injuries.

22. B: The nerve lesion involves the axons of the lower motor neuron.

19 Cranial Nerves V-VIII

SUGGESTED PLAN FOR REVIEW OF CHAPTER 19

1. The detail of all these cranial nerves must be learned.
2. The trigeminal nerve and its branches are frequently involved by trauma and disease. The nerve and its nuclei provide many good questions for examiners.
3. The abducent nerve only does one thing—it supplies the lateral rectus muscle of the eye. It would be a good opportunity now for the reader to review the gross anatomy of the extraocular muscles of the eye with their nerve supply and understand and learn their actions on the eyeball.
4. The facial nerve is frequently involved by disease, which may affect the lower or the upper motor neurons. Remember that the neurons in the main motor nucleus that supply the muscles of the lower part of the face receive cortico-bulbar fibers only from the opposite cerebral cortex.
5. The vestibulocochlear nerve is complicated but the details should be learned.

INTRODUCTION

The trigeminal nerve (V) is the largest cranial nerve. It is called the trigeminal nerve because it has three major branches: **ophthalmic (V1), maxillary (V2), and mandibular (V3).** The main trunk of the trigeminal nerve leaves the ventral surface of the pons as a large sensory root and a small motor root. The sensory fibers are largely distributed to the skin of the face and the motor fibers innervate the muscles of mastication.

The abducent nerve (VI) is a small motor nerve that leaves the ventral surface of the brain between the pons and the medulla oblongata. It innervates the lateral rectus muscle of the eye.

The facial nerve (VII) has two nerve roots that leave the ventral surface of the brain between the pons and medulla oblongata. The motor root is distributed mainly to the muscles of facial expression. The sensory root contains taste fibers from the mouth and palate and carries secretomotor fibers to the salivary glands, the nasal and palatine glands, and the lacrimal gland.

The vestibulocochlear nerve consists of two distinct parts, the **vestibular nerve** and the **cochlear nerve,** which leave the ventral surface of the brain between the pons and the medulla oblongata. They are concerned with the transmission of afferent information from the internal ear to the central nervous system.

The purpose of this chapter is to discuss the nuclei of these cranial nerves, their central connections, and their distribution.

TRIGEMINAL NERVE (CRANIAL NERVE V)

Trigeminal Nerve Nuclei. The trigeminal nerve contains both sensory and motor fibers. It has four nuclei: (1) the main sensory nucleus, (2) the spinal nucleus, (3) the mesencephalic nucleus, and (4) the motor nucleus.

MAIN SENSORY NUCLEUS. This lies in the posterior part of the pons, lateral to the motor nucleus (Fig. 19-1). It is continuous below with the spinal nucleus.

SPINAL NUCLEUS. This is continuous superiorly with the main sensory nucleus in the pons and extends inferiorly through the medulla oblongata and the upper part of the spinal cord, as far as the second cervical segment (Fig. 19-1).

MESENCEPHALIC NUCLEUS. This is situated in the lateral part of the gray matter around the cerebral aqueduct. It extends inferiorly into the pons as far as the main sensory nucleus (Fig. 19-1).

MOTOR NUCLEUS. This is situated in the pons medial to the main sensory nucleus (Fig. 19-1).

Sensory Components of the Trigeminal Nerve. The sensations of pain, temperature, touch, and pressure from the skin of the face and mucous membranes travel along axons whose cell bodies are situated in the **trigeminal sensory ganglion.** The central processes of these cells form the sensory root of the trigeminal nerve. The fibers divide into ascending and descending branches when they enter the pons or they ascend or descend without division (Fig. 19-1). The ascending branches terminate in the main sensory nucleus and the descending branches terminate in the spinal nucleus. The sensations of touch and pressure are conveyed by nerve fibers that terminate in the main sensory nucleus. The sensations of pain and temperature pass to the spinal nucleus (Fig. 19-1). The sensory fibers from the ophthalmic division of the trigeminal nerve terminate in the inferior part of the spinal nucleus; fibers from the maxillary division terminate in the middle of the spinal nucleus; and fibers from the mandibular division end in the superior part of the spinal nucleus.

Proprioceptive impulses from the muscles of mastication and from the facial and extraocular muscles are carried by fibers in the sensory root of the trigeminal nerve that have bypassed the semilunar or trigeminal ganglion (Fig. 19-1). The fibers' cell of origin are the unipolar cells of the mesencephalic nucleus (Fig. 19-1).

The axons of the neurons in the main sensory and spinal nuclei, and the cen-

Fig. 19-1

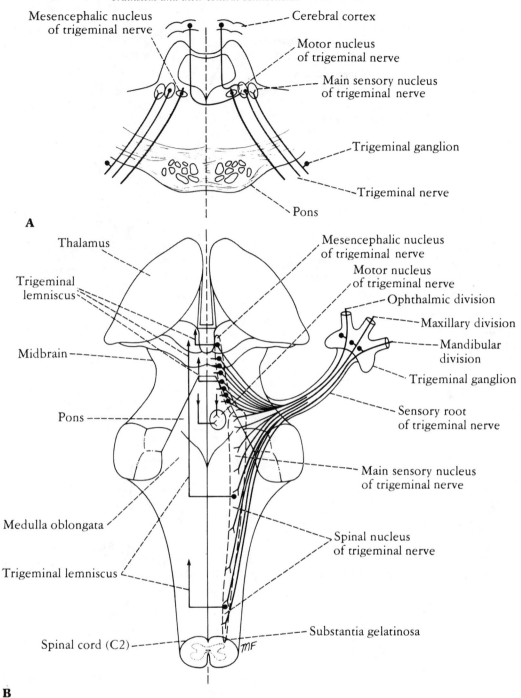

tral processes of the cells in the mesencephalic nucleus, now cross the median plane and ascend as the **trigeminal lemniscus** to terminate on nerve cells of the **ventral posteromedial nucleus of the thalamus.** The axons of these cells now travel through the internal capsule to the postcentral gyrus (areas 3, 1, and 2) of the cerebral cortex.

Motor Component of the Trigeminal Nerve. The motor nucleus receives corticonuclear fibers from both cerebral hemispheres (Fig. 19-1), fibers from the reticular formation, the red nucleus, the tectum, and the medial longitudinal fas-

Fig. 19-2

A and B. Diagrams showing the distribution of the sensory branches of the trigeminal nerve. Note that the skin area over the angle of the jaw is supplied by branches of the cervical plexus (B).

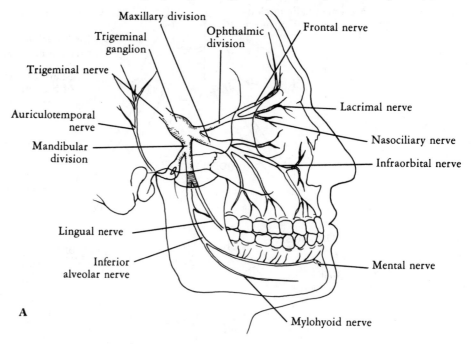

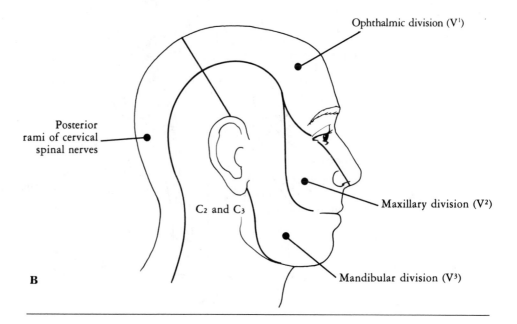

ciculus. In addition, it receives fibers from the mesencephalic nucleus, thereby forming a monosynaptic reflex arc.

The cells of the motor nucleus give rise to the axons that form the motor root. The motor nucleus supplies the **muscles of mastication,** the **tensor tympani,** the **tensor veli palatini,** and the **mylohyoid** and the **anterior belly of the digastric muscle.**

Trigeminal Nerve. The trigeminal nerve leaves the anterior aspect of the pons as a small motor root and a large sensory root. The nerve passes forward out of the posterior cranial fossa and rests on the upper surface of the apex of the petrous part of the temporal bone in the middle cranial fossa. The large sensory root now expands to form the crescent-shaped **trigeminal ganglion,** which lies within a pouch of dura mater called the **trigeminal or Meckel's cave.** The ophthalmic, maxillary, and mandibular nerves arise from anterior border of the ganglion. The ophthalmic nerve (V1) contains only sensory fibers and leaves the skull through the superior orbital fissure to enter the orbital cavity. The maxillary nerve (V2) also contains only sensory fibers and leaves the skull through the foramen rotundum. The mandibular nerve (V3) contains both sensory and motor fibers and leaves the skull through the foramen ovale.

The sensory fibers to the skin of the face from each division supply a distinct zone (Fig. 19-2), there being little or no overlap of the dermatomes. (Compare with the overlap of the dermatomes of the spinal nerves.) As noted previously, the motor fibers in the mandibular division are mainly distributed to the muscles of mastication.

Trigeminal Nerve Lesions. There will be sensory loss over each zone of the face supplied by the divisions of the trigeminal nerve. In addition, in lesions of the ophthalmic division, the cornea and conjunctiva will be insensitive to touch. Motor loss will be seen if the patient is asked to clench his teeth. The masseter and temporalis muscles can be palpated, and when the innervation is lost, they will fail to contract.

ABDUCENT NERVE (CRANIAL NERVE VI)

The abducent nerve is a small motor nerve that supplies the **lateral rectus muscle** of the eyeball. The motor nucleus is situated beneath the floor of the fourth ventricle, close to the midline and beneath the **colliculus facialis** (Fig. 19-3).

Abducent Nerve Nucleus. The nucleus receives afferent corticonuclear fibers from both cerebral hemispheres. It also receives the tectobulbar tract from the superior colliculus, by which the visual cortex is connected to the nucleus. In

Fig. 19-3   *Abducent nerve nucleus and its central connections.*

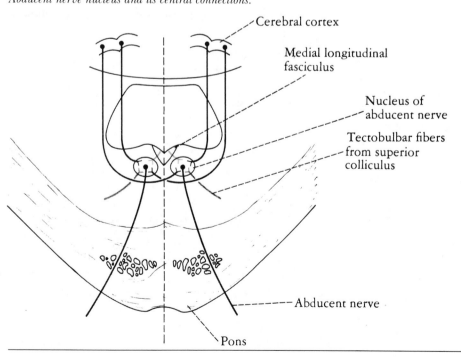

addition, it receives fibers from the medial longitudinal fasciculus, by which it is connected to the nuclei of the third, fourth, and eighth cranial nerves (Fig. 19-3).

Abducent Nerve. The fibers of the abducent nerve pass anteriorly through the pons and emerge in the groove between the lower border of the pons and the medulla oblongata. It passes forward through the cavernous sinus, lying below and lateral to the internal carotid artery. The nerve then enters the orbit through the superior orbital fissure. The abducent nerve is entirely a motor nerve and supplies the lateral rectus muscle and is, therefore, responsible for turning the eye laterally.

Abducent Nerve Lesion. A lesion of the abducent nerve causes a paralysis of the lateral rectus muscle of the eyeball and the patient is unable to turn the eye laterally. At rest the eye is turned medially (medial strabismus) by the unopposed action of the medial rectus muscle (supplied by the oculomotor nerve).

FACIAL NERVE (CRANIAL NERVE VII)

Facial Nerve Nuclei. The facial nerve has three nuclei: (1) the main motor nucleus, (2) the parasympathetic nuclei, and (3) the sensory nucleus.

MAIN MOTOR NUCLEUS. This lies in the reticular formation of the lower part of the pons (Fig. 19-4). The part of the nucleus that supplies the muscles of the upper part of the face receives corticonuclear fibers from both cerebral hemispheres. The part of the nucleus that supplies the muscles of the lower part of the face receives only corticonuclear fibers from the opposite cerebral hemisphere.

These pathways explain the voluntary control of facial muscles. However, another involuntary pathway exists, which is separate and controls **mimetic or emotional changes in facial expression.** The origin and course of this upper motor neuron pathway is unknown.

PARASYMPATHETIC NUCLEI. These lie posterolateral to the main motor nucleus. They are the **superior salivatory** and **lacrimal nuclei** (Fig. 19-4). The superior salivatory nucleus receives afferent fibers from the hypothalamus through the **descending autonomic pathways.** Information concerning taste also is received from the **nucleus of the solitary tract** from the mouth cavity.

The lacrimal nucleus receives afferent fibers from the hypothalamus for emotional responses and from the sensory nuclei of the trigeminal nerve for reflex lacrimation secondary to irritation of the cornea or conjunctiva.

SENSORY NUCLEUS. This is the upper part of the **nucleus of the tractus solitarius** and lies close to the motor nucleus (Fig. 19-4). Sensations of taste travel through the peripheral axons of nerve cells situated in the **geniculate ganglion** on the seventh cranial nerve. The central processes of these cells synapse on nerve cells in the nucleus. Efferent fibers cross the median plane and ascend to the ventral posterior medial nucleus of the opposite thalamus and also a number of hypothalamic nuclei. From the thalamus, the axons of the thalamic cells pass through the internal capsule and corona radiata to end in the taste area of the cortex in the lower part of the postcentral gyrus.

Facial Nerve. The facial nerve consists of a motor and a sensory root. The fibers of the motor root first travel posteriorly around the medial side of the abducent

Fig. 19-4   *Facial nerve nuclei and their central connections.*

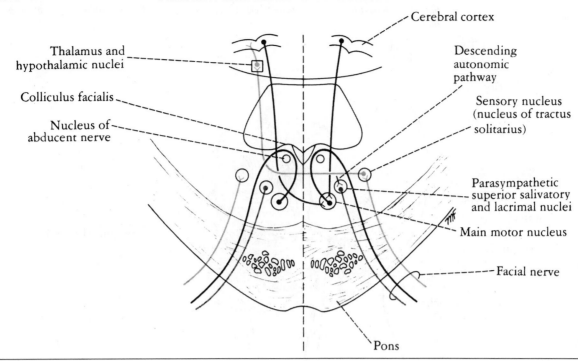

nucleus. Then they pass around the nucleus beneath the **colliculus facialis** in the floor of the fourth ventricle and finally pass anteriorly to emerge from the brainstem (Fig. 19-4).

The sensory root (**nervus intermedius**) is formed of the central processes of the unipolar cells of the geniculate ganglion. It also contains the efferent preganglionic parasympathetic fibers from the parasympathetic nuclei.

The two roots of the facial nerve emerge from the anterior surface of the brain between the pons and the medulla oblongata. They pass laterally in the posterior cranial fossa with the vestibulocochlear nerve and enter the internal acoustic meatus in the petrous part of the temporal bone. At the bottom of the meatus, the nerve enters the facial canal and runs laterally through the inner ear. On reaching the medial wall of the tympanic cavity, the nerve expands to form the sensory **geniculate ganglion** and turns sharply backward above the promontory. At the posterior wall of the tympanic cavity the facial nerve turns downward on the medial side of the aditus of the mastoid antrum, descends behind the pyramid, and emerges from the stylomastoid foramen.

Distribution of the Facial Nerve. The **motor nucleus** supplies the muscles of facial expression, the auricular muscles, the stapedius, the posterior belly of the digastric, and the stylohyoid muscles (Fig. 19-5).

The **superior salivatory nucleus** supplies the submandibular and sublingual salivary glands and the nasal and palatine glands. The **lacrimal nucleus** supplies the lacrimal gland.

The **sensory nucleus** receives taste fibers from the anterior two-thirds of the tongue, the floor of the mouth, and the soft palate.

Facial Nerve Lesions

UPPER MOTOR NEURON LESIONS. The part of the facial nucleus that controls the muscles of the upper part of the face receives corticonuclear fibers from both cerebral hemispheres, while the part of the nucleus that controls the muscles of

Fig. 19-5

Facial nerve. (A) Branches of facial nerve. (B) The branches of the facial nerve within the petrous part of the temporal bone. The taste fibers are shown in white. The glossopharyngeal nerve is also included.

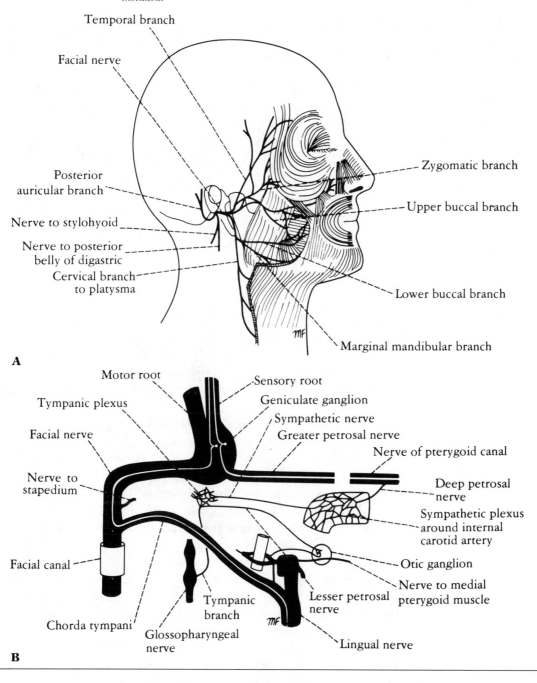

A

B

the lower part of the face receives corticonuclear fibers from only the opposite cerebral hemisphere. Therefore it follows that with a lesion involving the upper motor neurons on one side, the muscles of the lower part of the face on the opposite side will be paralyzed. The angle of the mouth will sag on that side.

LOWER MOTOR NEURON LESIONS. In lesions of the facial nerve nucleus or the facial nerve itself, all muscles of the face on the affected side will be paralyzed. The eyelid will droop, and the angle of the mouth will sag. Tears will flow over the lower eyelid, and saliva will dribble from the corner of the mouth. The patient will be unable to close the eye and will be unable to expose the teeth fully on the affected side.

SECRETOMOTOR LOSS. Secretory activity of the lacrimal, submandibular, and sublingual glands will be lost.

SENSORY LOSS. The sensation of taste for the anterior two-thirds of the tongue and the floor of the mouth will be lost.

VESTIBULO-COCHLEAR NERVE (CRANIAL NERVE VIII)

This nerve consists of two distinct parts, the **vestibular nerve** and the **cochlear nerve,** which are concerned with the transmission of afferent information from the internal ear to the central nervous system (Fig. 19-6).

Vestibular Nerve. The vestibular nerve conducts nerve impulses from the utricle and saccule that provide information concerning the position of the head; the nerve also conducts impulses from the semicircular canals that provide information concerning movements of the head.

The nerve fibers of the vestibular nerve are the central processes of nerve cells located in the **vestibular ganglion,** which is situated in the **internal acoustic meatus.** They enter the anterior surface of the brainstem in a groove between

Fig. 19-6   *Vestibular nerve nuclei and their central connections.*

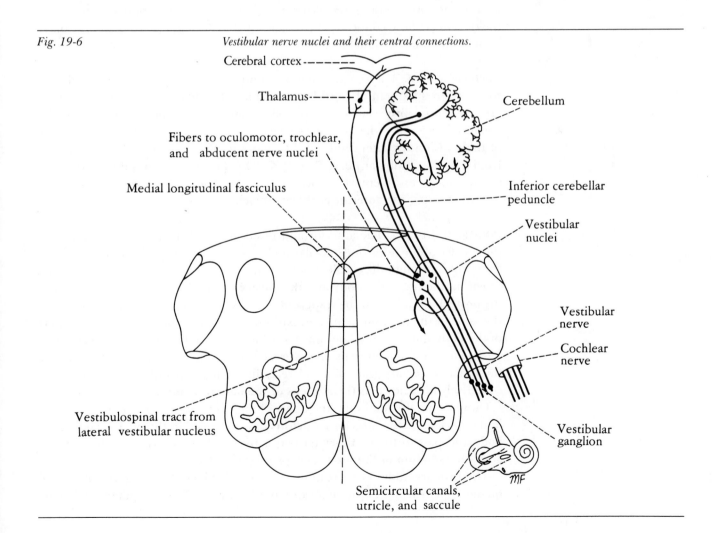

the lower border of the pons and the upper part of the medulla oblongata (Fig. 19-6). On entering the vestibular nuclear complex, the fibers divide into short ascending and long descending fibers; a small number of fibers pass directly to the cerebellum through the inferior cerebellar peduncle, thus bypassing the vestibular nuclei.

VESTIBULAR NUCLEAR COMPLEX. This complex consists of a group of four nuclei situated beneath the floor of the fourth ventricle (Fig. 19-7): (1) the **lateral vestibular nucleus,** (2) the **superior vestibular nucleus,** (3) the **medial vestibular nucleus,** and (4) the **inferior vestibular nucleus.**

The vestibular nuclei receive afferent fibers from the **utricle,** the **saccule,** and the **semicircular canals** through the vestibular nerve and fibers from the cerebellum through the inferior cerebellar peduncle. Efferent fibers from the nuclei pass to the cerebellum through the inferior cerebellar peduncle. Efferent fibers also descend uncrossed to the spinal cord from the lateral vestibular nucleus and form the **vestibulospinal tract** (Fig. 19-6). In addition, efferent fibers pass to the nuclei of the oculomotor, trochlear, and abducent nerves through the medial longitudinal fasciculus.

As the result of these connections the movements of the head and the eyes can be coordinated, so that visual fixation on an object may be maintained. The information received from the internal ear can assist in maintaining balance, by influencing the muscle tone of the limbs and trunk.

Ascending fibers also pass upward from the vestibular nuclei to the vestibular area in the postcentral gyrus. After relaying in the ventral posterior nuclei of the thalamus, these connections probably enable the cerebral cortex consciously to orientate the individual to space.

Cochlear Nerve. The cochlear nerve conducts nerve impulses concerned with sound from the organ of Corti in the cochlea. The fibers of the cochlear nerve are the central processes of nerve cells located in the **spiral ganglion of the cochlea.** They enter the anterior surface of the brainstem at the lower border of the pons on the lateral side of the emerging facial nerve and are separated from it by the vestibular nerve (Fig. 19-7). On entering the pons the nerve fibers divide, one branch entering the **posterior cochlear nucleus** and the other branch entering the **anterior cochlear nucleus.**

COCHLEAR NUCLEI. The anterior and posterior cochlear nuclei are situated on the surface of the inferior cerebellar peduncle. They receive afferent fibers from the cochlea through the cochlear nerve. The cochlear nuclei send axons medially to end in the trapezoid body and the olivary nucleus. Here they are relayed in the **posterior nucleus of the trapezoid body** and the superior olivary nucleus on the same or the opposite side. The axons now ascend through the posterior part of the pons and midbrain and form a tract known as the **lateral lemniscus** (Fig. 19-7). Each lateral lemniscus, therefore, consists of neurons from both sides. As these fibers ascend, some of them relay in small groups of nerve cells, which collectively are known as the **nucleus of the lateral lemniscus** (Fig. 19-7).

On reaching the midbrain, the fibers of the lateral lemniscus either terminate in the nucleus of the **inferior colliculus** or are relayed in the **medial geniculate body** and pass to the **auditory cortex** of the cerebral hemisphere through the **acoustic radiation of the internal capsule** (Fig. 19-7).

The primary auditory cortex (areas 41 and 42) includes the gyrus of Heschl on the upper surface of the superior temporal gyrus. The recognition and inter-

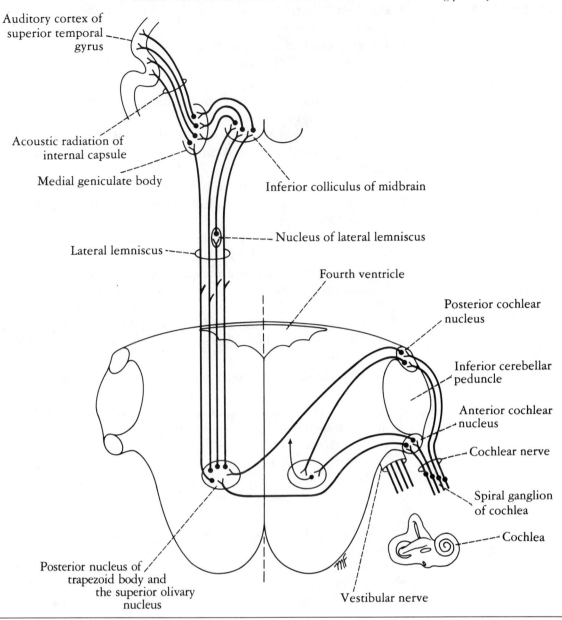

Auditory cortex of
superior temporal
gyrus

Acoustic radiation of
internal capsule

Medial geniculate body

Lateral lemniscus

Inferior colliculus of midbrain

Nucleus of lateral lemniscus

Fourth ventricle

Posterior cochlear
nucleus

Inferior cerebellar
peduncle

Anterior cochlear
nucleus

Cochlear nerve

Spiral ganglion
of cochlea

Cochlea

Posterior nucleus of
trapezoid body and
the superior olivary
nucleus

Vestibular nerve

pretation of sounds on the basis of past experience takes place in the secondary auditory area.

Vestibulocochlear Nerve. The vestibular and cochlear parts of the nerve leave the anterior surface of the brain between the lower border of the pons and the medulla oblongata and run laterally in the posterior cranial fossa entering the internal acoustic meatus with the facial nerve.

VESTIBULOCOCHLEAR NERVE LESIONS. The vestibular fibers are concerned with the sense of position and movement of the head. The cochlear fibers are concerned with the sense of hearing. Disturbances of vestibular function include giddiness (vertigo) and nystagmus. Disturbances of cochlear function include deafness and tinnitus.

In each of the following questions, answer:
A. If only (1) is correct
B. If only (2) is correct
C. If both (1) and (2) are correct
D. If neither (1) nor (2) is correct

1. Which of the following facts concerning the trigeminal nerve is (are) correct?
   (1) The trigeminal nerve has a large motor root and a small sensory root.
   (2) The trigeminal nerve leaves the brain on the anterior surface of the pons.
2. Which of the following facts concerning the nuclei of the trigeminal nerve is (are) correct?
   (1) The main sensory nucleus is continuous below with the spinal nucleus.
   (2) The spinal nucleus extends inferiorly as far as the second cervical segment of the spinal cord.
3. Which of the following facts concerning the mesencephalic nucleus of the trigeminal nerve is (are) correct?
   (1) It receives information from the muscles of facial expression and the extraocular muscles.
   (2) The afferent fibers from the muscles of mastication are the peripheral nerve processes of the unipolar cells in the mesencephalic nucleus.
4. Which of the following facts concerning the ascending sensory fibers from the trigeminal nuclei is (are) correct?
   (1) The trigeminal lemniscus terminates in the ventral posteromedial nucleus of the thalamus.
   (2) They ascend without crossing to the opposite side of the brainstem.
5. Which of the following facts concerning the motor nucleus of the trigeminal nerve is (are) correct?
   (1) It only receives fibers from the cerebral cortex of the opposite cerebral hemisphere.
   (2) The motor nucleus not only supplies the muscles of mastication but also the mylohyoid and the anterior belly of the digastric muscles.
6. Which of the following facts concerning the trigeminal ganglion is (are) correct?
   (1) The central processes of the nerve cells of the ganglion form the sensory root of the trigeminal nerve.
   (2) The afferent fibers of the mesencephalic nucleus bypass the ganglion.

In each of the following questions, answer:
A. If only (1), (2), and (3) are correct
B. If only (1) and (3) are correct
C. If only (2) and (4) are correct
D. If only (4) is correct
E. If all are correct

7. Which of the following statements concerning the ophthalmic division of the trigeminal nerve is (are) correct?
   (1) It contains only sensory fibers.
   (2) Its main branches leave the skull through the superior orbital fissure.
   (3) It supplies the skin of the forehead and the nose down as far as its tip.
   (4) The dermatome overlaps for some distance that of the maxillary nerve.
8. Which of the following statements concerning a lesion of the trigeminal nerve is (are) correct?

(1) The masseter muscle cannot be felt to contract.

(2) There is a loss of skin sensation over the angle of the jaw.

(3) The cornea and conjunctiva will be insensitive to touch.

(4) The temporalis muscle will be felt to contract.

9. Which of the following statements concerning the abducent nerve is (are) correct?

    (1) The motor nucleus has the motor root of the facial nerve winding around it.

    (2) The nucleus lies below the floor of the fourth ventricle.

    (3) The nerve leaves the brain on its anterior surface between the pons and the medulla oblongata.

    (4) The nerve supplies the lateral rectus muscle.

10. Which of the following statements concerning the facial nerve nuclei is (are) correct?

    (1) The part of the motor nucleus that supplies the muscles of the lower part of the face receives corticobulbar fibers only from the contralateral cerebral cortex.

    (2) The parasympathetic nuclei supply the lacrimal, submandibular, and parotid glands with secretomotor fibers.

    (3) The sensory nucleus receives taste fibers from the anterior two-thirds of the tongue.

    (4) The motor and parasympathetic nuclei are located in the upper part of the pons.

11. Which of the following statements concerning the facial nerve is (are) correct?

    (1) The facial nerve leaves the brain on the anterior surface between the pons and the medulla oblongata.

    (2) The facial nerve accompanies the vestibulocochlear nerve into the internal acoustic meatus.

    (3) The geniculate ganglion consists of nerve cells whose function is to conduct information of taste to the central nervous system.

    (4) The parasympathetic nerve fibers travel with the somatic nerve fibers in the motor root of the facial nerve.

12. Which of the following statements concerning a lesion of the facial nerve is (are) correct?

    (1) All the muscles of the face on the affected side will be paralyzed.

    (2) A lesion of the facial nerve produces identical signs and symptoms to a lesion of the facial motor nucleus.

    (3) There will be a loss of taste sensation on the anterior two-thirds of the tongue provided that the lesion is proximal to the point where the chorda tympani branch is given off.

    (4) The paralysis produced is that of the upper motor neuron type.

13. The nuclei associated with the facial nerve include the following:

    (1) Lacrimal nucleus.

    (2) Inferior salivatory nucleus.

    (3) Nucleus of the tractus solitarius.

    (4) Hypoglossal nucleus.

14. Which of the following nerve structure(s) participate(s) in the reception of sound?

    (1) Trigeminal nerve.

    (2) Lateral lemniscus.

    (3) Facial nerve.

    (4) Medial lemniscus.

15. Which of the following facts concerning the vestibular nuclei is (are) correct?
    (1) They are four in number.
    (2) They are located beneath the floor of the fourth ventricle.
    (3) They receive afferent fibers from the utricle and saccule of the internal ear.
    (4) They are connected to the third, fourth, and sixth cranial nerve nuclei by the medial longitudinal fasciculus.

16. Which of the following facts concerning the cochlear nerve is (are) correct?
    (1) The nerve fibers are the central processes of nerve cells in the spiral ganglion of the cochlea.
    (2) The nerve fibers end in the anterior and posterior cochlear nuclei.
    (3) Each lateral lemniscus consists of ascending nerve fibers concerned with the reception of sound from both ears.
    (4) The fibers of the lateral lemniscus terminate in the lateral geniculate body.

17. Which of the following facts concerning the reception of sound is (are) correct?
    (1) The nerve impulses pass through the acoustic radiation.
    (2) The primary auditory cortex is area 41 and 42.
    (3) The inferior colliculus is involved in the process.
    (4) The cochlear nuclei send axons to the trapezoid body.

Match the numbered structures in the pons shown in Figure 19-8 and listed below on the left with the appropriate lettered structures listed below on the right. An answer may be used more than once.

18. Number 1.   A. Nucleus of the tractus solitarius.
19. Number 2.   B. Superior salivatory nucleus.
20. Number 3.   C. Nucleus of abducent nerve.
21. Number 4.   D. Motor nucleus of facial nerve.
22. Number 5.   E. None of the above.

Fig. 19-8   *Transverse section through the caudal part of the pons.*

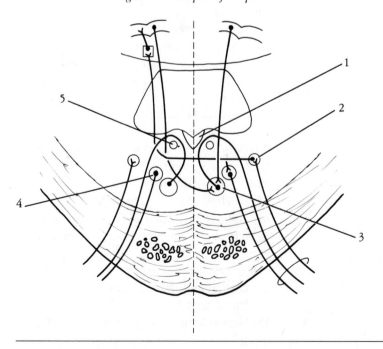

1. B: (1) The trigeminal nerve has a large sensory root and a small motor root.

2. C

3. C

4. A: (2) The ascending sensory fibers from the trigeminal nuclei cross to the opposite side of the brainstem.

5. B: (1) The motor nucleus of the trigeminal nerve receives descending fibers from the cerebral cortex on both sides.

6. C

7. A: (4) The dermatomes of the ophthalmic, maxillary, and mandibular divisions of the trigeminal nerve do not overlap.

8. B: (2) The skin over the angle of the jaw is supplied by the great auricular nerve (C2 and C3) and not by the trigeminal nerve. (4) The temporalis muscle is a muscle of mastication and is paralyzed if the trunk of the trigeminal nerve is cut.

9. E

10. B: (2) The parotid gland receives secretomotor fibers from the inferior salivatory nucleus of the glossopharyngeal nerve. (4) The motor and parasympathetic nuclei are located in the lower part of the pons.

11. A: (4) The parasympathetic secretomotor fibers travel in the sensory root (nervus intermedius) of the facial nerve.

12. A: (4) The paralysis produced by a lesion of the facial nerve is of the lower motor neuron type.

13. B: (2) The inferior salivatory nucleus is part of the glossopharyngeal nerve group of nuclei. (4) The hypoglossal nucleus is not associated in any way with the facial nerve.

14. A: (1) The trigeminal nerve supplies the tensor tympani muscle. (2) The lateral lemniscus conducts nervous impulses concerned with sound from the trapezoid body to the inferior colliculus or the medial geniculate body. (3) The facial nerve supplies the stapedius muscle in the middle ear, which is concerned with damping down the excessive oscillations of the stapes bone.

15. E

16. A: (4) The lateral geniculate body is concerned with light reflexes.

17. E

18. E

19. A

20. D

21. B

22. C

20 Cranial Nerves IX-XII

SUGGESTED PLAN FOR REVIEW OF CHAPTER 20

1. Learn the details of all these cranial nerves.
2. Note that the glossopharyngeal and vagus nerves form part of the cranial parasympathetic outflow (the oculomotor and the facial nerves are the other contributors).
3. Understand the lengthy distribution of the vagus nerve through the thorax and the abdomen. Realize that the abdominal part of the vagus nerve is distributed to the intestinal tract down as far as the splenic flexure of the colon. Appreciate that the branches of the vagus nerve below the stomach cannot be seen with the naked eye in dissected specimens; they run close to the sympathetic nerves along the arteries in the branches of the superior mesenteric plexus.
4. Remember that the accessory nerve has two parts, cranial and spinal. The cranial part is distributed within the branches of the vagus nerve.
5. Appreciate that the nuclei of cranial nerves IX to XII are located very close to one another in the medulla oblongata and that consequently disease usually affects more than one of these nerves.
6. Learn the hypoglossal nerve carefully. Understand the movements of the tongue, especially those involving the genioglossus muscles. When a patient is asked to protrude the tongue, the tongue is pulled forward by the equal contraction of both the right and left genioglossus muscles, which are attached in front to the mandible. If both muscles are acting normally with equal strength, the tongue will protrude forward in the midline. If, for example, the right genioglossus is weaker than the left, then the tip of the tongue will point to the right, i.e., it will be pulled forward and pushed over to the right by the stronger left muscle.

INTRODUCTION

The glossopharyngeal nerve (IX) is a sensory and a motor nerve. It receives sensations from the posterior third of the tongue, the pharynx, and the middle ear and has an afferent input from the carotid sinus and carotid body. It supplies one small muscle of the pharynx and contains parasympathetic secretomotor fibers to the parotid salivary gland.

The vague nerve (X) is the longest cranial nerve, having a course and distribution that extends through the neck, thorax, and abdomen. It is a sensory and a motor nerve and the fibers are distributed to the heart, great thoracic vessels; larynx, trachea, lungs; alimentary tract from the pharynx to the splenic flexure of the colon; liver, kidneys, and pancreas. Many of the motor fibers form part of the parasympathetic outflow.

The accessory nerve (XI) is entirely motor in function. It is an anatomical oddity in that it has a cranial root that resembles a true cranial nerve and arises from the brain inside the skull, and a spinal root that resembles an anterior root of a spinal nerve and arises from the upper five cervical segments; the spinal root then ascends through the foramen magnum to enter the skull and accompany the cranial root. A further peculiarity is that the cranial root joins the vagus nerve outside the skull and is distributed within its branches. The spinal root, as one would expect, supplies muscles in the neck, namely, the sternocleidomastoid and the trapezius.

The hypoglossal nerve (XII) is entirely motor in function and supplies the muscles of the tongue.

The purpose of this chapter is to discuss the nuclei of these cranial nerves, their central connections, and their distribution.

GLOSSOPHARYNGEAL NERVE (CRANIAL NERVE IX)

The glossopharyngeal nerve is a motor and a sensory nerve.

Glossopharyngeal Nerve Nuclei. The glossopharyngeal nerve has three nuclei: (1) the main motor nucleus, (2) the parasympathetic nucleus, and (3) the sensory nucleus.

MAIN MOTOR NUCLEUS. This is deeply placed in the medulla oblongata and is formed by part of the nucleus ambiguus (Fig. 20-1). It receives corticonuclear fibers from both cerebral hemispheres. The efferent fibers supply the stylopharyngeus muscle.

PARASYMPATHETIC NUCLEUS. This is called the **inferior salivatory nucleus** (Fig. 20-1). It receives afferent fibers from the hypothalamus through the descending autonomic pathways. It also receives information from the olfactory system through the reticular formation and information concerning taste from the nucleus of the solitary tract from the mouth cavity.

The efferent preganglionic parasympathetic fibers reach the otic ganglion through the **tympanic branch of the glossopharyngeal nerve,** the **tympanic plexus,** and the **lesser petrosal nerve.** The postganglionic fibers pass to the parotid salivary gland.

SENSORY NUCLEUS. This is part of the **nucleus of the tractus solitarius** (Fig. 20-1). Sensations of taste from the posterior one-third of the tongue and from the pharynx travel through the peripheral axons of nerve cells situated in the ganglion on the glossopharyngeal nerve. The central processes of these cells synapse on nerve cells in the nucleus. Efferent fibers cross the median plane and ascend to the ventral group of nuclei of the opposite thalamus and also a number

Fig. 20-1 *Glossopharyngeal nerve nuclei and their central connections.*

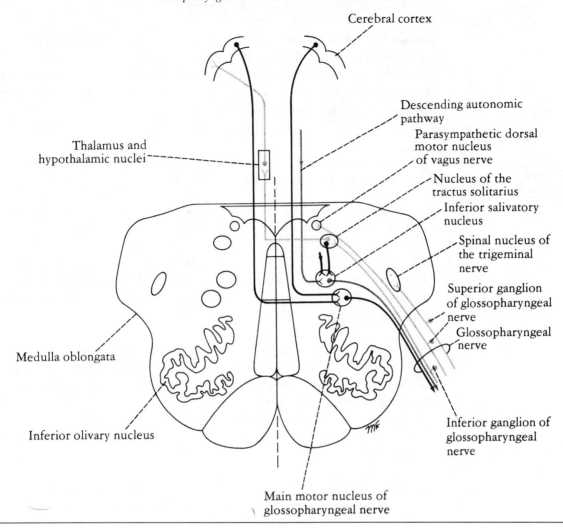

Cerebral cortex

Thalamus and hypothalamic nuclei

Descending autonomic pathway

Parasympathetic dorsal motor nucleus of vagus nerve

Nucleus of the tractus solitarius

Inferior salivatory nucleus

Spinal nucleus of the trigeminal nerve

Superior ganglion of glossopharyngeal nerve

Glossopharyngeal nerve

Medulla oblongata

Inferior olivary nucleus

Inferior ganglion of glossopharyngeal nerve

Main motor nucleus of glossopharyngeal nerve

of hypothalamic nuclei. From the thalamus, axons pass through the internal capsule and corona radiata to end in the lower part of the postcentral gyrus.

Note that afferent information that concerns common sensation from the posterior one-third of the tongue, the pharynx, and the ear enters the brainstem through the superior ganglion of the glossopharyngeal nerve, but ends in the spinal nucleus of the trigeminal nerve. Afferent impulses from the carotid sinus, a baroreceptor situated at the bifurcation of the common carotid artery, also travel with the glossopharyngeal nerve. They terminate in the **dorsal motor nucleus of the vagus nerve.** The carotid sinus reflex that involves the glossopharyngeal and vagus nerves assists in the regulation of arterial blood pressure.

Glossopharyngeal Nerve. The glossopharyngeal nerve emerges from the anterior surface of the medulla oblongata between the olive and the inferior cerebellar peduncle (Fig. 20-1). It passes laterally in the posterior cranial fossa and leaves the skull through the jugular foramen. The superior and inferior glossopharyngeal ganglia are situated on the nerve here. The nerve then descends through the upper part of the neck in company with the internal jugular vein and the internal carotid artery to reach the posterior border of the stylopharyngeus muscle, which it supplies. The nerve then passes forward between the superior and middle constrictor muscles to give sensory branches to the mucous membrane of the pharynx and the posterior third of the tongue.

Glossopharyngeal Nerve Lesions. The glossopharyngeal nerve supplies the stylopharyngeus muscle and sends secretomotor fibers to the parotid salivary gland. Sensory fibers innervate the posterior one-third of the tongue. The integrity of the nerve may be evaluated by the patient's sensation for touch and taste on the posterior one-third of the tongue.

| VAGUS NERVE (CRANIAL NERVE X) | The vagus nerve is a motor and a sensory nerve. |

VAGUS NERVE (CRANIAL NERVE X)

The vagus nerve is a motor and a sensory nerve.

Vagus Nerve Nuclei. The vagus nerve has three nuclei: (1) the main motor nucleus, (2) the parasympathetic nucleus, and (3) the sensory nucleus.

MAIN MOTOR NUCLEUS. This is deeply placed in the medulla oblongata and is formed by the nucleus ambiguus (Fig. 20-2). It receives corticonuclear fibers from both cerebral hemispheres. The efferent fibers supply the constrictor muscles of the pharynx and the intrinsic muscles of the larynx.

PARASYMPATHETIC NUCLEUS. This forms the **dorsal nucleus of the vagus** and lies beneath the floor of the lower part of the fourth ventricle (Fig. 20-2). It receives afferent fibers from the hypothalamus. It also receives other afferents, including those from the glossopharyngeal nerve (carotid sinus reflex). The efferent fibers are distributed to the involuntary muscle of the bronchi, heart, esophagus, stomach, small intestine, and large intestine as far as the distal one-third of the transverse colon.

SENSORY NUCLEUS. This is the lower part of the **nucleus of the tractus solitarius.** Sensations of taste from the pharynx travel through the peripheral axons of nerve cells situated in the **inferior ganglion of the vagus nerve.** The central processes of those cells synapse on nerve cells in the nucleus (Fig. 20-2). Efferent fibers cross the median plane and ascend to the ventral group of nuclei of the opposite thalamus and also to the hypothalamus. From the thalamus axons pass through the internal capsule and corona radiata to end in the postcentral gyrus.

Note that afferent information, concerning common sensation from the pharynx and larynx, enters the brainstem through the superior ganglion of the vagus nerve but ends in the **spinal nucleus of the trigeminal nerve.**

Vagus Nerve. The vagus nerve emerges from the anterior surface of the medulla oblongata between the olives and the inferior cerebellar peduncle (Fig. 20-2). The nerve passes laterally through the posterior cranial fossa and leaves the skull through the jugular foramen. The vagus nerve possesses two sensory ganglia, a rounded **superior ganglion,** situated on the nerve within the jugular foramen, and a cylindrical **inferior ganglion,** which lies on the nerve just below the foramen. Below the inferior ganglion, the cranial root of the accessory nerve joins the vagus nerve and is distributed mainly in its pharyngeal and recurrent laryngeal branches.

The vagus nerve descends vertically in the neck within the carotid sheath with the internal jugular vein and the internal and common carotid arteries.

The **right vagus nerve** enters the thorax and passes posterior to the root of the right lung contributing to the pulmonary plexus. It then passes on to the

Fig. 20-2   *Vagus nerve nuclei and their central connections.*

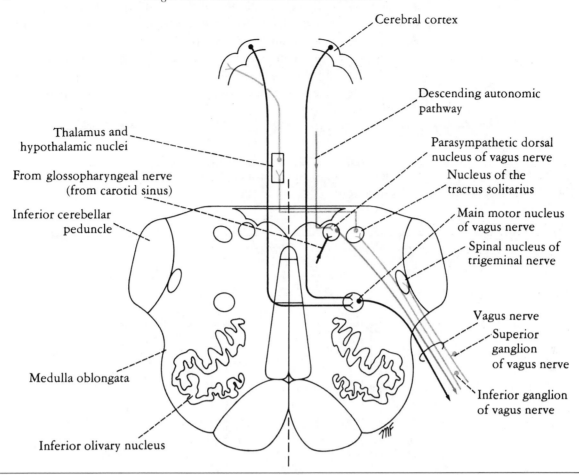

Cerebral cortex

Descending autonomic pathway

Thalamus and hypothalamic nuclei

Parasympathetic dorsal nucleus of vagus nerve

Nucleus of the tractus solitarius

From glossopharyngeal nerve (from carotid sinus)

Main motor nucleus of vagus nerve

Inferior cerebellar peduncle

Spinal nucleus of trigeminal nerve

Vagus nerve

Superior ganglion of vagus nerve

Medulla oblongata

Inferior ganglion of vagus nerve

Inferior olivary nucleus

posterior surface of the esophagus and contributes to the **esophageal plexus.** It enters the abdomen through the esophageal opening of the diaphragm. The posterior vagal trunk (which is the name now given to the right vagus) is distributed to the posterior surface of the stomach and by a large celiac branch to the duodenum, liver, kidneys, and small and large intestine as far as the distal third of the transverse colon. This wide distribution is accomplished through the celiac, superior mesenteric, and renal plexuses.

The **left vagus nerve** enters the thorax, crosses the left side of the aortic arch, and descends behind the root of the left lung contributing to the **pulmonary plexus.** The left vagus then descends on the anterior surface of the esophagus contributing to the **esophageal plexus.** It enters the abdomen through the esophageal opening of the diaphragm. The anterior vagal trunk (which is the name now given to the left vagus) divides into several branches, which are distributed to the stomach, liver, and upper part of the duodenum and head of the pancreas.

Vagus Nerve Lesions. The vagus nerve innervates many important organs, but the examination of this nerve depends on testing the function of the branches to the pharynx, soft palate, and larynx. The pharyngeal reflex may be tested by touching the lateral wall of the pharynx with a spatula. This should immediately cause the patient to gag; that is, the pharyngeal muscles will contract.

The innervation of the soft palate may be tested by asking the patient to say "ah." Normally, the soft palate rises and the uvula moves backward in the midline. For example, if there is a lesion of the right vagus nerve, the uvula will be pulled upward, backward, and to the left, since the right muscles are paralyzed.

All the muscles of the larynx are supplied by the recurrent laryngeal branch of the vagus, except the cricothyroid muscle, which is supplied by the external laryngeal branch of the superior laryngeal branch of the vagus. Hoarseness or absence of the voice may occur as a symptom of vagal nerve palsy. The movements of the vocal cords may be examined by means of a laryngoscope.

ACCESSORY NERVE (CRANIAL NERVE XI)

The accessory nerve is a motor nerve that is formed by the union of a cranial and a spinal root.

Fig. 20-3 *Cranial and spinal nuclei of the accessory nerve and their central connections.*

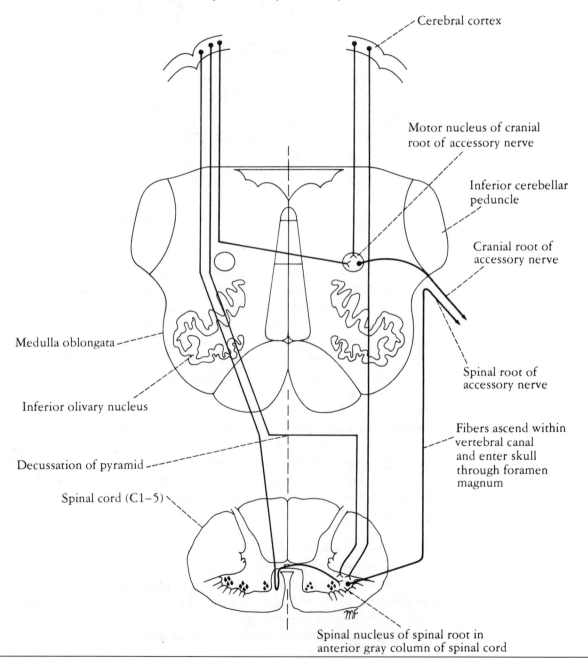

Cranial Root (Part). The cranial root is formed from the axons of nerve cells of the nucleus ambiguus (Fig. 20-3). The nucleus receives corticonuclear fibers from both cerebral hemispheres. The efferent fibers of the nucleus emerge from the anterior surface of the medulla oblongata between the olive and the inferior cerebellar peduncle. The nerve runs laterally in the posterior cranial fossa and joins the spinal root. The two roots unite and leave the skull through the jugular foramen. The roots then separate and the cranial root joins the vagus nerve and is distributed in its pharyngeal and recurrent laryngeal branches to the muscles of the soft palate, pharynx, and larynx.

Spinal Root (Part). The spinal root is formed from axons of nerve cells in the **spinal nucleus,** which is situated in the anterior gray column of the spinal cord in the upper five cervical segments (Fig. 20-3). The spinal nucleus is thought to receive corticospinal fibers from both cerebral hemispheres.

The nerve fibers emerge from the spinal cord midway between the anterior and posterior nerve roots of the cervical spinal nerves. The fibers form a nerve trunk that ascends into the skull through the foramen magnum. The spinal root passes laterally and joins the cranial root as they pass through the jugular foramen. After a short distance, the spinal part separates from the cranial root, runs downward and laterally, and enters the deep surface of the sternocleidomastoid muscle, which it supplies. The nerve then crosses the posterior triangle of the neck and passes beneath the trapezius muscle, which it supplies.

The accessory nerve thus brings about movements of the soft palate, pharynx, and larynx and controls the movements of two large muscles in the neck.

Accessory Nerve Lesions. The accessory nerve supplies the sternocleidomastoid and the trapezius muscles by means of its spinal root. A lesion of the accessory nerve will result in paralysis of these muscles.

HYPOGLOSSAL NERVE (CRANIAL NERVE XII)

The hypoglossal nerve is a motor nerve and supplies all the intrinsic muscles of the tongue and, in addition, the styloglossus, the hyoglossus, and the genioglossus muscles.

Hypoglossal Nucleus. The hypoglossal nucleus is situated close to the midline immediately beneath the floor of the lower part of the fourth ventricle (Fig. 20-4). It receives corticonuclear fibers from both cerebral hemispheres. However, the cells responsible for supplying the genioglossus muscle only receive corticonuclear fibers from the opposite cerebral hemisphere.

The hypoglossal nerve fibers emerge on the anterior surface of the medulla oblongata between the pyramid and the olive (Fig. 20-4). It crosses the posterior cranial fossa and leaves the skull through the hypoglossal canal. The nerve passes downward and forward in the neck between the internal carotid artery and the internal jugular vein until it reaches the lower border of the posterior belly of the digastric muscle. Here, it turns forward and crosses the internal and external carotid arteries and the loop of the lingual artery. It passes deep to the posterior margin of the mylohyoid muscle lying on the lateral surface of the hypoglossus muscle. In the upper part of its course, the hypoglossal nerve is joined by C1 fibers from the cervical plexus.

Hypoglossal Nerve Lesions. In lesions of the hypoglossal nerve, the tongue deviates toward the paralyzed side. The tongue will be smaller on the side of the

Fig. 20-4   *Hypoglossal nucleus and its central connections.*

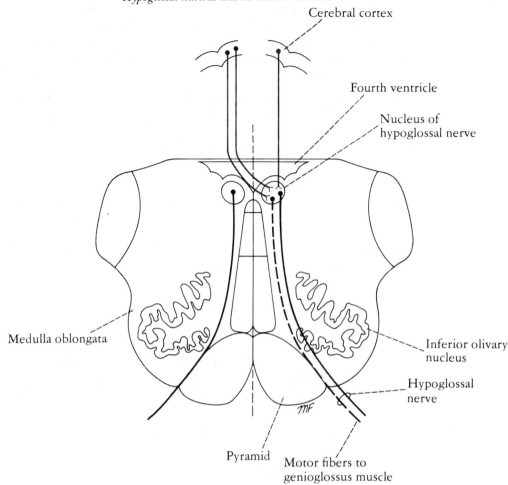

lesion, owing to muscle atrophy. The greater part of the hypoglossal nucleus receives corticonuclear fibers from both cerebral hemispheres. However, the part of the nucleus that supplies the genioglossus receives corticonuclear fibers only from the opposite cerebral hemisphere. If a patient has a lesion of the corticonuclear fibers, there will be no atrophy of the tongue and on protrusion the tongue will deviate to the side opposite the lesion. (Note that the genioglossus is the muscle that pulls the tongue forward.)

NATIONAL BOARD TYPE QUESTIONS

In each of the following questions, answer:
A. If only (1) is correct
B. If only (2) is correct
C. If both (1) and (2) are correct
D. If neither (1) nor (2) is correct

1. Which of the following statements concerning the glossopharyngeal nerve is (are) correct?
    (1) It emerges from the brainstem between the olive and the inferior cerebellar peduncle.
    (2) It possesses superior and inferior sensory ganglia.

2. Which of the following statements concerning the nuclei of the glossopharyngeal nerve is (are) correct?
   (1) The main motor nucleus is situated in the medulla oblongata and forms part of the nucleus ambiguus.
   (2) The parasympathetic nucleus controls the sublingual salivary gland.
3. Which of the following statements concerning the sensory nucleus of the glossopharyngeal nerve is (are) correct?
   (1) It forms part of the nucleus of the tractus solitarius.
   (2) It receives the sensations of taste from the posterior one-third of the tongue.
4. Which of the following statements concerning the sensory input of the glossopharyngeal nerve is (are) correct?
   (1) Common sensation impulses from the posterior one-third of the tongue end in the spinal nucleus of the trigeminal nerve.
   (2) Impulses from the carotid sinus end in the dorsal motor nucleus of the vagus nerve.
5. Which of the following statements concerning lesions of the glossopharyngeal nerve is (are) correct?
   (1) Loss of common sensation on the posterior one-third of the tongue.
   (2) Loss of taste sensation on the pharyngeal wall.
6. Which of the following statements concerning the nuclei of the vagus nerve is (are) correct?
   (1) The main motor nucleus supplies the constrictor muscles of the pharynx.
   (2) Efferent fibers from the sensory nucleus ascend to the nuclei of the ipsilateral thalamus and to the hypothalamus.

In each of the following questions, answer:
A. If only (1), (2), and (3) are correct
B. If only (1) and (3) are correct
C. If only (2) and (4) are correct
D. If only (4) is correct
E. If all are correct

7. Which of the following statements concerning the vagus nerve is (are) correct?
   (1) It forms part of the cranial parasympathetic outflow.
   (2) It innervates the alimentary tract from the pharynx down as far as the splenic flexure of the colon.
   (3) The nerve leaves the skull through the jugular foramen.
   (4) It possesses no sensory ganglia along its course.
8. Which of the following statements concerning a lesion of the vagus nerve is (are) correct?
   (1) The pharyngeal gag reflex will be lost.
   (2) The pupil will dilate.
   (3) The soft palate will be deviated to the contralateral side when the patient is instructed to say "ah."
   (4) There will be a loss of taste sensation from the anterior two-thirds of the tongue.
9. Which of the following statements concerning the spinal part of the accessory nerve is (are) correct?
   (1) It arises from the first three cervical segments of the spinal cord.
   (2) It enters the skull through the foramen magnum.
   (3) It leaves the skull through the foramen lacerum.
   (4) It supplies the sternocleidomastoid and trapezius muscles.

10. Which of the following statements concerning the cranial part of the accessory nerve is (are) correct?
    (1) It leaves the medulla oblongata between the olive and the inferior cerebellar peduncle.
    (2) It joins the spinal part of the accessory nerve within the posterior cranial fossa.
    (3) It is entirely motor in function.
    (4) It joins the vagus nerve and is distributed in its branches to the pharynx and larynx.

11. Which of the following statements concerning the hypoglossal nerve nucleus is (are) correct?
    (1) It is located beneath the floor of the lower part of the fourth ventricle.
    (2) It receives corticobulbar fibers from both cerebral hemispheres.
    (3) The neurons of the nucleus that supply the genioglossus muscle receive only corticobulbar fibers from the cerebral cortex of the contralateral side.
    (4) The motor nucleus forms part of the nucleus ambiguus.

12. Which of the following statements concerning the hypoglossal nerve is (are) correct?
    (1) It supplies all the intrinsic muscles of the tongue.
    (2) In lesions of the nerve, the tip of the tongue deviates to the same side when the tongue is protruded from the mouth.
    (3) It supplies the styloglossus and hyoglossus muscles.
    (4) It leaves the anterior surface of the brain between the pyramid and the olive.

Match the cranial nerves listed below on the left with an appropriate lettered function or structure listed below on the right. An answer may be used more than once.

13. Glossopharyngeal nerve.	A. Taste from the anterior two-thirds of the tongue.
14. Hypoglossal nerve.	B. Stylopharyngeus muscle.
15. Vagus nerve (parasympathetic fibers).	C. Opens the pyloric sphincter.
16. Spinal part of accessory nerve.	D. Muscles of the soft palate.
17. Cranial part of accessory nerve.	E. None of the above.

ANSWERS AND EXPLANATIONS

1. C
2. A: (2) The parasympathetic nucleus controls the parotid salivary gland.
3. C
4. C
5. C
6. A: (2) Efferent fibers from the sensory nucleus of the vagus cross the midline and ascend to the nuclei of the contralateral thalamus and the hypothalamus.
7. A: (4) The vagus nerve possesses a superior and an inferior sensory ganglion just within and below the jugular foramen, respectively.
8. B: (2) The pupil would dilate with a lesion of the oculomotor nerve. (4) A loss of taste sensation from the anterior two-thirds of the tongue occurs with lesions of the facial nerve or its chorda tympani branch.

9. C: (1) The spinal part of the accessory nerve arises from the upper five cervical segments of the spinal cord. (4) The spinal and cranial parts of the accessory nerve leave the skull through the jugular foramen.

10. E

11. A: (4) The motor nucleus of the hypoglossal nerve does not form part of the nucleus ambiguus.

12. E

13. B

14. E: The hypoglossal nerve supplies all the muscles of the tongue except the palatoglossus muscle (supplied by the cranial part of the accessory nerve via the branches of the vagus).

15. C

16. E: The spinal part of the accessory nerve supplies the sternocleidomastoid and trapezius muscles.

17. D

21 Autonomic Nervous System

SUGGESTED PLAN FOR REVIEW OF CHAPTER 21

1. The autonomic nervous system and the endocrine system control the internal environment of the body. The autonomic system is a difficult but important system to learn. Read the chapter slowly and commit the basic information to memory. The physiologists, the pharmacologists, and the clinicians require this information.

2. Have a precise knowledge about what is meant by the terms *sympathetic and parasympathetic outflows.*

3. Recognize that both the sympathetic and parasympathetic parts of the autonomic system have afferent and efferent fibers and higher centers of control. Appreciate that parts of the autonomic system are present in both the peripheral and central parts of the nervous system.

4. Be able to make a simple drawing of a transverse section of the spinal cord in the thoracic region showing the sympathetic outflow, the rami, and the ganglionated sympathetic trunk.

5. Be able to define: (a) gray ramus, (b) white ramus, (c) splanchnic nerve, and (d) sympathetic plexus. Understand the innervation of the suprarenal medulla.

6. Know the positions of the main parasympathetic ganglia in the head and neck.

7. Learn about neurotransmitters, ganglion blocking agents, and blocking agents concerned with cholinergic and adrenergic receptors.

8. Be able to compare the structure and functions of the sympathetic and parasympathetic parts of the autonomic system.

9. Understand the control of the autonomic nervous system and the role played by the hypothalamus.

10. Learn in detail the examples of autonomic innervations given in this chapter. These are commonly used by examiners to construct good questions.

INTRODUCTION

The autonomic nervous system, along with the endocrine system, exerts control over the functions of many organs and tissues in the body.

The autonomic nervous system, like the somatic nervous system, has afferent, connector, and efferent neurons. The afferent impulses originate in visceral receptors and travel via afferent pathways to the central nervous system where they are integrated through connector neurons at different levels and then leave via efferent pathways to visceral effector organs.

The efferent pathways of the autonomic system are made up of preganglionic and postganglionic neurons. The cell bodies of the preganglionic neurons are situated in the lateral gray column of the spinal cord and in the motor nuclei of the third, seventh, ninth, and tenth cranial nerves. The axons of these neurons synapse with the postganglionic neurons that are collected together to form **ganglia** outside the central nervous system.

The control exerted by the autonomic system is widespread since one preganglionic axon may synapse with several postganglionic neurons. Large collections of afferent and efferent nerve fibers and their associated ganglia form **autonomic plexuses** in the thorax, abdomen, and pelvis.

The visceral receptors include chemoreceptors, baroreceptors, and osmoreceptors. Pain receptors are present in viscera, and certain types of stimuli, such as oxygen lack or stretch, may cause extreme pain.

BASIC ANATOMY OF THE AUTONOMIC NERVOUS SYSTEM

The autonomic nervous system innervates involuntary structures such as the heart, the smooth muscles, and the glands. The system is distributed throughout the central and peripheral nervous systems; is divided into two parts, the **sympathetic** and the **parasympathetic;** and, as emphasized above, consists of both afferent and efferent fibers. This division between sympathetic and parasympathetic is made on the basis of anatomical differences, differences in the neurotransmitters, and differences in the physiological effects.

SYMPATHETIC PART OF THE AUTONOMIC NERVOUS SYSTEM

The sympathetic system is the larger of the two parts of the autonomic system and is widely distributed throughout the body, innervating the heart and lungs, the muscle in the walls of many blood vessels, the hair follicles and the sweat glands, and many abdominopelvic viscera.

The function of the sympathetic system is to prepare the body for an emergency. The heart rate is increased, arterioles of the skin and intestine are constricted, those of skeletal muscle are dilated, and blood pressure is raised. There is a redistribution of blood so that it leaves the skin and gastrointestinal tract and passes to the brain, heart, and skeletal muscle. In addition the sympathetic nerves dilate the pupils, inhibit smooth muscle of the bronchi, intestine, and bladder wall, and close the sphincters. The hair is made to stand on end, and sweating occurs.

The sympathetic system consists of the efferent outflow from the spinal cord, two ganglionated sympathetic trunks, important branches, plexuses, and regional ganglia.

Efferent Nerve Fibers (Sympathetic Outflow). The lateral gray columns (horns) of the spinal cord from the first thoracic segment to the second lumbar segment (sometimes third lumbar segment) possess the cell bodies of the sympathetic connector neurons (Fig. 21-1). The myelinated axons of these cells leave the cord in the anterior nerve roots and pass via the **white rami communicantes** to the **paravertebral ganglia** of the **sympathetic trunk.** Once these fibers (preganglionic) reach the ganglia in the sympathetic trunk, they are distributed as follows:

1. They synapse with an excitor neuron in the ganglion (Fig. 21-2). The gap between the two neurons is bridged by the neurotransmitter **acetylcholine.** The postganglionic nonmyelinated axons leave the ganglion and pass to the thoracic spinal nerves as **gray rami communicantes.** They are distributed in branches of the spinal nerves to smooth muscle in the blood vessel walls, sweat glands, and arrector pili muscles of the skin.
2. They travel cephalad in the sympathetic trunk to synapse in ganglia in the cervical region (Fig. 21-2). The postganglionic nerve fibers pass via gray rami communicantes to join the cervical spinal nerves. Many of the preganglionic fibers entering the lower part of the sympathetic trunk from the lower thoracic and upper two lumbar segments of the spinal cord travel caudal to synapse in ganglia in the lower lumbar and sacral regions. Here again, the postganglionic nerve fibers pass via gray rami communicantes to join the lumbar, sacral, and coccygeal spinal nerves (Fig. 21-2).

Fig. 21-1   *Arrangement of somatic part of nervous system (on left) and autonomic part of nervous system (on right).*

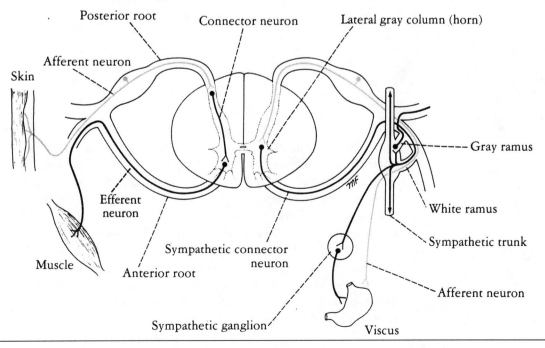

Fig. 21-2   *Efferent part of autonomic nervous system.*

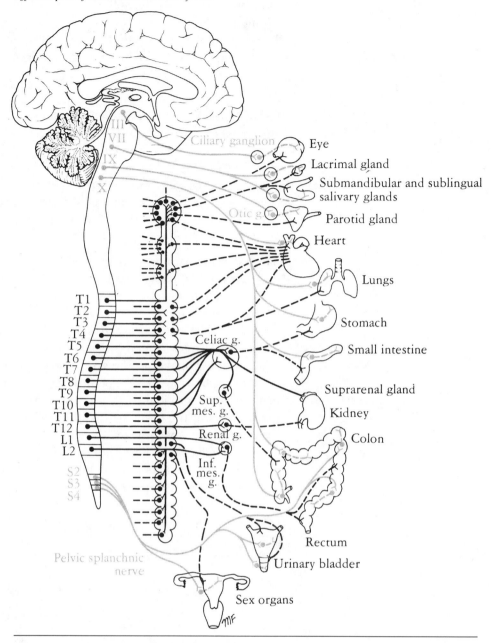

T1
T2
T3
T4
T5
T6
T7
T8
T9
T10
T11
T12
L1
L2
S2
S3
S4

Ciliary ganglion
Eye
Lacrimal gland
Submandibular and sublingual
salivary glands
Otic g
Parotid gland
Heart
Lungs
Stomach
Celiac g.
Small intestine
Suprarenal gland
Sup.
mes. g.
Kidney
Renal g.
Colon
Inf.
mes.
g.
Rectum
Pelvic splanchnic
nerve
Urinary bladder
Sex organs

3. They may pass through the ganglia of the sympathetic trunk without synapsing. These myelinated fibers leave the sympathetic trunk as the **greater splanchnic, lesser splanchnic,** and **lowest or least splanchnic nerves.** The greater splanchnic nerve is formed from branches from the fifth to the ninth thoracic ganglia. It descends obliquely on the side of the bodies of the thoracic vertebrae and pierces the crus of the diaphragm to synapse with excitor cells in the ganglia of the **celiac plexus,** the **renal plexus,** and the suprarenal medulla. The lesser splanchnic nerve is formed from branches of the tenth and eleventh thoracic ganglia. It descends with the greater splanchnic nerve and pierces the diaphragm to join excitor cells in ganglia in the lower part of the **celiac plexus.** The lowest splanchnic nerve (when present) arises from the twelfth thoracic ganglion, pierces the diaphragm, and synapses with excitor

neurons in the ganglia of the **renal plexus.** The splanchnic nerves, therefore, are formed of preganglionic fibers. The postganglionic fibers arise from the excitor cells in the peripheral plexuses and are distributed to the smooth muscle and glands of the viscera. A few preganglionic fibers, traveling in the greater splanchnic nerve, end directly on the cells of the **suprarenal medulla.**

Afferent Nerve Fibers. The afferent myelinated nerve fibers travel from the viscera through the sympathetic ganglia without synapsing. They pass to the spinal nerve via white rami communicantes and reach their cell bodies in the posterior root ganglion of the corresponding spinal nerve (Fig. 21-1). The central axons then enter the spinal cord and may form the afferent component of a local reflex arc or ascend to higher centers, such as the hypothalamus.

The Sympathetic Trunks. The sympathetic trunks are two ganglionated nerve trunks that extend the whole length of the vertebral column. (Fig. 21-2). In the neck each trunk has 3 ganglia, in the thorax there are 11 or 12, in the lumbar region 4 or 5, and in the pelvis 4 or 5.

PARASYMPATHETIC PART OF THE AUTONOMIC NERVOUS SYSTEM	The activities of the parasympathetic part of the autonomic system are directed toward conserving and restoring energy. The heart rate is slowed, pupils are constricted, peristalsis is increased and glandular activity is augmented, sphincters are opened, and the bladder wall is contracted.

Efferent Nerve Fibers (Craniosacral Outflow). The connector nerve cells of this part of the system are located in the brainstem and the sacral segments of the spinal cord (Fig. 21-2). Those nerve cells located in the brainstem form parts of the nuclei of origin of the following cranial nerves: the **oculomotor** (parasympathetic or Edinger-Westphal nucleus), the **facial** (superior salivatory nucleus and lacrimatory nucleus), the **glossopharyngeal** (inferior salivatory nucleus), and the **vagus** nerves (dorsal nucleus of vagus). The axons of these connector nerve cells emerge from the brain contained in the cranial nerves.

The sacral connector nerve cells are found in the gray matter of the **second, third, and fourth sacral segments of the cord.** These cells are not sufficiently numerous to form a lateral gray horn, as do the sympathetic connector neurons in the thoracolumbar region. The myelinated axons leave the spinal cord in the anterior nerve roots of the corresponding spinal nerves. They then leave the sacral nerves and form the **pelvic splanchnic nerves** (Fig. 21-2).

All the efferent fibers described so far are preganglionic, and they synapse with excitor neurons in the peripheral ganglia, which are usually situated close to the viscera they innervate. Here again acetylcholine is the transmitter. The cranial preganglionic fibers relay in the **ciliary, pterygopalatine, submandibular,** and **otic ganglia** (Fig. 21-2). The preganglionic fibers in the pelvic splanchnic nerves relay in ganglia in the **hypogastric** plexuses. In certain situations, the ganglion cells are diffusely arranged in nerve plexuses such as the **cardiac plexus,** the **pulmonary plexus,** and in the **myenteric** and **mucosal plexuses** of the gastrointestinal tract. The pelvic splanchnic nerves synapse in ganglia in the hypogastric plexuses. The postganglionic fibers are nonmyelinated and short in length.

Afferent Nerve Fibers. The afferent myelinated fibers leave the viscera and reach their cell bodies in the sensory ganglia of cranial nerves or in posterior root ganglia of the sacral spinal nerves. The central axons then enter the central nervous system and form regional reflex arcs or ascend to higher centers, such as the hypothalamus. Once the afferent fibers gain entrance to the spinal cord or brain, they are thought to travel alongside, or to be mixed with, the somatic afferent fibers.

THE LARGE AUTONOMIC PLEXUSES	Large collections of sympathetic and parasympathetic efferent nerve fibers and their associated ganglia, together with visceral afferent fibers, form autonomic nerve plexuses in the thorax, abdomen, and pelvis. Branches from these plexuses innervate the viscera. In the abdomen the plexuses are associated with the aorta and its branches and the subdivisions of these autonomic plexuses are named according to the branch of the aorta along which they are lying: cardiac, pulmonary, celiac, superior mesenteric, inferior mesenteric, aortic, and superior and inferior hypogastric plexus.

AUTONOMIC GANGLIA

The autonomic ganglion is the site where preganglionic fibers synapse on postganglionic neurons. Ganglia are situated along the course of efferent nerve fibers of the autonomic nervous system. Sympathetic ganglia form part of the sympathetic trunk or are prevertebral in position. Parasympathetic ganglia, on the other hand, are situated close to or within the walls of the viscera.

Preganglionic fibers are myelinated, small, and relatively slow conducting B fibers. The postganglionic fibers are unmyelinated, smaller, and slower conducting C fibers.

Preganglionic Transmitters. The synaptic transmitter that excites the postganglionic neurons in both sympathetic and parasympathetic ganglia is **acetylcholine** (Fig. 21-3). The action of acetylcholine in autonomic ganglia is terminated by **acetylcholinesterase.** The small ganglionic interneurons contain **dopamine,** which is thought to act as a transmitter.

Ganglion Blocking Agents. There are two types of ganglion blocking agents. **Nicotine** acts as a blocking agent in high concentrations, first by stimulating the postganglionic neuron by causing depolarization, and then by maintaining depolarization of the excitable membrane. **Hexamethonium** and **tetraethylammonium** block ganglia by competing with acetylcholine at the receptor sites (Fig. 21-3).

POSTGANGLIONIC NERVE ENDINGS

Postganglionic fibers terminate on the effector cells without special discrete endings. The axons run between the gland cells and the smooth and cardiac muscle cells and lose their covering of Schwann cells. At sites where transmission occurs, clusters of vesicles are present within the axoplasm. If the site on the axon is at some distance from the effector cell, transmission time may be slow. The diffusion of transmitter through large extracellular distances causes a given nerve to have an action on a large number of effector cells.

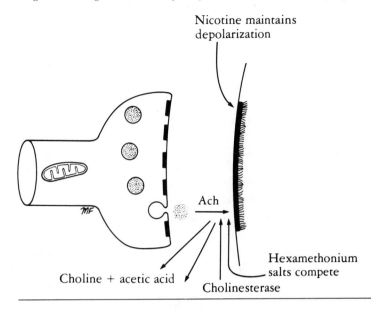

Nicotine maintains
depolarization

Ach

Choline + acetic acid

Cholinesterase

Hexamethonium
salts compete

Postganglionic Transmitters. Parasympathetic postganglionic nerve endings liberate **acetylcholine** as their transmitter substance. The acetylcholine traverses the synaptic cleft and binds reversibly with the cholinergic receptor on the postsynaptic membrane. Within 2 to 3 msec it is hydrolyzed into acetic acid and choline by the enzyme acetylcholinesterase, which is located on the surface of the nerve and receptor membranes. The choline is reabsorbed into the nerve ending and used again for synthesis of acetylcholine.

Most sympathetic postganglionic nerve endings liberate **norepinephrine** as their transmitter substance. In addition, some sympathetic postganglionic nerve endings, particularly those that end on cells of sweat glands, release **acetylcholine.**

Sympathetic endings that use norepinephrine are called **adrenergic endings.** There are two kinds of receptors in the effector organs, called **alpha** and **beta receptors.**

Two subgroups of alpha receptors (alpha-1 and alpha-2 receptors) and two subgroups of beta receptors (beta-1 and beta-2 receptors) have been described. Norepinephrine has a greater effect on alpha receptors than on beta receptors. On the other hand, beta receptors are more strongly stimulated by other adrenergic drugs such as **isoproterenol.** As a general rule alpha receptor sites are associated with most of the excitatory functions of the sympathetic system (e.g., smooth muscle contraction, vasoconstriction, diaphoresis), whereas the beta receptor sites are associated with most of the inhibitory functions (e.g., smooth muscle relaxation). Beta-2 receptors are predominant in the lung and stimulation results in bronchodilation. The myocardium, where beta receptors are associated with excitation, is an exception.

The action of norepinephrine on the receptor site of the effector cell is terminated by reuptake into the nerve terminal where it is stored in presynaptic vesicles. It is protected from inactivation by the enzyme **monoamine oxidase.**

Blocking of Cholinergic Receptors. In the case of the parasympathetic and the sympathetic postganglionic nerve endings that liberate acetylcholine as the transmitter substance, the receptors on the effector cells are **muscarinic.** This means that the action can be blocked by **atropine.** Atropine is a competitive antagonist to the muscarinic actions and it occupies the cholinergic receptor sites on the effector cells.

Blocking of Adrenergic Receptors. Phenoxybenzamine is an example of a drug that is capable of blocking norepinephrine receptors.

HIGHER CONTROL OF THE AUTONOMIC NERVOUS SYSTEM

The sympathetic outflow in the spinal cord (T1–L2[3]) and the parasympathetic craniosacral outflow (cranial nuclei 3, 7, 9, and 10; spinal S2, 3, and 4) are controlled by the hypothalamus. The hypothalamus appears to integrate the autonomic and neuroendocrine systems, thus preserving body homeostasis. It receives signals from all parts of the nervous system, afferent input from the viscera, and information concerning the hormone levels in the blood. This input is integrated within the hypothalamus and transmitted to the lower autonomic centers in the brainstem and spinal cord by descending tracts of the reticular formation. In a similar manner, **releasing factors** or **release-inhibiting factors** are liberated into the circulation, affecting hormone levels and endocrine secretions and thus influencing organ activity.

Stimulation of different parts of the cerebral cortex and the limbic system can produce autonomic effects that are brought about through the hypothalamus.

It is a known fact that during infancy, as a result of the process of learning, the sphincters of the bladder and rectum are brought under voluntary control. It is also recognized that many of the physical responses to an emotional reaction are brought about by the autonomic nervous system. These changes can be explained by the connections that exist between the cerebral cortex, the limbic system, and the hypothalamus.

FUNCTIONS OF THE AUTONOMIC NERVOUS SYSTEM

The autonomic nervous system, along with the endocrine system, maintains body homeostasis. The endocrine control is slower and exerts its influence by means of blood-borne hormones.

The sympathetic and parasympathetic components of the autonomic system cooperate in maintaining the stability of the internal environment. The sympathetic part prepares and mobilizes the body in an emergency, when there is sudden severe exercise, fear, or rage. The parasympathetic part aims at conserving and storing energy, for example, in the promotion of digestion and the absorption of food by increasing secretions of the glands of the gastrointestinal tract and stimulating peristalsis.

The sympathetic and parasympathetic parts of the system usually have antagonistic control over a viscus. For example, the sympathetic activity will increase the heart rate, whereas the parasympathetic will cause slowing of the heart rate. The sympathetic activity will make the bronchial smooth muscle relax but it is contracted by the parasympathetic.

It should be pointed out, however, that many viscera do not possess this fine dual control from the autonomic system; for example, the erector pili muscles have sympathetic innervation only.

The autonomic system should not be regarded as an isolated portion of the nervous system, for we know that it can play a role with somatic activity in expressing emotion, and that certain autonomic activities, such as micturition, can be brought under voluntary control.

For important anatomical, physiological, and pharmacological differences between the sympathetic and the parasympathetic parts of the autonomic system, see Table 21-1.

Note that the sympathetic part of the system has a widespread action on the body, as the result of the preganglionic fibers synapsing on many postganglionic neurons and the suprarenal medulla releasing norepinephrine and epinephrine into the bloodstream. The parasympathetic has a more discrete control, since the preganglionic fibers synapse on only a few postganglionic neurons and there is no comparable organ to the suprarenal medulla.

The effects of the autonomic nervous system on body organs are summarized in Table 21-2.

Table 21-1.	Comparison of Anatomical, Physiological, and Pharmacological Characteristics of the Sympathetic and Parasympathetic Parts of the Autonomic Nervous System	
	Sympathetic	Parasympathetic
Action	Prepares body for emergency	Conserves and restores energy
Outflow	T1–L2 (3)	CN 3, 7, 9, and 10; S2, 3, and 4
Preganglionic fibers	Myelinated	Myelinated
Ganglia	Paravertebral (sympathetic trunks); prevertebral (e.g., celiac, superior mesenteric, inferior mesenteric)	Small ganglia close to viscera (e.g., otic, ciliary) or ganglion cells in plexuses (e.g., cardiac, pulmonary)
Neurotransmitter within ganglia	Acetylcholine	Acetylcholine
Ganglion-blocking agents	Hexamethonium and tetraethylammonium by competing with acetylcholine	Hexamethonium and tetraethylammonium by competing with acetylcholine
Postganglionic fibers	Long, nonmyelinated	Short, nonmyelinated
Characteristic activity	Widespread due to many postganglionic fibers and liberation of epinephrine and norepinephrine from suprarenal medulla	Discrete action with few postganglionic fibers
Neurotransmitter at postganglionic endings	Norepinephrine at most endings and acetylcholine at few endings (sweat glands)	Acetylcholine at all endings
Blocking agents on receptors of effector cells	Alpha-adrenergic receptors—phenoxybenzamine; beta-adrenergic receptors—propranolol	Atropine, scopolamine
Agents inhibiting synthesis and storage of neurotransmitter at postganglionic endings	Reserpine	
Agents inhibiting hydrolysis of neurotransmitter at site of effector cells		Acetylcholinesterase blockers (e.g., neostigmine)
Drugs mimicking autonomic activity	Sympathomimetic drugs Phenylephrine: alpha receptors Isoproterenol: beta receptors	Parasympathomimetic drugs Pilocarpine Methacholine
Higher control	Hypothalamus	Hypothalamus

Table 21-2.   *Effects of Autonomic Nervous System on Organs of the Body*

Organ		Sympathetic action	Parasympathetic action
Eye	Pupil	Dilates	Constricts
	Ciliary muscle	Relaxes	Contracts
Glands	Lacrimal, parotid, submandibular, sublingual, nasal	Reduces secretion by causing vasoconstriction of blood vessels	Increases secretion
	Sweat	Increases secretion	
Heart	Cardiac muscle	Increases force of contraction	Decreases force of contraction
	Coronary arteries (mainly controlled by local metabolic factors)	Dilates (beta receptors), constricts (alpha receptors)	
Lung	Bronchial muscle	Relaxes (dilates bronchi)	Contracts (constricts bronchi), increases secretion
	Bronchial secretion		
	Bronchial arteries	Constricts	Dilates
Gastrointestinal tract	Muscle in walls	Decreases peristalsis	Increases peristalsis
	Muscle in sphincters	Contracts	Relaxes
	Glands	Reduces secretion by vasoconstriction of blood vessels	Increases secretion
Liver		Breaks down glycogen into glucose	
Gallbladder		Relaxes	Contracts
Kidney		Decreases output due to constriction of arteries	
Urinary bladder	Bladder wall (detrusor)	Relaxes	Contracts
	Sphincter vesicae	Contracts	Relaxes
Erectile tissue of penis and clitoris			Relaxes, causes erection
Ejaculation		Contracts smooth muscle of vas deferens, seminal vesicles, and prostate	
Systemic arteries			
Skin		Constricts	
Abdominal		Constricts	
Muscle		Constricts (alpha receptors), dilates (beta receptors), dilates (cholinergic)	
Erector pili muscles		Contracts	
Suprarenal			
Cortex		Stimulates	
Medulla		Liberates epinephrine and norepinephrine	

SOME IMPORTANT AUTONOMIC INNERVATIONS

Eye

UPPER LID. The smooth muscle fibers of the levator palpebrae superioris are innervated by sympathetic postganglionic fibers from the superior cervical sympathetic ganglion (Fig. 21-4). Division of the sympathetic innervation paralyzes the smooth muscle and causes drooping of the upper lid (ptosis).

IRIS. The sphincter pupillae is supplied by parasympathetic fibers from the parasympathetic nucleus (Edinger-Westphal nucleus) of the oculomotor nerve (Fig.

Fig. 21-4

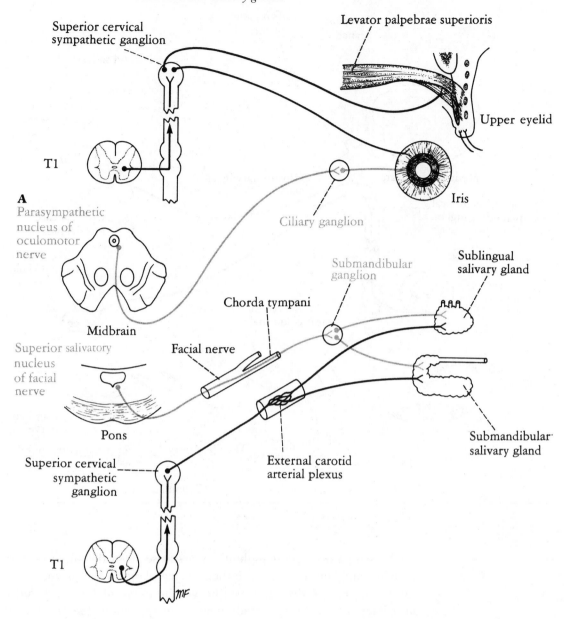

21-4). After synapsing in the **ciliary ganglion,** the postganglionic fibers pass forward to the eyeball in the **short ciliary nerves** to supply the sphincter pupillae. (Note that the ciliary muscle of the eye is also supplied by the same nerves.)

The dilator pupillae is supplied by postganglionic fibers from the superior cervical sympathetic ganglion (Fig. 21-4). The fibers reach the eyeball in the **short** and the **long ciliary nerves.**

LACRIMAL GLAND. The parasympathetic secretomotor nerves originate in the **lacrimatory nucleus** of the facial nerve (Fig. 21-5). The preganglionic fibers reach the **pterygopalatine ganglion** through the **great petrosal nerve** and the **nerve of the pterygoid canal.** The postganglionic fibers join the maxillary nerve and travel in its **zygomatic branch,** the **zygomaticotemporal nerve,** and the **lacrimal nerve** to reach the lacrimal gland.

Fig. 21-5

The autonomic innervation of the parotid salivary gland and the lacrimal gland.

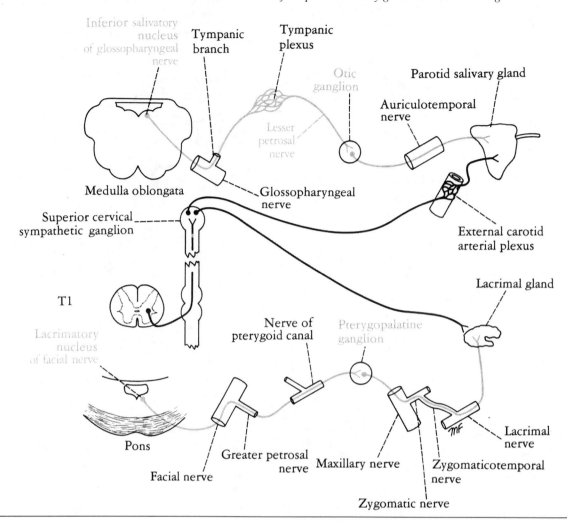

The sympathetic postganglionic fibers arise from the superior cervical sympathetic ganglion and travel to the lacrimal gland in the plexus of the internal carotid artery, the **deep petrosal nerve,** the **nerve of the pterygoid canal,** the **maxillary nerve,** the **zygomatic nerve,** the **zygomaticotemporal nerve,** and finally the **lacrimal nerve.**

Salivary Glands

SUBMANDIBULAR AND SUBLINGUAL GLANDS. Parasympathetic secretomotor fibers originate in the **superior salivatory nucleus** of the facial nerve (Fig. 21-4). The preganglionic fibers pass to the **submandibular ganglion** and other small ganglia close to the duct through the **chorda tympani nerve** and the **lingual nerve.** The postganglionic fibers pass to the glands.

Sympathetic postganglionic fibers arise from the superior cervical sympathetic ganglion and reach the glands along the arterial supply; they are vasoconstrictor in function.

PAROTID GLAND. Parasympathetic secretomotor fibers from the **inferior salivatory nucleus** of the glossopharyngeal nerve supply the gland (Fig. 21-5). The

Fig. 21-6   *The autonomic innervation of the heart and lungs.*

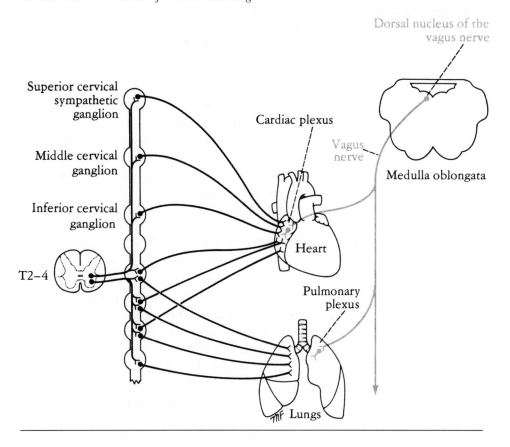

preganglionic fibers pass to the **otic ganglion** through the **tympanic branch of the glossopharyngeal nerve** and the **lesser petrosal nerve.** Postganglionic fibers pass to the gland through the auriculotemporal nerve.

Sympathetic postganglionic fibers arise from the superior cervical sympathetic ganglion and reach the gland along the external carotid artery.

Heart. The sympathetic postganglionic fibers pass from the cervical and upper thoracic portions of the sympathetic trunks (Fig. 21-6). Postganglionic fibers reach the heart by way of the **superior, middle,** and **inferior cardiac branches** of the cervical portion of the sympathetic trunk and a number of **cardiac branches** from the thoracic portion of the sympathetic trunk. The fibers pass through the **cardiac plexuses** and terminate on the **sinoatrial node** and the **atrioventricular nodes,** on cardiac muscle fibers, and on coronary arteries. Activation of these fibers results in cardiac acceleration, increased force of contraction of the cardiac muscle, and dilation of the coronary arteries.

The parasympathetic preganglionic fibers originate in the **dorsal nucleus of the vagus nerve** and descend into the thorax in the vagus nerves. The fibers end by synapsing in the **cardiac plexuses.** The postganglionic fibers terminate on the **sinoatrial** and **atrioventricular nodes** and on the coronary arteries. Activation of these nerves results in a reduction in the rate and force of contraction of the heart and a constriction of the coronaries.

Further examples of autonomic innervations are shown in Table 21-2.

In each of the following questions, answer:
A. If only (1) is correct
B. If only (2) is correct
C. If both (1) and (2) are correct
D. If neither (1) nor (2) is correct

1. Which of the following general statements concerning the autonomic nervous system is (are) correct?
   (1) It has afferent, connector, and efferent neurons.
   (2) The afferent impulses originate in visceral receptors.
2. Which of the following statements concerning the visceral receptors is (are) correct?
   (1) They include chemoreceptors, baroreceptors, and osmoreceptors.
   (2) The pain receptors can be stimulated by oxygen excess.
3. Which of the following statements concerning the general arrangement of the autonomic nervous system is (are) correct?
   (1) It innervates involuntary structures.
   (2) It is confined to the peripheral part of the nervous system.
4. Which of the following statements concerning the sympathetic part of the autonomic nervous system is (are) correct?
   (1) It prepares the body for relaxation.
   (2) It dilates the pupils.
5. Which of the following statements concerning the parasympathetic part of the autonomic nervous system is (are) correct?
   (1) The peristaltic waves of the gut are increased.
   (2) The urinary bladder wall is made to contract.
6. Which of the following statements concerning the efferent outflow of the autonomic system is (are) correct?
   (1) The sympathetic outflow is restricted to spinal cord segments T5–L1.
   (2) The parasympathetic outflow is present in cranial nerves 3, 7, 9, and 10.

In each of the following questions, answer:
A. If only (1), (2), and (3) are correct
B. If only (1) and (3) are correct
C. If only (2) and (4) are correct
D. If only (4) is correct
E. If all are correct

7. Which of the following statements concerning a lesion of the sympathetic innervation of the head and neck (Horner's syndrome) is (are) correct?
   (1) The patient has vasodilation of the arteries of the facial skin.
   (2) The pupil is constricted.
   (3) There is enophthalmos.
   (4) There is ptosis of the upper eyelid
8. Which of the following statements concerning the autonomic innervation of the heart is (are) correct?
   (1) The sympathetic nerves cause cardiac acceleration, increased force of contraction of the cardiac muscle, and dilation of the coronary arteries.
   (2) The postganglionic parasympathetic fibers terminate on the sinoatrial and atrioventricular nodes.

(3) The sympathetic preganglionic fibers originate in the upper four thoracic ganglia of the sympathetic trunk.

(4) The action of norepinephrine at sympathetic postganglionic nerve endings is terminated by monoamine oxidase.

9. Which of the following statements concerning the autonomic nervous system is (are) correct?

(1) White rami communicantes contain myelinated afferent fibers.

(2) Gray rami communicantes contain postganglionic parasympathetic fibers.

(3) The greater splanchnic nerve is formed of myelinated nerve fibers.

(4) The lesser splanchnic nerve arises from the fifth to the ninth ganglia of the thoracic part of the sympathetic trunk.

10. Norepinephrine is secreted by which of the following nerve endings?

(1) Preganglionic sympathetic nerve fibers.

(2) Preganglionic sympathetic fibers to the suprarenal medulla.

(3) Preganglionic parasympathetic nerve fibers.

(4) Postganglionic sympathetic nerve fibers.

11. Which of the following statements concerning the innervation of the submandibular salivary gland is (are) correct?

(1) The parasympathetic preganglionic fibers synapse in the otic ganglion.

(2) The secretomotor supply originates in the superior cervical sympathetic ganglion.

(3) The parasympathetic control is in the superior salivatory nucleus of the oculomotor nerve.

(4) The sympathetic preganglionic fibers arise from the first thoracic segment of the spinal cord.

12. Which of the following statements concerning the parasympathetic outflow in the spinal cord is (are) correct?

(1) T1–L2.

(2) L4, 5, and S1, 2, and 3.

(3) L2, 3, and 4.

(4) S2, 3, and 4.

13. Which of the following statements concerning the action of anticholinesterase drugs is (are) correct?

(1) They prevent the release of acetylcholine at the nerve endings.

(2) They increase the release of acetylcholine at the nerve endings.

(3) They mimic the action of acetylcholine at the receptor site.

(4) They inhibit the breakdown of acetylcholine.

14. Which of the following statements concerning sympathetic receptors is (are) correct?

(1) There are two kinds of receptors present.

(2) Norepinephrine has a greater effect on beta receptors than on alpha receptors.

(3) Beta receptors are predominant in the bronchial walls.

(4) Isoproterenol is a strong stimulant of alpha receptors.

15. Which of the following statements concerning autonomic postganglionic endings that liberate acetylcholine is (are) correct?

(1) The receptors on the effector organs are muscarinic.

(2) The action of acetylcholine at these endings is blocked by atropine.

(3) Atropine occupies the cholinergic receptor sites.

(4) Atropine blocks the release of acetylcholine.

Match the numbered autonomic ganglia listed below on the left with the most appropriate lettered viscus or muscle listed below on the right. The answers may be used more than once.

16. Middle cervical sympathetic ganglion.
17. Ciliary ganglion.
18. Pterygopalatine ganglion.
19. Submandibular ganglion.
20. Celiac ganglion.

A. Constrictor pupillae.
B. Parotid salivary gland.
C. Lacrimal gland.
D. Stomach.
E. None of the above.

Match the numbered cranial nerves listed below on the left with the most appropriate lettered nuclei listed below on the right. The answers may be used more than once.

21. Facial nerve.
22. Glossopharyngeal nerve.
23. Oculomotor nerve.
24. Vagus.
25. Abducent nerve.

A. Edinger-Westphal nucleus.
B. Dorsal motor nucleus.
C. Lacrimatory nucleus.
D. Inferior salivatory nucleus.
E. None of the above.

Match the numbered organs listed below on the left with the appropriate lettered actions of the sympathetic nerves on the smooth muscle listed below on the right. The answers may be used more than once.

26. Urinary bladder wall.
27. Bronchus.
28. Systemic arteries.
29. Pyloric sphincter of stomach.
30. Prostate.

A. Contracts.
B. Relaxes.
C. None of the above.

ANSWERS AND EXPLANATIONS

1. C
2. A: (2) Pain receptors can be stimulated by lack of oxygen.
3. A: (2) The autonomic nervous system is widely distributed throughout the central and peripheral parts of the nervous system.
4. B: (1) The sympathetic part of the autonomic nervous system prepares the body for an emergency.
5. C
6. B: (1) The sympathetic outflow is restricted to spinal cord segments T1–L2 (3).
7. E
8. A: (4) The action of norepinephrine at sympathetic postganglionic endings is terminated by reuptake into the nerve terminal.
9. B: (2) Gray rami communicantes contain nonmyelinated postganglionic sympathetic nerve fibers. (4) The lesser splanchnic nerve arises from the tenth and eleventh ganglia of the thoracic part of the sympathetic trunk.
10. D: (1) Preganglionic sympathetic nerve fibers liberate acetylcholine at their endings. (2) Preganglionic sympathetic nerve fibers to the suprarenal medulla liberate acetylcholine at their nerve endings. (3) Preganglionic parasympathetic nerve fibers liberate acetylcholine at their nerve endings.

11. D: (1) The parasympathetic preganglionic fibers synapse in the submandibular ganglion. (2) The secretomotor nerve supply is parasympathetic and originates in the superior salivatory nucleus of the facial nerve. (3) For the parasympathetic control, see (2).
12. D
13. D
14. B: (2) Norepinephrine has a greater effect on alpha receptors than on beta receptors. (4) Isoproterenol is a strong stimulant of beta receptors.
15. A: (4) Atropine does not block the release of acetylcholine.
16. E
17. A
18. C
19. E
20. D
21. C
22. D
23. A
24. B
25. E
26. B
27. B
28. A
29. A
30. A

22 Meninges

SUGGESTED PLAN FOR REVIEW OF CHAPTER 22

1. Understand the structure and arrangement of the dura, arachnoid, and pia mater.
2. Learn the vertebral level at which each of the meninges terminates inferiorly in the child and the adult.
3. Be able to define (a) subarachnoid space, (b) falx cerebri, (c) tentorium cerebelli, and (d) diaphragma sellae.
4. Know the structure of a venous sinus. How do the layers of the dura mater contribute to its walls?
5. Learn the location of the superior sagittal sinus, the inferior sagittal sinus, the straight sinus, the transverse sinus, and the sigmoid sinus.
6. Learn the location and general shape of the cavernous sinus. Know the names of the structures that pass through the sinus and the structures that lie within its lateral wall. What is the connection between this sinus and infections of the face? This sinus is a common source of questions.
7. Be able to define a cistern, an arachnoid villus, and an arachnoid granulation.

INTRODUCTION

The brain and spinal cord are enclosed within three concentric membranous sheaths, the meninges. The outermost is thick, tough, and fibrous and is called the **dura mater;** the middle membrane is thin and delicate and is known as the **arachnoid mater;** and the innermost is delicate and vascular and closely applied to the surfaces of the brain and spinal cord and is known as the **pia mater.**

The three meninges, together with the bones of the skull and the vertebral column, protect the nervous tissue from mechanical forces applied from the exterior. Further protection is afforded by the cerebrospinal fluid, which lies in the subarachnoid space between the arachnoid mater and the pia mater.

The purpose of this chapter is to give a brief overview of the arrangement of the meninges.

MENINGES OF THE SPINAL CORD	The meninges of the spinal cord have already been described in Chapter 6.

MENINGES OF THE BRAIN	The brain, like the spinal cord, has a covering of dura mater, arachnoid mater, and pia mater.

DURA MATER	The dura mater of the brain is formed of two layers, the endosteal layer and the meningeal layer. These are closely united except along certain lines, where they separate to form **venous sinuses.**

Endosteal Layer. The endosteal layer is periosteum covering the inner surface of the skull. At the foramen magnum it does **not** become continuous with the dura mater of the spinal cord. Around the margins of all the foramina in the skull it becomes continuous with the **periosteum** on the outside of the skull. At the sutures, it is continuous with the **sutural ligaments.** It is most strongly adherent to the bones over the base of the skull.

Meningeal Layer. The meningeal layer is the dura mater proper. It is a dense, strong fibrous membrane covering the brain and is continuous through the foramen magnum with the dura mater of the spinal cord. It provides tubular sheaths for the cranial nerves as the latter pass through the foramina in the skull. Outside the skull, the sheaths fuse with the epineurium of the nerves.

The meningeal layer gives rise to four septa, which divide the cranial cavity into spaces that lodge the subdivisions of the brain (Figs. 22-1 and 22-2). The function of these septa is to restrict the displacement of the brain during head movements.

FALX CEREBRI. The falx cerebri is a sickle-shaped fold of dura mater that lies in the midline between the two cerebral hemispheres (Figs. 22-1 and 22-2). It is attached in front to the crista galli and posteriorly to the upper surface of the **tentorium cerebelli** and the internal surface of the skull. The **superior sagittal sinus** runs in its upper fixed border and the **inferior sagittal sinus** runs in its lower free margin; the **straight sinus** runs along its attachment to the tentorium cerebelli.

TENTORIUM CEREBELLI. The tentorium cerebelli is a crescent-shaped fold of dura mater placed between the upper surface of the cerebellum and the occipital lobes of the cerebral hemispheres (Figs. 22-1, 22-2, and 22-3). In the anterior edge there is a gap, the **tentorial notch,** for the passage of the midbrain. The

Fig. 22-1

Interior of skull, showing dura mater and its contained venous sinuses.

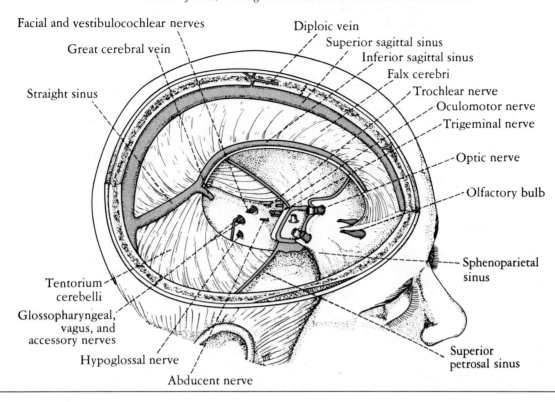

Facial and vestibulocochlear nerves
Great cerebral vein
Straight sinus
Diploic vein
Superior sagittal sinus
Inferior sagittal sinus
Falx cerebri
Trochlear nerve
Oculomotor nerve
Trigeminal nerve
Optic nerve
Olfactory bulb
Sphenoparietal sinus
Tentorium cerebelli
Glossopharyngeal, vagus, and accessory nerves
Hypoglossal nerve
Abducent nerve
Superior petrosal sinus

Fig. 22-2

The falx cerebri and the tentorium cerebelli. Note the continuity between the meningeal layer of dura mater within the skull and the dura mater of the spinal cord at the foramen magnum.

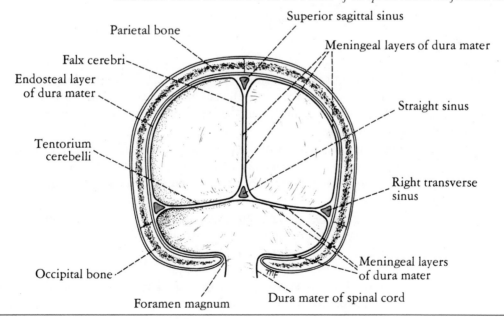

Parietal bone
Falx cerebri
Endosteal layer of dura mater
Tentorium cerebelli
Occipital bone
Foramen magnum
Superior sagittal sinus
Meningeal layers of dura mater
Straight sinus
Right transverse sinus
Meningeal layers of dura mater
Dura mater of spinal cord

fixed border is attached to the posterior clinoid processes, the petrous part of the temporal bone, and the inner surface of the occipital bone. The free border is attached to the anterior clinoid process on each side. At the point where the two borders cross, the third and fourth cranial nerves pass forward to enter the lateral wall of the cavernous sinus.

The falx cerebri and the falx cerebelli are attached to the upper and lower

Fig. 22-3

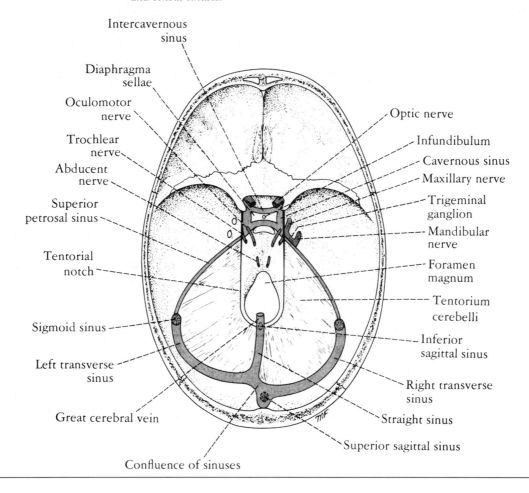

Intercavernous sinus

Diaphragma sellae

Oculomotor nerve

Trochlear nerve

Abducent nerve

Superior petrosal sinus

Tentorial notch

Sigmoid sinus

Left transverse sinus

Great cerebral vein

Confluence of sinuses

Optic nerve

Infundibulum

Cavernous sinus

Maxillary nerve

Trigeminal ganglion

Mandibular nerve

Foramen magnum

Tentorium cerebelli

Inferior sagittal sinus

Right transverse sinus

Straight sinus

Superior sagittal sinus

surfaces of the tentorium, respectively. The **straight sinus** runs along its attachment to the falx cerebri, the **superior petrosal sinus** runs along its attachment to the petrous bone, and the **transverse sinus** runs along its attachment to the occipital bone.

Close to the apex of the petrous part of the temporal bone, the lower layer of the tentorium is pouched forward beneath the superior petrosal sinus, to form a **recess for the trigeminal nerve and the trigeminal ganglion.**

FALX CEREBELLI. The falx cerebelli is a small, vertical fold of dura mater that projects forward between the two cerebellar hemispheres. Its posterior fixed margin contains the **occipital sinus.**

DIAPHRAGMA SELLAE. The diaphragma sellae is a small, circular fold of dura mater that forms the roof of the sella turcica (Fig. 22-3). A small hole in its center is for the passage of the stalk of the **hypophysis cerebri.**

Dural Nerve Supply. The dural nerve supply is mainly derived from branches of the **trigeminal nerve,** the **upper three cervical nerves,** the **cervical part of the sympathetic trunk,** and the **vagus nerve.**

Dural Arterial Supply. Numerous arteries supply the dura mater from the **internal carotid, ascending pharyngeal, occipital,** and **vertebral arteries.** From the clinical standpoint, the most important is the **middle meningeal artery**, which is commonly damaged in head injuries.

MIDDLE MENINGEAL ARTERY. The middle meningeal artery arises from the maxillary artery in the infratemporal fossa. It enters the cranial cavity through the foramen spinosum and then lies between the meningeal and endosteal layers of dura. The artery then runs forward and laterally in a groove on the upper surface of the squamous part of the temporal bone. The anterior (frontal) branch deeply grooves or tunnels the anterior-inferior angle of the parietal bone, and its course corresponds roughly to the line of the underlying precentral gyrus of the brain. The posterior (parietal) branch curves backward and supplies the posterior part of the dura mater.

Dural Venous Drainage. The middle meningeal vein follows the branches of the middle meningeal artery and drains into the pterygoid venous plexus or the sphenoparietal sinus. The veins lie lateral to the arteries.

DURAL VENOUS SINUSES

The venous sinuses of the cranial cavity are situated between the layers of the dura mater (Figs. 22-3 and 22-4). They receive blood from the brain, from the diploë of the skull, from the orbit, and from the internal ear; they also receive the cerebrospinal fluid from the subarachnoid space through the **arachnoid villi**. The blood in the dural sinuses ultimately drains into the internal jugular veins in the neck. The dural sinuses are lined by endothelium, and their walls are devoid of muscular tissue. They contain no valves. **Emissary veins,** which are also valveless, connect the dural venous sinuses with the **diploic veins** of the skull and with the veins of the scalp.

Superior Sagittal Sinus. The superior sagittal sinus lies in the upper fixed border of the falx cerebri (Figs. 22-1 and 22-2). It begins anteriorly at the foramen cecum, where it occasionally receives a vein from the nasal cavity. It runs posteriorly, and at the internal occipital protuberance it usually becomes continuous with the right **transverse sinus.** On each side the sinus communicates with two or three irregularly shaped **venous lacunae.** Numerous arachnoid villi and granulations project into the lacunae.

The superior sagittal sinus receives in its course the **superior cerebral veins.** At the internal occipital protuberance it is dilated to form the **confluence of the sinuses** and receives the **occipital sinus.**

Inferior Sagittal Sinus. The inferior sagittal sinus lies in the lower free margin of the falx cerebri (Figs. 22-1 and 22-2). It runs backward and joins the **great cerebral vein** to form the straight sinus. It receives cerebral veins from the medial surface of the cerebral hemispheres.

Straight Sinus. The straight sinus lies at the junction of the falx cerebri with the tentorium cerebelli (Fig. 22-1). It is formed by the union of the **inferior sagittal sinus** with the **great cerebral vein.** It drains usually into the left transverse sinus. It receives some of the superior cerebellar veins.

Transverse Sinus. The transverse sinuses are paired structures (Figs. 22-2 and 22-3). The right sinus begins at the internal occipital protuberance as a continuation of the superior sagittal sinus. The left sinus is usually a continuation of the straight sinus. Each sinus runs forward along the attached margin of the

Fig. 22-4

Coronal section through the body of the sphenoid bone, showing the hypophysis cerebri and cavernous sinuses. Note the position of the internal carotid artery and the cranial nerves.

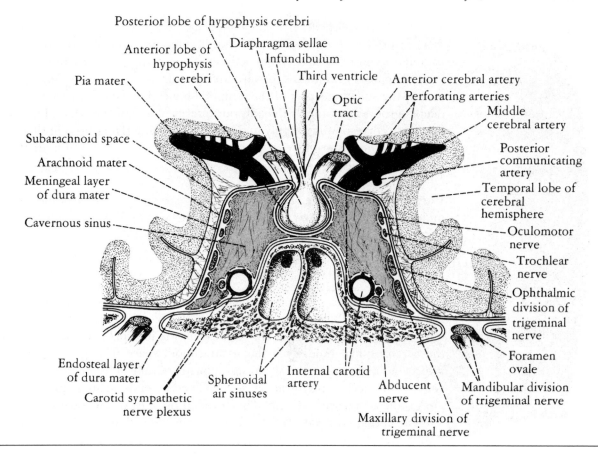

tentorium cerebelli. They end on each side by becoming the **sigmoid sinus.** The transverse sinuses receive the **superior petrosal sinuses** and the **inferior cerebral** and the **cerebellar veins.**

Sigmoid Sinus. The sigmoid sinuses are a direct continuation of the transverse sinuses (Fig. 22-3). Each sinus curves downward behind the mastoid antrum and leaves the skull through the posterior part of the jugular foramen to become the internal jugular vein.

Occipital Sinus. The occipital sinus lies in the attached margin of the falx cerebelli. It begins near the foramen magnum, where it communicates with the **vertebral veins** and drains into the confluence of sinuses.

Cavernous Sinuses. The cavernous sinuses are situated in the middle cranial fossa on each side of the body of the sphenoid bone (Fig. 22-4) and extend from the superior orbital fissure in front to the apex of the petrous part of the temporal bone behind. The sinus receives the inferior ophthalmic vein, the sphenoparietal sinus, the central vein of the retina, and the cerebral veins. The cavernous sinus drains into the transverse sinus through the superior petrosal sinus.

The **internal carotid artery,** surrounded by its **sympathetic nerve plexus,** runs forward through the sinus (Fig. 22-4). The **abducent nerve** also passes through the sinus. The **third and fourth cranial nerves** and the **ophthalmic and maxillary divisions of the trigeminal nerve** run forward in the lateral wall of the sinus (Fig. 22-4).

Intercavernous Sinuses. The intercavernous sinuses connect the two cavernous sinuses through the sella turcica (Fig. 22-3).

Superior and Inferior Petrosal Sinuses. The superior and inferior petrosal sinuses are small sinuses situated on the superior and inferior borders of the petrous part of the temporal bone on each side of the skull. Each superior sinus drains the cavernous sinus into the transverse sinus, and each inferior sinus drains the cavernous sinus into the internal jugular vein.

ARACHNOID MATER	The arachnoid mater is a delicate, impermeable membrane covering the brain and lying between the pia mater internally and the dura mater externally. It is separated from the dura by a potential space, the **subdural space,** filled by a film of fluid; it is separated from the pia by the **subarachnoid space,** which is filled with **cerebrospinal fluid.** The outer and inner surfaces of the arachnoid are covered with flattened mesothelial cells.

The arachnoid bridges over the sulci on the surface of the brain, and in certain situations the arachnoid and pia are widely separated to form the **subarachnoid cisternae.** The **cisterna cerebellomedullaris** lies between the inferior surface of the cerebellum and the roof of the fourth ventricle. The **cisterna interpeduncularis** lies between the two cerebral peduncles. All the cisternae are in free communication with one another and with the remainder of the subarachnoid space.

The arachnoid projects into the venous sinuses (especially the superior sagittal) to form **arachnoid villi** and **arachnoid granulations.** These are sites where the cerebrospinal fluid diffuses into the bloodstream.

The subarachnoid space is filled with cerebrospinal fluid and contains the cerebral arteries and the cranial nerves. At certain sites there are extensions of the subarachnoid space, and these are described on page 200.

PIA MATER	The pia mater is a vascular membrane that closely covers the surface of the brain and descends into the sulci. As a two-layered fold, called the **tela choroidea,** it projects into the ventricles to form the **choroid plexuses.**

NATIONAL BOARD TYPE QUESTIONS	Select the **best** response.

1. The following statements concerning the dura mater of the brain are correct **except:**
   A. The meningeal layer of dura is continuous through the foramen magnum with the dura mater covering the spinal cord.
   B. The endosteal layer of dura mater is continuous through the foramina in the skull with the periosteum outside the skull.
   C. The cranial venous sinuses are located between the endosteal and meningeal layers of dura mater.
   D. Each cranial nerve pierces the meningeal layer of dura inside the skull before it leaves the skull.
   E. The meningeal layer of dura extends through the optic canal to fuse with the sclera of the eyeball.

2. The following statements concerning the falx cerebri are correct **except:**
   A. It is a sickle-shaped fold of the meningeal layer of dura mater.
   B. It is attached anteriorly to the crista galli of the ethmoid bone.
   C. The straight sinus runs along its lower free border.
   D. The superior sagittal sinus runs along its upper fixed border.
   E. It is attached to the tentorium cerebelli.

3. The following statements concerning the tentorium cerebelli are correct **except:**
   A. The tentorial notch allows the passage of the midbrain.
   B. The free border is attached anteriorly to the posterior clinoid processes.
   C. It separates the occipital lobes of the brain from the cerebellum.
   D. The transverse venous sinus lies in its attached lateral border.
   E. The superior petrosal sinus runs along its attached border to the petrous part of the temporal bone.

4. The following statements concerning the blood supply to the dura mater within the skull are correct **except:**
   A. The arteries include branches of the internal carotid, maxillary, and vertebral arteries.
   B. The middle meningeal artery arises from the maxillary artery.
   C. The middle meningeal artery enters the skull through the foramen spinosum.
   D. The middle meningeal artery runs between the bone and the endosteal layer of dura.
   E. The anterior branch of the middle meningeal artery grooves the anterior inferior angle of the parietal bone and it is here that it is commonly injured.

5. The following general statements concerning the dural venous sinuses are correct **except:**
   A. They possess no valves.
   B. They have thick muscular walls.
   C. They receive blood from the brain and the internal ear.
   D. They are connected to the scalp veins by valveless emmissary veins.
   E. They drain cerebrospinal fluid through the arachnoid granulations.

6. The following statements concerning the cavernous venous sinus are correct **except:**
   A. It is situated in the middle cranial fossa.
   B. It receives the central vein of the retina and the inferior ophthalmic vein.
   C. The internal carotid artery and the trochlear nerve run through the sinus.
   D. The oculomotor and the ophthalmic and maxillary divisions of the trigeminal nerves run forward in its lateral wall.
   E. It is drained posteriorly into the transverse sinus through the superior petrosal sinus.

In each of the following questions, answer:
A. If only (1), (2), and (3) are correct
B. If only (1) and (3) are correct
C. If only (2) and (4) are correct
D. If only (4) is correct
E. If all are correct

7. Which of the following nerves is (are) sensory to the dura mater?
   (1) Hypoglossal nerve.
   (2) Upper three cervical nerves.

(3) Glossopharyngeal nerve.

(4) Trigeminal nerve.

8. Which of the following statements is (are) correct concerning the sigmoid venous sinus?

(1) It is a direct continuation of the transverse sinus.

(2) It lies in the posterior cranial fossa.

(3) It is related anteriorly to the mastoid antrum.

(4) It passes through the jugular foramen to become the internal jugular vein.

9. Which of the following statements is (are) correct concerning the arachnoid mater?

(1) It is a delicate, impermeable membrane.

(2) It is separated from the dura mater by a film of fluid in the subdural space.

(3) Beneath it lies the subarachnoid space filled with cerebrospinal fluid.

(4) It does not extend through foramina in the skull to provide sheaths for the cranial nerves.

10. Which of the following statements is (are) correct concerning the pia mater?

(1) It is a vascular membrane.

(2) It dips into the sulci of the brain.

(3) It projects into the ventricles of the brain to form the choroid plexuses.

(4) In places it is separated from the brain to form the important cisterns.

11. The following statements concerning the subarachnoid space is (are) correct **except:**

(1) It extends inferiorly as far as the second sacral vertebra.

(2) It contains the cerebral arteries and veins.

(3) The cranial nerves lie within the subarachnoid space.

(4) It dips into the sulci of the cerebral hemispheres.

12. Which of the following structures restrict the movements of the brain within the skull?

(1) The falx cerebelli.

(2) The falx cerebri.

(3) The tentorium cerebelli.

(4) The diaphragma sellae.

13. Which of the following general statements concerning the meninges of the brain is (are) correct?

(1) At the sutures the sutural ligaments connect the endosteal layer of the dura to the periosteum outside the skull.

(2) The fibrous tissue in the walls of the dural venous sinuses resists the outside pressure of the cerebrospinal fluid.

(3) The inner and outer surfaces of the arachnoid mater are covered with mesothelial cells.

(4) The sympathetic nerves do not supply the meninges.

14. Which of the following general statements concerning the subarachnoid cisternae is (are) correct?

(1) The cisterna cerebellomedullaris lies between the inferior surface of the cerebellum and the roof of the fourth ventricle.

(2) The foramena of Magendie and Luschka open into the cisterna cerebellomedullaris.

(3) There is a cistern on the ventral surface of the midbrain.

(4) One unique characteristic about the cisterns is that they have no communication with one another.

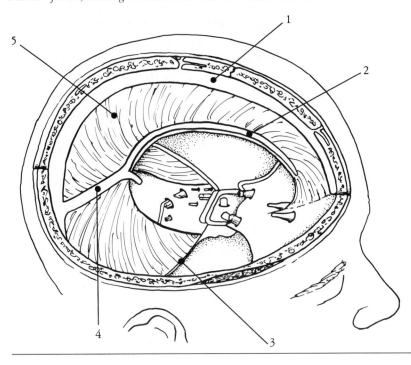

15. Which of the following general statements concerning the arachnoid mater is (are) correct?
    (1) The arachnoid villi project into the venous blood as minute outpouchings of the subarachnoid space.
    (2) Groups of arachnoid villi are known as arachnoid granulations.
    (3) The superior sagittal sinus possesses large numbers of arachnoid granulations.
    (4) The arachnoid mater and the subarachnoid space extend forward into the orbital cavity to the back of the optic disc of the eye.

Match the numbered structures in Figure 22-5 and listed below on the left with appropriate lettered structures listed below on the right. The answers may be used more than once.

16. Number 1.   A. Falx cerebri.
17. Number 2.   B. Straight sinus.
18. Number 3.   C. Superior sagittal sinus.
19. Number 4.   D. Tentorium cerebelli.
20. Number 5.   E. None of the above.

ANSWERS AND EXPLANATIONS

1. D: The meningeal layer of dura mater extends through each foramina in the skull and provides a short sheath for the cranial nerves; the sheath fuses with the epineurium of each cranial nerve outside the skull.
2. C: The straight sinus runs along the border of the falx cerebri that is attached to the upper surface of the tentorium cerebelli. The inferior sagittal sinus runs along the lower free border of the falx.
3. B: The free border of the tentorium cerebelli is attached anteriorly to the anterior clinoid processes.

4. D: The middle meningeal artery inside the skull runs between the meningeal and endosteal layers of the dura mater. Hemorrhage from this artery is called an extradural hemorrhage because the blood will lie outside the true meningeal layer of the dura.

5. B: Dural venous sinuses have thick fibrous walls but the walls contain no muscle.

6. C: The cavernous sinus has running through its cavity (covered with endothelium) the internal carotid artery and its sympathetic plexus and the abducent nerve.

7. C: (1) The hypoglossal nerve is a pure motor nerve. (3) The glossopharyngeal nerve does not supply the dura mater with sensory fibers.

8. E

9. A: (4) The arachnoid mater, along with the dura and pia, extend through each foramen, providing the cranial nerves with a short sheath; the meninges end by fusing with the epineurium of each cranial nerve.

10. A: (4) The cisterns are formed under the arachnoid mater and form part of the subarachnoid space; the pia mater is closely adherent to the outer surface of the brain and spinal cord.

11. E

12. A: (4) The diaphragma sellae covers over the sella turcica and protects the underlying hypophysis cerebri.

13. A: (4) The sympathetic fibers do supply the dura mater and are distributed to the meningeal arteries.

14. A: (4) All the subarachnoid cisterns communicate with each other via the subarachnoid space.

15. E

16. C

17. E

18. E

19. B

20. A

Index